Advances in Diagnosis and Management of Ovarian Cancer

Samir A. Farghaly
Editor

Advances in Diagnosis and Management of Ovarian Cancer

Springer

Editor
Samir A. Farghaly, MD, PhD
Department of Obstetrics
and Gynecology
Weill Cornell Medical College
The New York Presbyterian
Hospital-Weill Cornell Medical Center
Cornell University
New York, NY
USA

ISBN 978-1-4614-8270-3 ISBN 978-1-4614-8271-0 (eBook)
DOI 10.1007/978-1-4614-8271-0
Springer New York Heidelberg Dordrecht London

Library of Congress Control Number: 2013954553

Printed on acid-free paper

Springer is part of Springer Science+Business Media (www.springer.com)

This book is dedicated to the memory of my mother, Amina, and my father, Aly, who had a great influence on me and my academic and professional medical career. To my late siblings, Nabil and Magdy, and their families. Also, to my sisters, Sorya and Nadia, my brother, Raafat and their families. In addition, to my beloved children, Raied and Tamer.

Moreover, I dedicate this book to the memory of Hugh R.K. Barber, M.D., who passed away in 2006. He was a leader in the field of Gynecologic Oncology and was internationally renowned for his seminal work in ovarian cancer. He was Chairman of the Department of Obstetrics and Gynecology at Lenox Hill Hospital Medical Center, New York, NY, USA. I had the pleasure of meeting him in 2005, and having several extensive discussions about the topic of ovarian cancer, he was an inspiration to me and my current book.

Samir A. Farghaly, MD, PhD

Foreword

The importance of this book is included in its very theme, as it presents gynecological cancer of the most unfavorable prognosis. In fact, despite the numerous advances in surgery, chemotherapy, and molecular therapies, the survival rates have only slightly improved. Selecting ovarian tumors as the object of study, as assessed by a multi-specialized team, can assist the gynecological oncologists, and also refine the approach to the disease and increase their professional standard.

This book, written by 32 international acknowledged experts, with rich and clear illustrations, offers an expert guide to all aspects of this neoplasia.

From the epidemiology, through risk, management in early and advanced stages, pediatric neoplasia, to the quality of life, the author explores all the possible aspects of this disease and all the implications that affect the outcome.

The chapters are all written very clearly, allowing anyone from the student to the expert to fully benefit from consultation of the manual, and the in-depth information makes it easier to understand its contents.

In conclusion, I believe that the comprehensive text conveys a significant progress in understanding this complex neoplasia.

Montreal, Canada — Dr. (Med) Maria Marchetti

Preface

Worldwide, 204,449 new cases of ovarian cancer are diagnosed each year, with an estimated 124,860 disease-related deaths. There are notable differences in ovarian cancer incidence across the world. In Europe, in 2012, there were 65,538 cases with a mortality rate of 42,704 women. The American Cancer Society's estimates for ovarian cancer in the USA for 2013 are: about 22,240 women will receive a new diagnosis of ovarian cancer and about 14,230 women will die from the disease. The ovarian cancer statistics for incidence indicates it is highest in the USA and Northern Europe and lowest in Africa and Asia. Ovarian cancer is the ninth most common cancer among women, excluding nonmelanoma skin cancers. It ranks fifth in cancer deaths among women. It accounts for about 3 % of all cancers in women. A woman's risk of getting ovarian cancer during her lifetime is about 1 in 72. Her lifetime chance of dying from ovarian cancer is about 1 in 100. Incidence rates of ovarian cancer increase with age, becoming more prevalent in the eighth decade of life. Patients are typically diagnosed when the disease has metastasized (stage III or IV) which has an overall survival rate between 5 and 25 %.

Five-year survival in ovarian cancer has doubled over the past 30 years, increasing from approximately 25 % to 50 %. This is a result of developments in diagnosis and more efficient management. Clearly, there is more room to increase this rate to a higher number. This could be achieved by developing novel tests for early detection and diagnosis and innovative medical therapy and surgical techniques. The ideal approach to women with ovarian cancer is a multidisciplinary one, with many professionals contributing to the excellent care and outcome that we wish to see for those individuals we are privileged to look after.

This book discusses a range of early diagnostic and therapeutic considerations, including epidemiologic, molecular genetic testing, histopathologic, open surgical, minimally invasive surgical, and targeted molecular therapy for patients with hereditary and nonhereditary ovarian cancer.

The importance of updated knowledge of the epidemiology of ovarian cancer as it affects primary prevention, early detection, and possibly therapeutic strategies is discussed in Chap. 1. The risk of developing breast/ovarian cancer in women with BRAC1 and BRAC2 mutant genes and the molecular genetic testing of these genes and others are discussed in Chap. 2. The risk management of hereditary ovarian cancer such as surveillance, chemoprevention, and prophylactic surgery is detailed in Chap. 3. The development and evaluation of improved biomarker-based tests and recent advances in this arena are discussed in Chap. 4.

The origin, histopathologic, and molecular genetic aspects of surface epithelial tumors of the ovary are detailed in Chap. 5. The immunohistochemical and molecular pathological aspects of non-epithelial ovarian cancer, as it presents unique clinical diagnostic and therapeutic challenges, are outlined in Chap. 6. The management strategies in early-stage, late-stage, and recurrent ovarian cancer are detailed in Chap. 7. The recent advances in diagnosis and management of ovarian neoplasms in the pediatric female population of less than 17 years old are discussed in Chap. 8. Comprehensive current management of patients with early-stage ovarian cancer, including the role of minimally invasive surgery and fertility sparing surgery for young women, is detailed in Chap. 9. The importance of aggressive surgical debunking and novel chemotherapy regimens, including intraperitoneal chemotherapy in patients with late-stage ovarian cancer is outlined in Chap. 10. The intraperitoneal chemotherapy administration and its complication in patients with peritoneal carcinomatosis secondary to epithelial ovarian cancer are detailed in Chap. 11. As a novel therapeutic option, targeted molecular genetic therapy for patients with ovarian cancer is detailed in Chap. 12. Variety of quantities and qualitative assessment of the psychological impact of ovarian cancer and the positive impact of cancer experience are outlined in Chap. 13. Finally, the importance of quality of life (QOL) as an outcome on both disease and treatment decision making in patients affected with ovarian cancer is detailed in Chap. 14.

This book is intended for all clinicians caring for women with ovarian cancer, including attending surgeons and physicians, fellows, and residents in the disciplines of gynecologic oncology, surgical oncology, medical oncology, and primary care. Allied medical staff, palliative services, and nurse specialists will also find it a useful adjunct to getting current information on diagnosis and management of ovarian cancer.

I hope that you enjoy this book and benefit from the extensive experience of the internationally renowned contributors to this book from the USA, UK, and Italy who have authored its contents.

New York, NY, USA Samir A. Farghaly, MD, PhD

Contents

Contributors

Kate Absolom, PhD, BSc (Hons) Psychosocial Oncology and Clinical Practice Research Group, Leeds Institute of Molecular Medicine, Division of Cancer Studies and Pathology, University of Leeds, Leeds, UK

Caterina Accettura, MD Department of Oncology, Vito Fazzi Hospital, Lecce, Italy

Andrea Besharat, MPH Division of Population Sciences, Department of Cancer Epidemiology, H. Lee Moffitt Cancer Center and Research Institute, Tampa, FL, USA

John Butler, MD Department of Gynaecological Oncology, St Bartholomew's Hospital, West Smithfield, London, UK

David Cella, PhD Department of Medical Social Sciences, Northwestern University Feinberg School of Medicine, Chicago, IL, USA

Samir A. Farghaly, MD, PhD Department of Obstetrics and Gynecology, The Weill Cornell Medical College/Weill Cornell Graduate School of Medical Sciences, and The New York Presbyterian Hospital-Weill Cornell Medical Center, Cornell University, New York, NY, USA

Anne C. Fischer, MD, PhD Department of Pediatric Surgery, William Beaumont Hospital, Royal Oak, MI, USA

Department of Surgery, Oakland University William Beaumont Medical School, Royal Oak, MI, USA

Christopher A. Friedrich, MD, PhD Division of Oncology, Department of Medicine, University of Mississippi Medical Center, Jackson, MS, USA

Marianna Giampaglia, MD Department of Oncology, Vito Fazzi Hospital, Lecce, Italy

Marilena Greco, PhD, BSc Laboratory of Medical Genetics, Giovanni Paolo II Oncological Centre, Lecce Hospital, Lecce, Italy

Sarah Gustapane, MD Department of Obstetrics and Gynecology, SS. Annunziata Hospital, Chieti, Italy

Geoff Hall, MB, ChB, MRCP, PhD, FRCP Department of Oncology, University of Leeds/St James's Institute of Oncology, Leeds, UK

Cyril W. Helm, MB.BChir Northern Gynaecological Oncology Centre, Queen Elizabeth Hospital, Gateshead, Tyne and Wear, UK

Eleni Ieremia, FRCPath Department of Cellular Pathology, Barts Health NHS Trust, London, UK

Sally E. Jensen, PhD Department of Medical Social Sciences and Department of Surgery, Division of Organ Transplantation, Northwestern University Feinberg School of Medicine, Chicago, IL, USA

Alexandra Lawrence, MD, MRCOG Department of Gynaecological Oncology, St. Bartholomew's Hospital, West Smithfield, London, UK

Queen's Hospital, Rom Valley Way, Romford, UK

Silvana Leo, MD Department of Oncology, Vito Fazzi Hospital, Lecce, Italy

Anna E. Lokshin, PhD University of Pittsburgh Cancer Institute, Hillman Cancer Center, Pittsburgh, PA, USA

Departments of Medicine, Pathology, and Ob/Gyn, School of Medicine, University of Pittsburgh, Pittsburgh, PA, USA

Vito Lorusso, MD Department of Medical Oncology, National Institute for Cancer Research, Istituto Tumori Giovanni Paolo II, Bari, Italy

Michele Maffia, PhD Department of Biological and Environmental Sciences and Technologies, University of Salento, Lecce, Italy

Purnima Makhija, MD Department of Cellular Pathology, Barts Health NHS Trust, London, England, UK

Antonio Malvasi, MD Department of Obstetrics and Gynecology, Santa Maria Hospital, Bari, Italy

Tim Mould, MD, FRCOG, MBBS, MA, DM, FRCOG Department of Gynaecological Oncology, University College London, London, UK

Brian M. Nolen, PhD University of Pittsburgh Cancer Institute, Hillman Cancer Center, Pittsburgh, PA, USA

Jennifer Permuth-Wey, PhD Division of Population Sciences, Department of Cancer Epidemiology, H. Lee Moffitt Cancer Center and Research Institute, Tampa, FL, USA

Thomas A. Sellers, PhD Division of Population Sciences, Department of Cancer Epidemiology, H. Lee Moffitt Cancer Center and Research Institute, Tampa, FL, USA

Naveena Singh, MBBS, FRCPath Department of Cellular Pathology, Barts Health NHS Trust, London, England, UK

Paul H. Sugarbaker, MD, FACS, FRCS Department of Center for Gastrointestinal Malignancies, Washington Cancer Institute, MedStar Washington Hospital Center, Washington, DC, USA

Elena Takeuchi, MB ChB, MRCP Psychosocial Oncology and Clinical Practice Research Group, St. James's Institute of Oncology, Leeds, UK

Andrea Tinelli, MD Department of Obstetrics and Gynecology, Vito Fazzi Hospital, Lecce, Italy

Galina Velikova, BMBS(MD), PhD, FRCP Department of Oncology, University of Leeds/St James's Institute of Oncology, Leeds, UK

Daniele Vergara, BSc, PhD Department of Biological and Environmental Sciences and Technologies, University of Salento, Lecce, Italy

Epidemiology of Ovarian Cancer: An Update

1

Jennifer Permuth-Wey, Andrea Besharat, and Thomas A. Sellers

Introduction

Ovarian cancer (OC) is the eighth most commonly diagnosed cancer among women in the world, accounting for nearly 4 % of all female cancers [1]. OC also represents the third leading gynecologic cancer, following cancer of the cervix and uterine corpus, and causes more deaths per year than any other cancer of the female reproductive system [1, 2]. On a worldwide basis, an estimated 225,000 new cases are diagnosed and 140,000 women die of OC annually [1]. In 2011, approximately 22,000 new cases of OC were diagnosed and 15,500 OC-related deaths occurred in the United States [3]. A woman's risk of developing OC in her lifetime is 1 in 71, and her chance of dying of the disease is 1 in 95 [3]. Mortality is high because women typically present with late stage disease when the overall 5-year relative survival rate is 44 % [4]. Thus, the public health burden is significant.

Despite the high incidence and mortality rates, the etiology of this lethal disease is not completely understood. Research to identify the causes of OC is sorely needed; such knowledge could inform strategies for risk assessment, prevention, surveillance, early detection, and treatment. The purpose of this chapter is to review some of the established and suspected epidemiologic risk factors for OC. We divide this chapter into four sections: the pathologic classification of OC, descriptive epidemiology, risk factors and protective factors, and summary and conclusions.

J. Permuth-Wey, PhD • A. Besharat, MPH
T.A. Sellers, PhD (✉)
Division of Population Sciences,
Department of Cancer Epidemiology,
H. Lee Moffitt Cancer Center and Research Institute,
12902 Magnolia Drive, MRC CAN-CONT,
Tampa, FL 33612, USA
e-mail: jenny.wey@moffitt.org;
andrea.besharat@rmpdc.org;
thomas.sellers@moffitt.org

Pathologic Classification of Ovarian Cancer

Nearly all benign and malignant ovarian tumors originate from one of three cell types: epithelial cells, stromal cells, and germ cells. In developed countries, more than 90 % of malignant ovarian tumors are epithelial in origin, 5–6 % of tumors constitute sex cord-stromal tumors, and 2–3 % are germ cell tumors [2]. The pathology and classification of ovarian tumors are described in detail by Chen et al. [5]. Epidemiologic studies have suggested etiologic differences in these three cell types [6]. Most epidemiologic research, including the present review, focuses on epithelial OC because they are the predominant subtype. Malignant epithelial OCs, also known as carcinomas, are comprised of four main histologic subtypes: serous, clear cell, endometrioid, and mucinous [7]. Based on two population-based studies [8, 9], the relative frequencies of these four subtypes are 68–71, 12–13, 9–11, and 3 %, respectively. Within each of these categories

S.A. Farghaly (ed.), *Advances in Diagnosis and Management of Ovarian Cancer*,
DOI 10.1007/978-1-4614-8271-0_1, © Springer Science+Business Media New York 2014

are tumors of uncertain malignant behavior (known as "borderline tumors" or "tumors of low malignant potential") that contain microscopic features of malignancy without frank invasion into surrounding stroma. Such borderline tumors are usually not included in the published statistics of most cancer-reporting systems [6]. However, the risk factors for OC seem to apply similarly for borderline and invasive epithelial tumors, although mean age at diagnosis is earlier among women with borderline tumors [10, 11].

It is important to point out that epithelial OCs themselves reflect a heterogeneous group of diseases. As reviewed by McCluggage [7], histologic subtypes differ in their cellular origin, the molecular alterations that mark their initiation and progression, and their natural behavior and prognosis. Furthermore, epidemiologic studies suggest that the major histotypes of epithelial OC also have different risk factor profiles [10–17]. We will comment on some of these study findings throughout this chapter. Thus, it seems prudent to consider the histologic distribution of cases when designing, conducting, and interpreting OC research.

Descriptive Epidemiology

OC incidence exhibits wide geographic variation, as shown in Fig. 1.1 [1]. The highest age-adjusted incidence rates are observed in developed parts of the world, including North America and Western and Northern Europe, with rates in most of these areas exceeding 8 per 100,000. Rates are intermediate in South America (6.2 per 100,000)

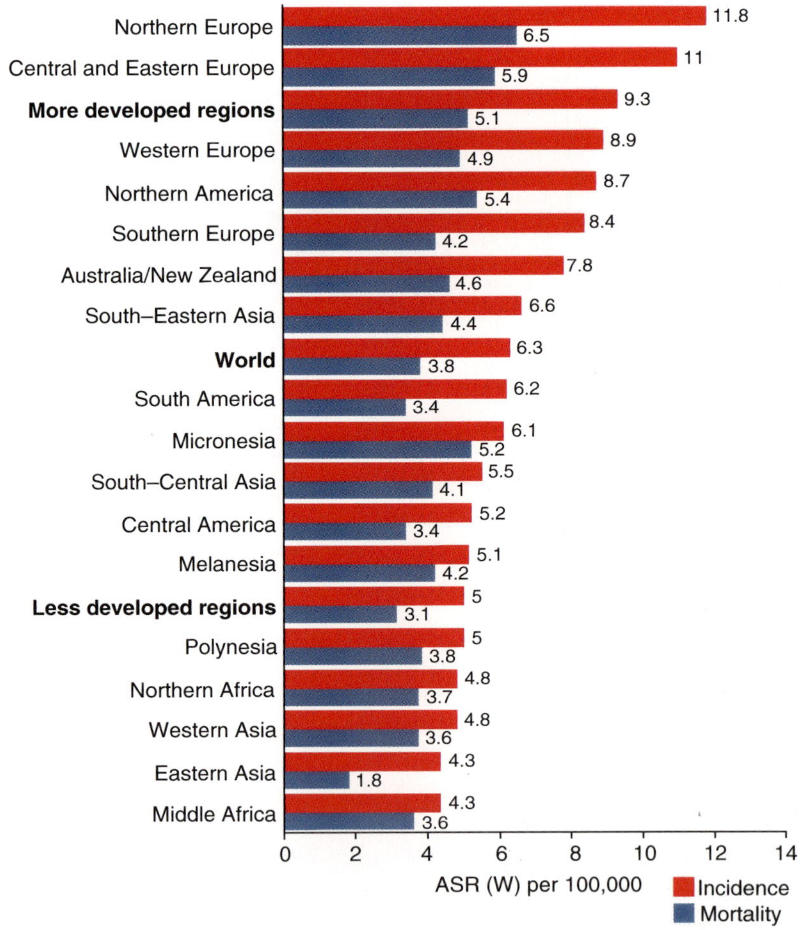

Fig. 1.1 Worldwide ovarian cancer incidence and mortality rates. Rates are per 100,000 and represent age-standardized rates according to the world standard population (ASR (W)) (From the International Agency for Research on Cancer [1])

Table 1.1 Age-adjusted ovarian cancer incidence and mortality rates in the United States by race

Race/ethnicity	Incidence rates[a] by race per 100,000 women	Death rates[a] by race per 100,000 women
All races	12.8	8.6
White	13.5	8.9
Black	10.0	7.2
Asian/Pacific Islander	9.9	4.9
American Indian/ Alaska Native	10.6	6.8
Hispanic	10.6	6.0

[a]Age-standardized rates (world) per 100,000 women are based on cases diagnosed in 2004–2008 from 17 SEER Registries [4]

and lowest in Asia and Africa. Migration from countries with low rates to those with high rates results in greater risk [18, 19], underscoring the importance of nongenetic factors. However, even within the United States, racial differences in incidence and mortality are apparent that mimic the observed international variation (Table 1.1). Rates are highest among Whites, intermediate for Hispanics, and lowest among Blacks and Asians [4]. In most parts of North America and Europe, the incidence of OC was constant in the decades prior to the 1990s and has gradually declined since that time [4, 20–22]. The incidence of OC increases with age, with a median age at diagnosis of 63 years [4]. Approximately 88 % of OCs occur after age 45. In the United States, there has also been a gradual decline in OC-related mortality for all races combined [22].

Risk Factors and Preventive Factors

Inherited Susceptibility

One of the most significant risk factors for OC is a family history of the disease, which occurs among approximately 7 % of women with OC [23]. First-degree relatives of OC probands have a three- to sevenfold increased risk, especially if multiple relatives are affected and at early age at onset [24–28].

It is clear that a subset of OCs occurs as part of a hereditary cancer syndrome that is inherited in an autosomal dominant pattern. The majority of hereditary OCs can be attributed to mutations in the *BRCA1* and *BRCA2* genes [29]. According to data from the Breast Cancer Linkage Consortium, the risk of OC through age 70 years is up to 44 % in *BRCA1* families [30] and approaches 27 % in *BRCA2* families [31]. Mutation screening of population-based series of OC cases has shown that 10–15 % of epithelial OCs can be attributed to mutations in either *BRCA1* or *BRCA2* [32–40]. In addition, OC occurs in families with hereditary nonpolyposis colorectal cancer syndrome (HNPCC), also known as Lynch syndrome [41]. The genetic defects underlying HNPCC (the mismatch repair genes *hMLH1, hMSH2, hPMS1, hPMS2,* and *hMSH6)* may account for at least 2 % of epithelial OC and confer up to a 20 % lifetime risk [4, 29, 42–45]. Overall, mutations in highly penetrant genes account for 10–15 % of epithelial OCs [46, 47]. Candidate gene studies such as those reviewed by Fasching et al. [48]. and genome-wide association studies [49–51] involving non-familial OC cases have identified more common, low-penetrant variants that may be associated with OC risk will be covered in Chap. 2.

Hormonal Risk Factors

Hormones such as estrogen and progesterone are believed to be involved in promoting ovarian carcinogenesis. An extensive review of the hormonal etiology of epithelial OC [52] concluded that there are two, not necessarily mutually exclusive, hypotheses that reflect what is currently known about the disease. The "incessant ovulation" hypothesis proposes that the number of ovulatory cycles increases the rate of cellular division associated with the repair of the surface epithelium after each ovulation, thereby increasing the likelihood of spontaneous mutations that may promote carcinogenesis [53]. Indeed, positive correlations exist between increasing numbers of lifetime ovulations and OC risk [54–57]. The second hypothesis, often referred to as the "gonadotropin hypothesis," posits that gonadotropins such as luteinizing hormone and follicle-stimulating hormone overstimulate the ovarian epithelium, causing increased proliferation and subsequent malignant transformation [58]. The epidemiology of OC does not help clearly distinguish between these two hypotheses.

The following sections review the epidemiologic data on both endogenous correlates of reproductive hormone exposure and exogenous sources of hormones, specifically oral contraceptives and hormone replacement therapy (HRT). For a more detailed summary of the hormonal aspects of OC, the reader is referred to a review by Riman et al. [59].

Age at Menarche and Age at Menopause

According to the incessant ovulation hypothesis, early age at menarche and late age at menopause could increase the risk for OC through an increased number of ovulatory cycles. Conversely, according to the gonadotropin hypothesis, a late age at menopause delays the surge of postmenopausal gonadotropin hormones, possibly reducing OC risk. Numerous epidemiologic studies have examined the relation between lifetime menstrual history and OC risk. Results of studies that have examined the age at onset of menses are not terribly consistent [60–70]. For example, in a collaborative analysis of 12 US case-control studies conducted between 1956 and 1986, data from 2,197 White OC cases and 8,893 White controls detected no elevation in risk among women with onset of menses before 12 years of age [66]. Similarly, no statistically significant association was detected in the prospective Nurses' Health Study cohort of 121,700 female registered nurses aged 30–55 years when the study began [69]. One Chinese study identified a significant protection with late age at menarche (after age 18) [71], while another study observed a slight increased risk with late age at menarche [72]. Additional research has failed to clarify the literature [53, 61, 73–78]. Data on age at natural menopause and OC risk are also inconsistent. Numerous case-control studies have identified an association between late age at menopause and the risk of OC, with odds ratios ranging from 1.4 to 4.6 in the highest category of age at menopause [60, 61, 63, 67, 71, 72, 76]. In the European Prospective Investigation into Cancer and Nutrition (EPIC) cohort, age at menopause (>52 vs ≤45 years) was associated with an increased OC risk (HR = 1.57, 95 % CI: 1.16–2.13); however, after women diagnosed with OC within the first 2 years of follow-up were excluded, the risk was slightly attenuated and marginally statistically significant (HR = 1.40, 95 % CI: 0.98–2.00) [77]. The authors speculated that older women in the subclinical stage of OC may mistake bleeding for menses, which is why risk was attenuated when recently diagnosed cases were removed from the analysis. Other case–control studies [66, 68, 74, 75, 79–81] and several cohort studies [69, 73] found no such association. The collaborative analysis by Whittemore et al., for example, calculated an OR of 1.1 (95 % CI: 0.71–1.3) for menopause occurring after the age of 55 [66].

A recent study report from the Nurses' Health Study and Nurses' Health Study II found that age at natural menopause was associated with an increased risk of endometrioid tumors (RR = 1.13, 95 % CI: 1.04–1.22), but not serous invasive or mucinous tumors [17]. There are various explanations for the conflicting results regarding the relationship between ages at menarche and menopause and OC risk [82]. Besides the role of chance, it has been proposed that these differences may be explained through real differences between populations. Additionally, it is possible that the definition of menarche and menopause can be subject to recall and misclassification bias. It has also been pointed out that various populations have different age distributions and that some studies may have failed to adjust for age or other covariates in the analysis. In summary, it can be inferred from the available evidence that if early age at menarche and late age at menopause increase the risk of OC, the magnitude is likely small.

Pregnancy, Parity, and Infertility

The association between pregnancy and OC risk has been studied extensively. Pregnancy causes anovulation and suppresses secretion of pituitary gonadotropins. Both the "incessant ovulation" and the "gonadotropin" hypotheses would predict that pregnancy reduces the risk of OC. Indeed, one of the most consistent findings is that parous women have a 30–60 % lower risk for OC than nulliparous women [53, 60, 67, 71–75, 80, 82–86]. Furthermore, each additional full-term pregnancy is estimated to lower risk by approximately 15 % [66, 73, 87]. While many case-control studies with hospital controls have shown positive associations with late age at first birth (≥30 years of age) [60, 65, 66, 74, 76, 83, 88–91], a reduced risk with late age at first birth has been identified in some case-control studies with population controls [64, 66, 92]. Recent data also suggests that OC risk does not vary by the time interval between the first and last birth [93].

It is unclear whether spontaneous or induced abortions impact OC risk. Although many investigations have found that an increased number of incomplete pregnancies may slightly decrease risk [53, 60, 65, 66, 72, 73, 94–96], others have reported risk to be increased among women with one or more incomplete pregnancies [75, 86], and a sizeable number of studies have yielded null results [64, 67, 68, 70, 74, 80, 83, 85, 97]. Induced abortions have been associated with lower risk in several studies [73, 95, 96], but not others [64, 76, 94]. With regard to spontaneous abortions and OC risk, positive [68, 83, 94], inverse [70], and null associations [71, 85, 95] have been reported. Interpretation of this literature is difficult because of the recognized potential for recall bias of spontaneous or induced pregnancies [59].

It is yet to be determined whether nulliparity and low parity per se, rather than difficulty becoming pregnant due to female infertility, is the relevant factor. Infertility is a term that is used to describe a heterogeneous group of biologically distinct conditions ranging from genital tract infections and tubal disturbances to medical conditions such as endometriosis and polycystic ovarian syndrome [98, 99]. Infertility appears to be associated with increased OC risk in most studies [60, 66, 70, 74, 80, 83, 85, 86, 91, 98], but not all [73, 100]. Infertility seems to pose the greatest risk among women who remain nulliparous, while periods of temporary infertility among parous women are of little concern [60, 66, 70, 74, 85]. For example, in a large Canadian case-control study in which most nulliparous women were so by choice, infertility was not associated with OC risk among parous women, but there was a trend towards elevated risk among a small group of infertile nulliparous women (OR = 2.5, 95 % CI: 0.6–4.1) [70].

Possible reasons for the inconsistent results may include the failure to examine the various types of infertility separately. Furthermore, it has been reported that some factors such as a personal history of endometriosis [101–103] or polycystic ovarian syndrome [104] may influence both infertility and OC risk. The definition of infertility used across studies is variable, including physician-diagnosed infertility, self-reported infertility, and periods of unprotected intercourse without becoming pregnant [59]. A particular challenge is trying to distinguish an influence of infertility from an adverse effect of fertility drug exposure. Although some studies report that women with a prior history of fertility drug use who remain nulliparous are at an elevated risk for ovarian tumors, particularly tumors of low malignant potential [66, 105], the results are not consistent [98–100, 106–108]. Early detection bias may explain the discrepant findings, as early stage cancers may be overdiagnosed in infertile women due to the close medical surveillance [109].

Lactation

Lactation suppresses secretion of pituitary gonadotropins and leads to anovulation, particularly in the initial months after delivery [6]. If the incessant ovulation and gonadotropin hypotheses are true, lactation should reduce the risk of OC. Although the majority of studies have identified a slight decrease in OC risk with lactation, with odds ratios approximating 0.6–0.7 [66, 67, 70, 84–86, 110–113], some have not [64, 68, 80]. Despite the conflicting results, the overall impression is that lactation protects against epithelial OC, especially in the first few months following delivery.

Benign Gynecologic Conditions and Gynecologic Surgery

Several gynecologic conditions have been examined as risk factors for OC, including polycystic ovarian syndrome (PCOS), endometriosis, and pelvic inflammatory disease (PID). PCOS is a heterogeneous disease often characterized by obesity, hirsutism, infertility, and menstrual abnormalities. The association between PCOS and OC risk was investigated using data from the Cancer and Steroid Hormone Study, a population-based case-control study [104]. Among 476 histologically confirmed epithelial OC cases and 4,081 controls, 7 cases (1.5 %) and 24 controls (0.06 %) reported a history of PCOS (OR = 2.5-fold, 95 % CI: 1.1–5.9) [104]. The association appeared to be stronger among women who never used oral contraceptives (OR = 10.5, 95 % CI: 2.5–44.2) and women in the first quartile of body mass index (13.3–18.5 kg/m^2) at age 18 (OR = 15.6, 95 % CI: 3.4–71.0), but these estimates have wide confidence intervals. Larger studies that adjust for potential confounders of the PCOS-OC association are needed before conclusions can be drawn regarding these findings.

Endometriosis is one of the most common gynecologic disorders, affecting 10–15 % of women in reproductive years [114]. Even though endometriosis is considered a benign condition, it has been linked with OC in the medical literature since 1925. Sayasneh and colleagues [114] recently reported a systematic review of eight studies; seven found an increased risk of OC, with effect sizes ranging from 1.3 to 1.9. The strongest associations were evident among endometrioid and clear cell histologies, consistent with molecular data that supports the uterus as the origin of these subtypes [7]. However, the authors suggest that the association between endometriosis and endometrioid and clear cell ovarian carcinomas may represent sharing of similar risk factors rather than a causal association [114], a topic that merits further research.

PID causes inflammation of the endometrium, fallopian tubes, and ovaries. Previous studies from the 1990s that evaluated the association between PID and OC risk yielded inconsistent results [115, 116]. Recently, Lin and colleagues [117] evaluated this association in a large nationwide cohort from Taiwan that included 67,936 women with PID (42 of whom later developed OC) and 135,872 women without a history of PID (48 of whom developed OC). A history of PID was found to be a risk factor (adjusted HR = 1.92 (95 % CI: 1.27–2.92)), especially among subjects diagnosed with PID before the age of 35 and women who had at least five episodes of PID. Note, however, that the absolute rates of OC among women with PID are clearly low overall.

Several gynecologic procedures appear to influence the risk for OC. It is well established that among high risk women, bilateral prophylactic oophorectomy decreases OC risk by at least 90 % [118]. Numerous studies have identified a reduced risk of OC associated with either a hysterectomy or tubal ligation (without oophorectomy), with the protective effect for each of these procedures ranging from 30 to 40 % [60, 70, 119–124]. For example, a recent meta-analysis estimated that tubal ligation reduced OC risk by 34 % [125]. Furthermore, the risk reduction from these procedures appears to last for at least 10–15 years, which argues against screening bias (due to selective removal of subclinical ovarian tumors) as the basis for the findings [81, 120, 126, 127]. Although it is uncertain how these procedures reduce the risk of OC, removal of the uterus and/or blockage of the tubes may prevent potential carcinogens from ascending the genital tract [62] and decreases blood flow to the ovaries [127]. In particular, Vercillini and colleagues [128] hypothesize that retrograde menstruation (i.e., menstrual fluid flows backwards into the fallopian tubes instead of leaving the body through the vagina) may promote iron-induced oxidative stress and subsequent cancer development in the fallopian tubes and ovaries.

Oral Contraceptives (OC) and Other Forms of Contraception

The 30–40 % lower risk of ovarian cancer among women who ever used oral contraceptives is firmly established. The findings are consistent over the past several decades, even as the drug formulations evolved from high estrogen and progestin content popular in the 1960s to decreasing hormone content in the mid-1970s, and in the early 1980s when the sequential compounds (biphasic and triphasic) were introduced [129]. The risk reduction increases with duration of use

[66, 70, 130–133] by at least 5 % per year, with about a 50 % reduction in risk for long-term use of 10 years or greater, [134] and persists long after use has ceased [80, 84, 132, 135–138]. Moreover, the risk reduction is not confined to any particular type of combined oral contraceptive formulation [139, 140] or to any histologic type of ovarian cancer, although the inverse relation is less consistent for mucinous cancers [11, 13, 16, 141]. There are few epidemiologic studies that have evaluated progestin-only contraceptives, mostly due to the rarity of this exposure, but the existing data suggest they too lower risk of ovarian cancer [84, 132, 142].

Oral contraceptive use corresponds to the avoidance of approximately 3,000–5,000 ovarian cancer cases and 2,000–3,000 deaths per year in both Europe [20] and in North America [143]. The use of OCs therefore has implications for individual risk assessment and on a public health scale.

Few recent studies have examined methods of contraception other than oral contraceptives and tubal ligation. In a population-based case-control study of 902 epithelial OC/tubal/peritoneal cases and 1,800 controls, Ness and colleagues [124] found that ever use of an intrauterine device (IUD) was associated with lower risk of OC (adjusted OR = 0.75, 95 % CI: 0.59–0.95). The benefit was evident with short duration of IUD use (≤4 years), but risk progressively increased with longer duration of IUD use (albeit nonsignificantly). The authors suggested that shorter use may reduce upper genital tract inflammation by killing sperm, while longer use may imply more insertions and greater risk of infection and inflammation. IUD use has previously been associated with an increased OC risk (RR = 1.76, 95 % CI: 1.08–2.85) among women in the Nurses' Health Study [144]; however, most IUD use in their study occurred in the 1970s–1980s prior to the newer IUD formulations. Contrary to results from the Nurses' Health Study [144] in which spousal vasectomy was not associated with OC risk (multivariate adjusted OR = 0.87, 95 % CI: 0.63–1.19), Ness and colleagues [124] observed vasectomy to be protective (adjusted OR = 0.77, 95 % CI: 0.61–0.99). The authors [124] speculated that vasectomy may confer a slight risk reduction from reduced exposure to sperm. Given that contraceptive methods are modifiable, these findings need to be replicated.

Hormone Replacement Therapy (HRT)

The benefit of oral contraceptives on OC risk is well established; however, the data on another exogenous hormone, HRT, is less clear. It has been postulated that HRT may reduce OC risk by decreasing the secretion of gonadotropins. However, the reduced levels are still above those of premenopausal women [145]. Conversely, postmenopausal HRT may increase OC risk due to increased estrogen-induced proliferation of ovarian cells [146].

Initial studies on the topic focused on unopposed estrogen therapy. In the collaborative reanalysis of 12 US case-control studies, no association was identified with duration of HRT use in either hospital-based (OR = 0.90 for a 5-year increment of use, $p = 0.37$) or population-based (OR = 1.10 for a 5-year increment of use, $p = 0.21$) studies [66]. Several case-control studies [147, 148], cohort studies, [149] and meta-analyses [150, 151] found no association with duration of use, although two have observed either a significant increase or a suggestive trend towards increased risk [13, 152]. Data from recent studies, including four meta-analyses, now indicate an increased OC risk for ever users of HRT [153–156]. Furthermore, several prospective studies have found that longer durations of HRT use are associated with OC risk or death [157–160]. For example, in the Nurses' Health Study cohort, both current and past HRT users of 5 or more years had a significantly higher risk for OC than never users current users (RR = 1.41, 95 % CI: 1.07–1.86) and past users (RR = 1.52, 95 % CI: 1.01–2.27) [161]. Based on their statistical modeling, the authors concluded that the elevated risk appeared to be driven largely by duration rather than by status of use. Additionally, in the UK Million Women Study [153], 2,273 incident ovarian cancers were observed among 948,576 postmenopausal women who did not have a prior cancer history or a bilateral oophorectomy. For current users of HRT, incidence of OC increased with increasing duration of use, but did not differ significantly by type of preparation used and its constituents or mode of administration.

Only recently have studies had sufficient statistical power to evaluate associations between combined estrogen and progestin use and OC risk. The effects of unopposed estrogen therapy (ET) are thought to be more detrimental to the ovaries than estrogen plus progestin (EPT) [162]. It is postulated that progestins promote apoptosis, while estrogen promotes proliferation of ovarian epithelial cells [162]. Most studies that investigated the association between EPT use and OC risk have found no association or a weak association [141, 153, 154, 156, 159, 161–164]; however, not all studies support a protective role for EPT. A few prospective studies [153, 158, 165] and meta-analysis [155] have reported a small increased risk for EPT users. In support of a weaker association for EPT, a recent meta-analysis of 14 population-based studies found that ET is associated with an increased risk of OC (RR = 1.22 for a 5-year increment of use, $p < 0.0001$); however, the risk among women who used EPT was attenuated (RR = 1.10 for a 5-year increment of use, $p = 0.001$) [154]. The authors suggest that the addition of progestin mitigates the effect of estrogen, because the increased risk of OC among EPT users was statistically significantly lower than the risk among ET users, $p = 0.004$ [154]. However, a large nationwide prospective cohort study of Danish women observed an increased risk both for ET users (RR = 1.31, 95 % CI: 1.11–1.54) and for EPT users (RR = 1.50, 95 % CI: 1.34–1.68) [165].

A recent cohort study investigated the association between HRT use and obesity on OC risk [166]. Among HRT nonusers, weight gain, waist circumference, and waist-to-hip ratio but not BMI increased the risk of OC [166]. HRT use of more than 5 years increased OC risk, but risk was not further increased for women who were overweight and used HRT. For example, while substantial weight gain (greater than 40 lbs) and HRT use of more than 5 years individually increased the risk of OC, the joint effect did not further increase the risk, which may imply a threshold effect [166]. Some studies have pointed to an increased risk only for certain histologic subtypes of OC. For example, the Nurses' Health Study cohort observed that the association with ET was slightly stronger for endometrioid tumors, which is consistent with other studies [17, 148, 167]. A link between ET and the development of endometrioid ovarian tumors is biologically plausible because endometrioid tumors are histologically similar to endometrial tissue [168], and ET use increases the risk of endometrial cancer [146]. However, although risks associated with HRT use varied significantly according to tumor histology ($p < 0.0001$) in the UK Million Women Study [153], the relative risk for current versus never users of HRT was greater for serous than for mucinous, endometrioid, or clear cell tumors (1.53 (1.31–1.79), 0.72 (0.52–1.00), 1.05 (0.77–1.43), or 0.77 (0.48–1.23), respectively).

It can be concluded from the available evidence that if an association exists between HRT use and OC, the magnitude is probably moderate, but women should be counseled about the potential increase in risk with long-term use of unopposed estrogen. Evidence suggests that the OC risk with ET alone is higher than the risk associated with EPT. Since many women are exposed to HRT several years before the peak age-specific incidence of OC, even a small change in risk may have a significant impact on disease rates at the population level.

Anthropometric Factors

The previous sections highlighting the importance of hormonal factors raise questions about other potential influences on circulating levels of estrogens. One area of great interest is body mass index (BMI), calculated as weight in kilograms divided by height in meters squared. In postmenopausal women the predominant source of circulating estrogens is aromatization of androgens in adipose tissue [52, 169]. The compelling role of obesity in the pathogenesis of hormone-related cancers has prompted research on the potential association with OC [170]. Despite a growing body of literature, the association between BMI and OC risk remains unresolved.

A 2007 meta-analysis of 28 population based studies reported an increased risk of OC for overweight women (BMI of 25–29.9 kg/m^2) and obese women (BMI ≥ 30 kg/m^2) compared with normal weight (BMI of 18.5–24.9 kg/m^2), pooled RR = 1.2 and 1.3, respectively [171]. A more recent report from the EPIC study obtained very similar results [172]. In a 2008 analysis of 12 prospective cohort studies, an increased OC risk was seen among premenopausal obese women compared to normal weight women (RR = 1.72. 95 % CI: 1.02–2.89); however, this increased risk was not apparent among postmenopausal women (RR = 1.07, 95 % CI: 0.87–1.33) [173].

Recent studies have investigated the relationship between obesity and OC risk stratified by hormone therapy (HT) use [166, 172, 174, 175]. In the EPIC study, higher BMI (HR per 2 kg/m^2 = 1.05, 95 % CI: 1.01–1.08) and hip circumference (highest vs lowest quartile), RR = 1.3 (95 % CI: 1.04–1.70), were associated with increased OC risk, [172] but waist circumference and waist-to-hip ratio (WHR) were not. In the Nurses' Health Study (NHS), greater hip circumference was a risk factor among postmenopausal women, but WHR, waist circumference, and BMI were not [175]. The results for BMI did not differ by hormone therapy use in the NHS or EPIC study. In contrast, two studies found an increased OC risk among obese never HT users (RR 1.8, 95 % CI: 1.2–2.8) [174] and an increased risk for greater weight gain since age 18 (RR = 1.8, 95 % CI: 1.0–3.0 for ≥40 lbs. vs stable weight), a larger waist circumference (RR = 1.8, 95 % CI: 1.1–3.0 for ≥35 vs <35 in.), and a larger waist-to-height ratio (RR = 1.8, 95 % CI: 1.1–3.1 for ≥35 vs <35 in.) [166].

It is hypothesized that different histologic subtypes of OC have different etiologies, and thus, recent studies have investigated the association between obesity and subtypes of epithelial OC. An increased risk for OC has been observed between WHR and risk of mucinous tumors (HR per 0.05 unit increment = 1.19, 95 % CI: 1.02–1.38), but not with serous, endometrioid, or clear cell tumors [172]. The large prospective NIH-AARP Diet and Health Study reported that endometrioid OC risk was increased among obese women (RR = 1.64, 95 % CI: 1.00–2.70), but no association was seen for serous OC [176]. Similarly, in the NHS, obesity was associated with increased endometrioid risk [17]; however, in a systematic review only the pooled analysis and one case–control study found BMI to be associated with an increased risk of endometrioid OC [171]. In another pooled analysis, no association between BMI and risk of endometrioid, mucinous, or serous tumors was evident [173].

The findings to date suggest BMI may confer a slight increased risk of OC, but considering adiposity is a modifiable risk factor, future studies on different anthropometric measures are warranted. Additionally, the possible relationship between OC risk and BMI among women who have never used HT should be investigated in future studies.

Diet and Nutrition

The previous section on anthropometric factors raises questions about the role of dietary factors, especially energy intake (balance) in the etiology of OC. Ecological studies have generated a number of hypotheses about the association between diet and OC risk [177]. Despite numerous analytical epidemiologic studies on various aspects of diet, the findings for most exposures remain inconsistent. The notable exception is intake of vegetables, for which the evidence that higher intakes are associated with lower risk is emerging [177], and to a certain extent also for consumption of whole grain foods and low-fat milk. However, the association between specific fats and oils, fish and meats, and certain milk products is inconsistent and awaits further investigation before firm conclusions can be made. Recent epidemiologic studies on meat consumption and OC do not provide further clarification [178–180]; however, a large prospective study found that women in the highest intake quartile of dietary nitrate had an increased risk of OC (HR = 1.31, 95 % CI: 1.01–1.68, and p-value for trend = 0.02). Similarly, the association between coffee intake and OC risk has been inconclusive to date, and a recent systematic review found no significant associations [72, 76, 181–185]. Although several studies including a recent systematic review noted a trend towards lower risk among tea drinkers, the findings remain inconsistent [181, 186, 187].

Since vitamin D levels are derived in part from our diet or dietary supplements, the literature on vitamin D is included in this section, even though the main source is production in the skin from sun exposure [188]. Vitamin D is converted to 25-hydroxyvitamin (25(OH)D) in the liver and further metabolized to the active form in the kidney, 1,25-dihydroxyvitamin D ($1,25(OH)_2D_3$) [188]. Experimental studies have shown that $1,25(OH)_2D_3$ inhibits cell proliferation in OC cell lines and induces apoptosis [189]. However, a recent systematic review of the epidemiologic literature concluded that there is no consistent or strong evidence that vitamin D decreases OC risk [190]. A meta-analysis of ten longitudinal studies reached a similar conclusion [191]. Although seven of the ten studies found a 17 % reduced risk of OC with increasing 25(OH)D levels, the pooled estimate was not statistically significant (RR=0.83, 95 % CI: 0.63–1.08) [191]. There is some evidence that the beneficial effect of vitamin D may be more pronounced among overweight or obese women [189, 192], perhaps reflecting differential bioavailability of circulating 25(OH)D levels [189].

Exercise and Physical Activity

The potential general health benefits of exercise are well established, and a specific effect on OC might be expected, at least indirectly, through exercise effects on reduction of adipose tissue (and therefore estrogen levels), lower ovulation frequency, and reduced chronic inflammation [193]. To date, 23 epidemiologic studies have investigated the association between physical activity and OC risk, including ten prospective cohort studies [194–203], two historical cohort studies [204, 205], eight population-based case-control studies [183, 206–212], and three hospital-based case-control studies [213–215]. Results are not entirely consistent, but a 2007 meta-analysis estimated a nearly 20 % lower risk for the most active women compared to the least active (pooled relative risk=0.81, 95 % CI: 0.72–0.92) [210]. Most studies that measured physical activity across the lifespan reported consistent null findings [200, 201, 208, 210] or risk reductions [183, 207, 209, 213] in each age period; however, one study [211] reported that strenuous recreational activity early in life may increase OC risk. Similarly, prolonged sedentary behavior, greater than 6 h compared to less than 3 h, was associated with an increased risk of OC (HR=1.55; 95 % CI: 1.08, 2.22; p for trend=0.01) [200]. An increased risk of OC was also found for high level versus low level of total sitting duration, OR=1.77 (95 % CI: 1.0–3.1) [216]. Because each OC subtype has different clinical and morphological features, the association between OC risk and physical activity may vary by histologic type [209, 212], but there is insufficient data to draw firm conclusions. Even though questions remain unanswered regarding the relationship between exercise and physical activity and OC risk, when considering the additional benefits of exercise on weight control, bone density, and heart disease, the promotion of regular activity to women should be encouraged.

Other Lifestyle and Environmental Factors

Cigarette Smoking

The majority of early reports concluded that smoking was not associated with an increased risk of OC [85, 184, 217, 218]. Based on results from more contemporary studies, this may have been because analyses were not stratified by histologic subtype. In fact, smoking appears to increase the risk for invasive mucinous tumors in a dose-response manner, but not other subtypes [12, 15, 219]. In 2006, a systematic literature review and meta-analysis [220] concluded that there is a doubling of risk of mucinous OC among current smokers compared to never smokers (summary RR 2.1, 95 % CI: 1.7–2.7), but no increased risk of serous (1.0, 95 % CI: 0.8–1.2) or endometrioid (0.8, 95 % CI: 0.6–1.1) cancers, and a significant risk reduction for clear cell cancers (0.6, 95 % CI: 0.3–0.9). The risk of mucinous cancer increased in a dose-response relationship but returned to that of never smokers within 20–30 years of stopping smoking. A population-based study of 812 women with OC diagnosed in Washington State and 1,313 controls published since that meta-analysis also showed that the incidence of borderline and invasive mucinous ovarian tumors was increased among women with a cigarette smoking history (OR = 1.8; 95 % CI: 1.2–2.9 and 0.8–4.3, respectively) [221]. The risk of invasive serous cancers was slightly increased among those who had smoked within the previous 15 years (OR = 1.4, 95 % CI: 1.1–1.9), but the risk for endometrioid and clear cell tumors was not elevated among smokers [221]. Histologically, mucinous ovarian tumors resemble mucinous gastrointestinal cancers, some of which (pancreatic cancer, gastric cancer) have been classified as smoking-related cancers [220]. Collectively, these findings suggest that risk of OC is one more reason to avoid cigarette smoking.

Alcohol Consumption

Alcohol consumption, a common and modifiable exposure, has been investigated as a possible cause of OC in numerous case-control and cohort studies with conflicting results. Most have observed null associations [67, 85, 183, 184, 222, 223], but there is an equal number that have found increased risk [72, 224, 225] and decreased risk [226–228]. There have been efforts to resolve the observed inconsistency by quantifying risk by the type of alcohol consumed (wine, beer, or alcohol) [225, 226] or histologic subtype of the tumor [225, 226, 228]. In a large population-based case-control study [229], consumption of beer (not liquor or wine) during early adulthood (20–30 years of age) was associated with a moderately increased risk of invasive OC, with the association limited to serous tumors (OR 1.52, 95 % CI: 1.01–2.30), though results for other histologic subtypes were based on sparse data. This risk was associated with regular consumption (one or more drinks per day), and there was no evidence of a dose-response relationship. Data from the Netherlands Cohort Study on Diet and Cancer found no association between alcohol consumption in the form of wine, beer, or liquor and OC risk [230]. A recently published pooled analysis of 10 cohort studies that included over 500,000 women and 2001 incident OC cases also found no association between total alcohol intake (pooled multivariate RR = 1.12, 95 % CI: 0.86–1.44 comparing ≥30–0 g day of alcohol) or alcohol intake from wine, beer, or spirits and OC [231]. There was no association (OR = 1.13, 95 % CI: 0.92–1.38; random effects) between wine consumption and OC risk in a recent meta-analysis of 10 studies (3 cohort and 7 case-control studies) with 135,871 women, including 65,578 wine drinkers [232]. Based on these data, it seems reasonable to conclude that if alcohol intake does influence risk of OC, the magnitude is small and possibly limited to particular histologic subtypes.

Occupational Exposures

Assessment of occupational risk factors for OC has been challenging due to a lack of well-designed epidemiologic studies adequately powered to detect associations; however, there is some evidence for excess risk among women employed in dry cleaning, telecommunications, paper packaging, and textile industries [233, 234], perhaps implicating exposures to organic dusts, aromatic amines, and hydrocarbons.

Asbestos and Talcum Powder

Both human [235, 236] and animal studies [237] have found asbestos fibers in the ovaries. The link between asbestos exposure and OC is less firmly established, in part due to small numbers of women who have been exposed to asbestos and disease misclassification (i.e., peritoneal mesothelioma, an asbestos-related disease, is often misdiagnosed as OC on death certificates). A recent systematic review and meta-analysis of fourteen cohort and two case-control studies [238] noted a statistically significant excess mortality in four of the cohort studies, all of which relied on death certificates for reports of the outcome. After including all studies in the meta-analysis, there was a 75 % excess risk of OC in women who had been exposed to asbestos (effect size=1.75 (95 % CI: 1.45–2.10)). However, the association was attenuated (effect size=1.29 (95 % CI: 0.97–1.73)) among studies that examined cancer incidence based upon pathologically confirmed OCs [238]. Despite the lack of consistency, the International Agency for Research on Cancer (IARC) has declared that evidence is "sufficient" in humans that exposure to asbestos causes OC [239].

Similar to asbestos, talcum powder is a silicate that has been studied extensively in relation to cancer risk. A meta-analysis of 16 studies reported an approximately 30 % increase in risk of OC with regular genital exposure to talc [240], and more recent studies suggest that women with certain variants in glutathionine S-transferase M1 (*GSTM1*) and/or glutathionine S-transferase T1 (*GSTT1*) may have a higher risk of OC associated with talc use [241]. However, as summarized by Muscat and Huncharek [242], mechanistic, pathology, and animal studies do not support evidence for the carcinogenicity of talc on the ovarian epithelium.

Asthma

Epidemiologic studies have identified inverse associations between the presence of allergies and the development of certain cancers [243]. Using the presence of asthma as an indicator for an allergy, El Masri and colleagues [244] conducted a hospital-based study of 1,582 cases and two large series of controls with bone fractures (n=4,744) and acute myocardial infarction (n=21,830). After adjusting for age, race-ethnicity, Medicaid status, obesity, and smoking, cases were 30 % less likely than controls with fractures to be asthmatics (adjusted OR=0.70, 95 % CI: 0.49–0.99). Similarly, when compared to controls with acute myocardial infarction, cases were less likely to have asthma (adjusted OR=0.62, 95 % CI: 0.45–0.87). These intriguing findings merit replication efforts.

Drug Use

Several recent prospective studies [245, 246] have investigated the association between aspirin and nonaspirin nonsteroidal anti-inflammatory drugs (NSAIDS) and OC incidence. Using data from the Nurses' Health Study and the Nurses' Health Study II, Pinheiro and colleagues [245] found that regular use of aspirin and NSAIDS was associated with hazard ratios of 1.11 (95 % CI: 0.92–1.33) and 0.81 (95 % CI: 0.64–1.01), respectively. No dose-response relationship with increased frequency or duration of use was observed, and results did not differ when stratifying by tumor histology [245]. Prizment and colleagues [246] investigated these drugs using data from a prospective cohort of approximately 20,000 women who were part of the Iowa Women's Health Study. Compared to women who reported no use of aspirin, the relative risks of OC for those who used aspirin <2, 2–5 times, and ≥6 times per week were 0.83, 0.77, and 0.61, respectively (p trend=0.04). No association was observed between NSAID use and OC risk.

As summarized recently by Li and colleagues [247], a growing body of evidence supports a role for the antidiabetic agent, metformin, in cancer prevention and treatment. To evaluate the association between use of metformin or other antidiabetic drugs and OC risk, a case-control study including 1,611 incident OC cases was performed using the UK-based General Practice Research Database [248]. Long-term use (≥30 prescriptions) of metformin (and not sulfonylureas) was associated with a trend towards reduced OC risk (OR=0.61, 95 % CI: 0.30–1.25), although results were not statistically significant. Further large-scale studies are needed before initiating prospective trials to investigate metformin as a chemopreventive (or therapeutic) agent.

Summary and Conclusions

Ovarian cancer is a leading cause of cancer incidence and mortality among women worldwide. This chapter describes the magnitude of the problem and summarizes epidemiologic studies that have provided clues on factors that may increase and decrease risk of this heterogeneous disease. Although many of the risk factors in Table 1.2 cannot be modified, reflecting the contribution of genetics and unavoidable exposures, a number of others can be altered. Increasing parity and oral

Table 1.2 Summary of established and suspected risk and protective factors for ovarian cancer

Risk factors	Protective factors
Age	Oral contraceptive use
Family history	Oophorectomy
Nulliparity	Hysterectomy
Increased numbers of lifetime ovulatory cycles	Tubal Ligation
Hormone replacement therapy	Lactation
Dietary Fat	High vegetable intake
Obesity	
Infertility	
Sedentary lifestyle	
Cigarette smoking	
Alcohol consumption	

contraceptive use lower risk of ovarian cancer. The same is probably true, but to a weaker degree, from lactation, incomplete pregnancies, regular physical activity, and avoidance of cigarettes. Infertility contributes to ovarian cancer risk among nulliparous women, while temporary fertility problems in parous women do not. Risks associated with postmenopausal HRT use require further investigation, especially since several studies suggest use may increase risk.

It is important to emphasize that the established risk factors aside from highly penetrant gene mutations neither confer large increases in risk nor account for all the variability in the incidence of this disease. Thus, many of the causes of ovarian cancer are yet to be identified. Additional research is needed to better understand the etiology of this deadly disease. This knowledge is necessary to reduce the public health burden from ovarian cancer.

References

1. Ferlay J, Shin H, Bray F, Forman D, Mathers C, Parkin DM. GLOBOCAN 2008 v 1.2: Cancer incidence, mortality, and prevalence worldwide: IARC CancerBase No. 10 [Internet]. Lyon, France: International Agency for Research on Cancer. Available from: http://globocan.iarc.fr. Accessed on 12/18/11. 2008.
2. Sankaranarayanan R, Ferlay J. Worldwide burden of gynaecological cancer: the size of the problem. Best Pract Res Clin Obstet Gynaecol. 2006;20(2):207–25.
3. Ahlgren JD. Epidemiology and risk factors in pancreatic cancer. Semin Oncol. 1996;23(2):241–50.
4. Howlader NNA, Krapcho M, Neyman N, Aminou R, Waldron W, Altekruse SF, Kosary CL, Ruhl J, Tatalovich Z, Cho H, Mariotto A, Eisner MP, Lewis DR, Chen HS, Feuer EJ, Cronin KA, Edwards BK (eds). SEER cancer statistics review, 1975–2008, National Cancer Institute. Bethesa, MD, http://seer.cancer.gov/csr/1975_2008/. Based on November 2010 SEER data submission, posted to the SEER website, 2011.
5. Chen VW, Ruiz B, Killeen JL, Cote TR, Wu XC, Correa CN. Pathology and classification of ovarian tumors. Cancer. 2003;97(10 Suppl):2631–42.
6. Weiss NS, Cook LS, Farrow DC, Rosenblatt KA. Ovarian cancer. In: Schottenfeld D, Fraumeni JF, editors. Cancer epidemiology and prevention. New York: Oxford University Press; 1996. p. 1040–57.
7. McCluggage WG. Morphological subtypes of ovarian carcinoma: a review with emphasis on new developments and pathogenesis. Pathology. 2011;43(5):420–32.
8. Seidman JD, Horkayne-Szakaly I, Haiba M, Boice CR, Kurman RJ, Ronnett BM. The histologic type and stage distribution of ovarian carcinomas of surface epithelial origin. Int J Gynecol Pathol. 2004;23(1):41–4.
9. Kobel M, Kalloger SE, Huntsman DG, et al. Differences in tumor type in low-stage versus high-stage ovarian carcinomas. Int J Gynecol Pathol. 2010;29(3):203–11.
10. Eltabbakh GH, Natarajan N, Piver MS, Mettlin CJ. Epidemiologic differences between women with borderline ovarian tumors and women with epithelial ovarian cancer. Gynecol Oncol. 1999;74(1):103–7.
11. Tung KH, Goodman MT, Wu AH, et al. Reproductive factors and epithelial ovarian cancer risk by histologic type: a multiethnic case-control study. Am J Epidemiol. 2003;158(7):629–38.
12. Marchbanks PA, Wilson H, Bastos E, Cramer DW, Schildkraut JM, Peterson HB. Cigarette smoking and epithelial ovarian cancer by histologic type. Obstet Gynecol. 2000;95(2):255–60.
13. Risch HA, Marrett LD, Jain M, Howe GR. Differences in risk factors for epithelial ovarian cancer by histologic type. Results of a case-control study. Am J Epidemiol. 1996;144(4):363–72.
14. Chiaffarino F, Parazzini F, Bosetti C, et al. Risk factors for ovarian cancer histotypes. Eur J Cancer. 2007;43(7):1208–13.
15. Kurian AW, Balise RR, McGuire V, Whittemore AS. Histologic types of epithelial ovarian cancer: have they different risk factors? Gynecol Oncol. 2005;96(2):520–30.
16. Parazzini F, Chiaffarino F, Negri E, et al. Risk factors for different histological types of ovarian cancer. Int J Gynecol Cancer. 2004;14(3):431–6.
17. Gates MA, Rosner BA, Hecht JL, Tworoger SS. Risk factors for epithelial ovarian cancer by histologic subtype. Am J Epidemiol. 2010;171(1):45–53.

18. Herrinton LJ, Stanford JL, Schwartz SM, Weiss NS. Ovarian cancer incidence among Asian migrants to the United States and their descendants. J Natl Cancer Inst. 1994;86(17):1336–9.
19. Kliewer EV, Smith KR. Ovarian cancer mortality among immigrants in Australia and Canada. Cancer Epidemiol Biomarkers Prev. 1995;4(5):453–8.
20. Bray F, Loos AH, Tognazzo S, La Vecchia C. Ovarian cancer in Europe: cross-sectional trends in incidence and mortality in 28 countries, 1953–2000. Int J Cancer. 2005;113(6):977–90.
21. Coleman MP, Esteve J, Damiecki P, Arslan A, Renard H. Trends in cancer incidence and mortality. IARC Sci Publ. 1993;121:1–806.
22. Howe HL, Wu X, Ries LA, et al. Annual report to the nation on the status of cancer, 1975–2003, featuring cancer among U.S. Hispanic/Latino populations. Cancer. 2006;107(8):1711–42.
23. Nguyen HN, Averette HE, Janicek M. Ovarian carcinoma. A review of the significance of familial risk factors and the role of prophylactic oophorectomy in cancer prevention. Cancer. 1994;74(2):545–55.
24. Parazzini F, Negri E, La Vecchia C, Restelli C, Franceschi S. Family history of reproductive cancers and ovarian cancer risk: an Italian case-control study. Am J Epidemiol. 1992;135(1):35–40.
25. Stratton JF, Pharoah P, Smith SK, Easton D, Ponder BA. A systematic review and meta-analysis of family history and risk of ovarian cancer. Br J Obstet Gynaecol. 1998;105(5):493–9.
26. Sutcliffe S, Pharoah PD, Easton DF, Ponder BA. Ovarian and breast cancer risks to women in families with two or more cases of ovarian cancer. Int J Cancer. 2000;87(1):110–7.
27. Ziogas A, Gildea M, Cohen P, et al. Cancer risk estimates for family members of a population-based family registry for breast and ovarian cancer. Cancer Epidemiol Biomarkers Prev. 2000;9(1):103–11.
28. Negri E, Pelucchi C, Franceschi S, et al. Family history of cancer and risk of ovarian cancer. Eur J Cancer. 2003;39(4):505–10.
29. Lynch HT, Casey MJ, Snyder CL, et al. Hereditary ovarian carcinoma: heterogeneity, molecular genetics, pathology, and management. Mol Oncol. 2009;3(2):97–137.
30. Ford D, Easton DF, Bishop DT, Narod SA, Goldgar DE. Risks of cancer in BRCA1-mutation carriers. Breast Cancer Linkage Consortium. Lancet. 1994;343(8899):692–5.
31. Antoniou A, Pharoah PD, Narod S, et al. Average risks of breast and ovarian cancer associated with BRCA1 or BRCA2 mutations detected in case Series unselected for family history: a combined analysis of 22 studies. Am J Hum Genet. 2003;72(5): 1117–30.
32. Malander S, Ridderheim M, Masback A, et al. One in 10 ovarian cancer patients carry germ line BRCA1 or BRCA2 mutations: results of a prospective study in Southern Sweden. Eur J Cancer. 2004;40(3): 422–8.
33. Menkiszak J, Gronwald J, Gorski B, et al. Hereditary ovarian cancer in Poland. Int J Cancer. 2003;106(6): 942–5.
34. Pal T, Permuth-Wey J, Betts JA, et al. BRCA1 and BRCA2 mutations account for a large proportion of ovarian carcinoma cases. Cancer. 2005;104(12): 2807–16.
35. Risch HA, McLaughlin JR, Cole DE, et al. Prevalence and penetrance of germline BRCA1 and BRCA2 mutations in a population series of 649 women with ovarian cancer. Am J Hum Genet. 2001;68(3): 700–10.
36. Stratton JF, Gayther SA, Russell P, et al. Contribution of BRCA1 mutations to ovarian cancer. N Engl J Med. 1997;336(16):1125–30.
37. Takahashi H, Behbakht K, McGovern PE, et al. Mutation analysis of the BRCA1 gene in ovarian cancers. Cancer Res. 1995;55(14):2998–3002.
38. Anton-Culver H, Cohen PF, Gildea ME, Ziogas A. Characteristics of BRCA1 mutations in a population-based case series of breast and ovarian cancer. Eur J Cancer. 2000;36(10):1200–8.
39. Bjorge T, Lie AK, Hovig E, et al. BRCA1 mutations in ovarian cancer and borderline tumours in Norway: a nested case-control study. Br J Cancer. 2004;91(10): 1829–34.
40. Van Der Looij M, Szabo C, Besznyak I, et al. Prevalence of founder BRCA1 and BRCA2 mutations among breast and ovarian cancer patients in Hungary. Int J Cancer. 2000;86(5):737–40.
41. Lynch HT, Smyrk T. Hereditary nonpolyposis colorectal cancer (Lynch syndrome). An updated review. Cancer. 1996;78(6):1149–67.
42. Aarnio M, Mecklin JP, Aaltonen LA, Nystrom-Lahti M, Jarvinen HJ. Life-time risk of different cancers in hereditary non-polyposis colorectal cancer (HNPCC) syndrome. Int J Cancer. 1995;64(6):430–3.
43. Aarnio M, Sankila R, Pukkala E, et al. Cancer risk in mutation carriers of DNA-mismatch-repair genes. Int J Cancer. 1999;81(2):214–8.
44. Prat J, Ribe A, Gallardo A. Hereditary ovarian cancer. Hum Pathol. 2005;36(8):861–70.
45. Bonadona V, Bonaiti B, Olschwang S, et al. Cancer risks associated with germline mutations in MLH1, MSH2, and MSH6 genes in Lynch syndrome. JAMA. 2011;305(22):2304–10.
46. Boyd J, Rubin SC. Hereditary ovarian cancer: molecular genetics and clinical implications. Gynecol Oncol. 1997;64(2):196–206.
47. Lynch HT, Casey MJ, Shaw TG, Lynch JF. Hereditary factors in gynecologic cancer. Oncologist. 1998;3(5): 319–38.
48. Fasching PA, Gayther S, Pearce L, et al. Role of genetic polymorphisms and ovarian cancer susceptibility. Mol Oncol. 2009;3(2):171–81.
49. Bolton KL, Tyrer J, Song H, et al. Common variants at 19p13 are associated with susceptibility to ovarian cancer. Nat Genet. 2010;42:880–4.
50. Goode EL, Chenevix-Trench G, Song H, et al. A genome-wide association study identifies

susceptibility loci for ovarian cancer at 2q31 and 8q24. Nat Genet. 2010;42:874–9.
51. Song H, Ramus SJ, Tyrer J, et al. A genome-wide association study identifies a new ovarian cancer susceptibility locus on 9p22.2. Nat Genet. 2009;41(9):996–1000.
52. Risch HA. Hormonal etiology of epithelial ovarian cancer, with a hypothesis concerning the role of androgens and progesterone. J Natl Cancer Inst. 1998;90(23):1774–86.
53. Casagrande JT, Louie EW, Pike MC, Roy S, Ross RK, Henderson BE. "Incessant ovulation" and ovarian cancer. Lancet. 1979;2(8135):170–3.
54. Tung KH, Wilkens LR, Wu AH, et al. Effect of anovulation factors on pre- and postmenopausal ovarian cancer risk: revisiting the incessant ovulation hypothesis. Am J Epidemiol. 2005;161(4):321–9.
55. Moorman PG, Schildkraut JM, Calingaert B, Halabi S, Vine MF, Berchuck A. Ovulation and ovarian cancer: a comparison of two methods for calculating lifetime ovulatory cycles (United States). Cancer Causes Control. 2002;13(9):807–11.
56. Schildkraut JM, Moorman PG, Bland AE, et al. Cyclin E overexpression in epithelial ovarian cancer characterizes an etiologic subgroup. Cancer Epidemiol Biomarkers Prev. 2008;17(3):585–93.
57. Terry KL, Titus-Ernstoff L, McKolanis JR, Welch WR, Finn OJ, Cramer DW. Incessant ovulation, mucin 1 immunity, and risk for ovarian cancer. Cancer Epidemiol Biomarkers Prev. 2007;16(1):30–5.
58. Cramer DW, Welch WR. Determinants of ovarian cancer risk. II. Inferences regarding pathogenesis. J Natl Cancer Inst. 1983;71(4):717–21.
59. Riman T, Persson I, Nilsson S. Hormonal aspects of epithelial ovarian cancer: review of epidemiological evidence. Clin Endocrinol (Oxf). 1998;49(6):695–707.
60. Booth M, Beral V, Smith P. Risk factors for ovarian cancer: a case-control study. Br J Cancer. 1989;60(4):592–8.
61. Franceschi S, La Vecchia C, Booth M, et al. Pooled analysis of 3 European case-control studies of ovarian cancer: II. Age at menarche and at menopause. Int J Cancer. 1991;49(1):57–60.
62. Parazzini F, Franceschi S, La Vecchia C, Fasoli M. The epidemiology of ovarian cancer. Gynecol Oncol. 1991;43(1):9–23.
63. Parazzini F, La Vecchia C, Negri E, Gentile A. Menstrual factors and the risk of epithelial ovarian cancer. J Clin Epidemiol. 1989;42(5):443–8.
64. Purdie D, Green A, Bain C, et al. Reproductive and other factors and risk of epithelial ovarian cancer: an Australian case-control study. Survey of Women's Health Study Group. Int J Cancer. 1995;62(6):678–84.
65. Tavani A, Negri E, Franceschi S, Parazzini F, La Vecchia C. Risk factors for epithelial ovarian cancer in women under age 45. Eur J Cancer. 1993;29A(9):1297–301.
66. Whittemore AS, Harris R, Itnyre J. Characteristics relating to ovarian cancer risk: collaborative analysis of 12 US case-control studies. II. Invasive epithelial ovarian cancers in white women. Collaborative Ovarian Cancer Group. Am J Epidemiol. 1992;136(10):1184–203.
67. Wu ML, Whittemore AS, Paffenbarger Jr RS, et al. Personal and environmental characteristics related to epithelial ovarian cancer. I. Reproductive and menstrual events and oral contraceptive use. Am J Epidemiol. 1988;128(6):1216–27.
68. Wynder EL, Dodo H, Barber HR. Epidemiology of cancer of the ovary. Cancer. 1969;23(2):352–70.
69. Hankinson SE, Colditz GA, Hunter DJ, et al. A prospective study of reproductive factors and risk of epithelial ovarian cancer. Cancer. 1995;76(2):284–90.
70. Risch HA, Marrett LD, Howe GR. Parity, contraception, infertility, and the risk of epithelial ovarian cancer. Am J Epidemiol. 1994;140(7):585–97.
71. Shu XO, Brinton LA, Gao YT, Yuan JM. Population-based case-control study of ovarian cancer in Shanghai. Cancer Res. 1989;49(13):3670–4.
72. Tzonou A, Day NE, Trichopoulos D, et al. The epidemiology of ovarian cancer in Greece: a case-control study. Eur J Cancer Clin Oncol. 1984;20(8):1045–52.
73. Kvale G, Heuch I, Nilssen S, Beral V. Reproductive factors and risk of ovarian cancer: a prospective study. Int J Cancer. 1988;42(2):246–51.
74. McGowan L, Norris HJ, Hartge P, Hoover R, Lesher L. Risk factors in ovarian cancer. Eur J Gynaecol Oncol. 1988;9(3):195–9.
75. Newhouse ML, Pearson RM, Fullerton JM, Boesen EA, Shannon HS. A case control study of carcinoma of the ovary. Br J Prev Soc Med. 1977;31(3):148–53.
76. Polychronopoulou A, Tzonou A, Hsieh CC, et al. Reproductive variables, tobacco, ethanol, coffee and somatometry as risk factors for ovarian cancer. Int J Cancer. 1993;55(3):402–7.
77. Tsilidis KK, Allen NE, Key TJ, et al. Oral contraceptive use and reproductive factors and risk of ovarian cancer in the European Prospective Investigation into Cancer and Nutrition. Br J Cancer. 2011;105(9):1436–42.
78. Moorman PG, Palmieri RT, Akushevich L, Berchuck A, Schildkraut JM. Ovarian cancer risk factors in African-American and white women. Am J Epidemiol. 2009;170(5):598–606.
79. Annegers JF, Strom H, Decker DG, Dockerty MB, O'Fallon WM. Ovarian cancer: incidence and case-control study. Cancer. 1979;43(2):723–9.
80. Cramer DW, Hutchison GB, Welch WR, Scully RE, Ryan KJ. Determinants of ovarian cancer risk. I. Reproductive experiences and family history. J Natl Cancer Inst. 1983;71(4):711–6.
81. Hartge P, Hoover R, McGowan L, Lesher L, Norris HJ. Menopause and ovarian cancer. Am J Epidemiol. 1988;127(5):990–8.
82. La Vecchia C. Epidemiology of ovarian cancer: a summary review. Eur J Cancer Prev. 2001;10(2):125–9.

83. Joly DJ, Lilienfeld AM, Diamond EL, Bross ID. An epidemiologic study of the relationship of reproductive experience to cancer of the ovary. Am J Epidemiol. 1974;99(3):190–209.
84. Centers for Disease Control Cancer and Steroid Hormone Study. The reduction in risk of ovarian cancer associated with oral-contraceptive use. N Engl J Med. 1987;316(11):650–5.
85. Hartge P, Schiffman MH, Hoover R, McGowan L, Lesher L, Norris HJ. A case-control study of epithelial ovarian cancer. Am J Obstet Gynecol. 1989;161(1):10–6.
86. Nasca PC, Greenwald P, Chorost S, Richart R, Caputo T. An epidemiologic case-control study of ovarian cancer and reproductive factors. Am J Epidemiol. 1984;119(5):705–13.
87. Adami HO, Hsieh CC, Lambe M, et al. Parity, age at first childbirth, and risk of ovarian cancer. Lancet. 1994;344(8932):1250–4.
88. La Vecchia C, Decarli A, Franceschi S, Regallo M, Tognoni G. Age at first birth and the risk of epithelial ovarian cancer. J Natl Cancer Inst. 1984;73(3): 663–6.
89. Negri E, Franceschi S, Tzonou A, et al. Pooled analysis of 3 European case-control studies: I. Reproductive factors and risk of epithelial ovarian cancer. Int J Cancer. 1991;49(1):50–6.
90. Franceschi S, La Vecchia C, Helmrich SP, Mangioni C, Tognoni G. Risk factors for epithelial ovarian cancer in Italy. Am J Epidemiol. 1982;115(5): 714–9.
91. Hildreth NG, Kelsey JL, LiVolsi VA, et al. An epidemiologic study of epithelial carcinoma of the ovary. Am J Epidemiol. 1981;114(3):398–405.
92. John EM, Whittemore AS, Harris R, Itnyre J. Characteristics relating to ovarian cancer risk: collaborative analysis of seven U.S. case-control studies. Epithelial ovarian cancer in black women. Collaborative Ovarian Cancer Group. J Natl Cancer Inst. 1993;85(2):142–7.
93. Bevier M, Sundquist J, Hemminki K. Does the time interval between first and last birth influence the risk of endometrial and ovarian cancer? Eur J Cancer. 2011;47(4):586–91.
94. Chen MT, Cook LS, Daling JR, Weiss NS. Incomplete pregnancies and risk of ovarian cancer (Washington, United States). Cancer Causes Control. 1996;7(4):415–20.
95. Mori M, Harabuchi I, Miyake H, Casagrande JT, Henderson BE, Ross RK. Reproductive, genetic, and dietary risk factors for ovarian cancer. Am J Epidemiol. 1988;128(4):771–7.
96. Negri E, Franceschi S, La Vecchia C, Parazzini F. Incomplete pregnancies and ovarian cancer risk. Gynecol Oncol. 1992;47(2):234–8.
97. Dick ML, Siskind V, Purdie DM, Green AC. Incomplete pregnancy and risk of ovarian cancer: results from two Australian case-control studies and systematic review. Cancer Causes Control. 2009; 20(9):1571–85.
98. Mosgaard BJ, Lidegaard O, Kjaer SK, Schou G, Andersen AN. Infertility, fertility drugs, and invasive ovarian cancer: a case-control study. Fertil Steril. 1997;67(6):1005–12.
99. Modan B, Ron E, Lerner-Geva L, et al. Cancer incidence in a cohort of infertile women. Am J Epidemiol. 1998;147(11):1038–42.
100. Franceschi S, La Vecchia C, Negri E, et al. Fertility drugs and risk of epithelial ovarian cancer in Italy. Hum Reprod. 1994;9(9):1673–5.
101. Brinton LA, Sakoda LC, Sherman ME, et al. Relationship of benign gynecologic diseases to subsequent risk of ovarian and uterine tumors. Cancer Epidemiol Biomarkers Prev. 2005;14(12):2929–35.
102. Edmondson RJ, Monaghan JM. The epidemiology of ovarian cancer. Int J Gynecol Cancer. 2001;11(6):423–9.
103. Vigano P, Somigliana E, Parazzini F, Vercellini P. Bias versus causality: interpreting recent evidence of association between endometriosis and ovarian cancer. Fertil Steril. 2007;88:588–93.
104. Schildkraut JM, Schwingl PJ, Bastos E, Evanoff A, Hughes C. Epithelial ovarian cancer risk among women with polycystic ovary syndrome. Obstet Gynecol. 1996;88(4 Pt 1):554–9.
105. Rossing MA, Daling JR, Weiss NS, Moore DE, Self SG. Ovarian tumors in a cohort of infertile women. N Engl J Med. 1994;331(12):771–6.
106. Ness RB, Cramer DW, Goodman MT, et al. Infertility, fertility drugs, and ovarian cancer: a pooled analysis of case-control studies. Am J Epidemiol. 2002; 155(3):217–24.
107. Potashnik G, Lerner-Geva L, Genkin L, Chetrit A, Lunenfeld E, Porath A. Fertility drugs and the risk of breast and ovarian cancers: results of a long-term follow-up study. Fertil Steril. 1999;71(5): 853–9.
108. Venn A, Watson L, Lumley J, Giles G, King C, Healy D. Breast and ovarian cancer incidence after infertility and in vitro fertilisation. Lancet. 1995; 346(8981):995–1000.
109. Ayhan A, Salman MC, Celik H, Dursun P, Ozyuncu O, Gultekin M. Association between fertility drugs and gynecologic cancers, breast cancer, and childhood cancers. Acta Obstet Gynecol Scand. 2004;83(12):1104–11.
110. Gwinn ML, Lee NC, Rhodes PH, Layde PM, Rubin GL. Pregnancy, breast feeding, and oral contraceptives and the risk of epithelial ovarian cancer. J Clin Epidemiol. 1990;43(6):559–68.
111. Rosenblatt KA, Thomas DB. Lactation and the risk of epithelial ovarian cancer. The WHO Collaborative Study of Neoplasia and Steroid Contraceptives. Int J Epidemiol. 1993;22(2):192–7.
112. Schneider 2nd AP. Risk factor for ovarian cancer. N Engl J Med. 1987;317(8):508–9.
113. Jordan SJ, Siskind V, C Green A, Whiteman DC, Webb PM. Breastfeeding and risk of epithelial ovarian cancer. Cancer Causes Control. 2010;21(1): 109–16.

114. Sayasneh A, Tsivos D, Crawford R. Endometriosis and ovarian cancer: a systematic review. ISRN Obstet Gynecol. 2011;2011:140310.
115. Risch HA, Howe GR. Pelvic inflammatory disease and the risk of epithelial ovarian cancer. Cancer Epidemiol Biomarkers Prev. 1995;4(5):447–51.
116. Parazzini F, La Vecchia C, Negri E, Moroni S, Pino D, Fedele L. Pelvic inflammatory disease and risk of ovarian cancer. Cancer Epidemiol Biomarkers Prev. 1996;5(8):667–9.
117. Lin HW, Tu YY, Lin SY, et al. Risk of ovarian cancer in women with pelvic inflammatory disease: a population-based study. Lancet Oncol. 2011;12(9): 900–4.
118. Domchek SM, Rebbeck TR. Prophylactic oophorectomy in women at increased cancer risk. Curr Opin Obstet Gynecol. 2007;19(1):27–30.
119. Green A, Purdie D, Bain C, et al. Tubal sterilisation, hysterectomy and decreased risk of ovarian cancer. Survey of Women's Health Study Group. Int J Cancer. 1997;71(6):948–51.
120. Hankinson SE, Hunter DJ, Colditz GA, et al. Tubal ligation, hysterectomy, and risk of ovarian cancer. A prospective study. JAMA. 1993;270(23): 2813–8.
121. Kreiger N, Sloan M, Cotterchio M, Parsons P. Surgical procedures associated with risk of ovarian cancer. Int J Epidemiol. 1997;26(4):710–5.
122. Miracle-McMahill HL, Calle EE, Kosinski AS, et al. Tubal ligation and fatal ovarian cancer in a large prospective cohort study. Am J Epidemiol. 1997;145(4): 349–57.
123. Rosenblatt KA, Thomas DB. Reduced risk of ovarian cancer in women with a tubal ligation or hysterectomy. The World Health Organization Collaborative Study of Neoplasia and Steroid Contraceptives. Cancer Epidemiol Biomarkers Prev. 1996;5(11):933–5.
124. Ness RB, Dodge RC, Edwards RP, Baker JA, Moysich KB. Contraception methods, beyond oral contraceptives and tubal ligation, and risk of ovarian cancer. Ann Epidemiol. 2011;21(3):188–96.
125. Cibula D, Widschwendter M, Majek O, Dusek L. Tubal ligation and the risk of ovarian cancer: review and meta-analysis. Hum Reprod Update. 2011;17(1):55–67.
126. Weiss NS, Harlow BL. Why does hysterectomy without bilateral oophorectomy influence the subsequent incidence of ovarian cancer? Am J Epidemiol. 1986;124(5):856–8.
127. Chiaffarino F, Parazzini F, Decarli A, et al. Hysterectomy with or without unilateral oophorectomy and risk of ovarian cancer. Gynecol Oncol. 2005;97(2):318–22.
128. Vercellini P, Crosignani P, Somigliana E, et al. The 'incessant menstruation' hypothesis: a mechanistic ovarian cancer model with implications for prevention. Hum Reprod. 2011;26(9):2262–73.
129. Gerstman BB, Gross TP, Kennedy DL, Bennett RC, Tomita DK, Stadel BV. Trends in the content and use of oral contraceptives in the United States, 1964–88. Am J Public Health. 1991;81(1):90–6.
130. Franceschi S, Parazzini F, Negri E, et al. Pooled analysis of 3 European case-control studies of epithelial ovarian cancer: III. Oral contraceptive use. Int J Cancer. 1991;49(1):61–5.
131. La Vecchia C, Franceschi S. Oral contraceptives and ovarian cancer. Eur J Cancer Prev. 1999;8(4): 297–304.
132. Rosenberg L, Palmer JR, Zauber AG, et al. A case-control study of oral contraceptive use and invasive epithelial ovarian cancer. Am J Epidemiol. 1994;139(7):654–61.
133. Vessey M, Painter R. Oral contraceptive use and cancer. Findings in a large cohort study, 1968–2004. Br J Cancer. 2006;95(3):385–9.
134. La Vecchia C. Estrogen-progestogen replacement therapy and ovarian cancer: an update. Eur J Cancer Prev. 2006;15(6):490–2.
135. Epithelial ovarian cancer and combined oral contraceptives. The WHO Collaborative Study of Neoplasia and Steroid Contraceptives. Int J Epidemiol. 1989;18(3):538–45.
136. Beral V, Hannaford P, Kay C. Oral contraceptive use and malignancies of the genital tract. Results from the Royal College of General Practitioners' Oral Contraception Study. Lancet. 1988;2(8624):1331–5.
137. La Vecchia C, Altieri A, Franceschi S, Tavani A. Oral contraceptives and cancer: an update. Drug Saf. 2001;24(10):741–54.
138. Rosenblatt KA, Thomas DB, Noonan EA. High-dose and low-dose combined oral contraceptives: protection against epithelial ovarian cancer and the length of the protective effect. The WHO Collaborative Study of Neoplasia and Steroid Contraceptives. Eur J Cancer. 1992;28A(11): 1872–6.
139. Ness RB, Grisso JA, Klapper J, et al. Risk of ovarian cancer in relation to estrogen and progestin dose and use characteristics of oral contraceptive. SHARE Study Group. Steroid Hormones and Reproductionss. Am J Epidemiol. 2000;152(3):233–41.
140. La Vecchia C. Oral contraceptives and ovarian cancer: an update, 1998–2004. Eur J Cancer Prev. 2006;15(2):117–24.
141. Riman T, Dickman PW, Nilsson S, et al. Risk factors for invasive epithelial ovarian cancer: results from a Swedish case-control study. Am J Epidemiol. 2002; 156(4):363–73.
142. Liang AP, Levenson AG, Layde PM, et al. Risk of breast, uterine corpus, and ovarian cancer in women receiving medroxyprogesterone injections. JAMA. 1983;249(21):2909–12.
143. Wingo PA, Cardinez CJ, Landis SH, et al. Long-term trends in cancer mortality in the United States, 1930–1998. Cancer. 2003;97(12 Suppl): 3133–275.
144. Tworoger SS, Fairfield KM, Colditz GA, Rosner BA, Hankinson SE. Association of oral contraceptive use, other contraceptive methods, and infertility

with ovarian cancer risk. Am J Epidemiol. 2007; 166(8):894–901.
145. Mathur RS, Landgrebe SC, Moody LO, Semmens JP, Williamson HO. The effect of estrogen treatment on plasma concentrations of steroid hormones, gonadotropins, prolactin and sex hormone-binding globulin in post-menopausal women. Maturitas. 1985;7(2):129–33.
146. Fraser IS. Estrogens and progestogens in clinical practice. London/New York: Churchill Livingstone; 1998.
147. Riman T, Dickman PW, Nilsson S, et al. Hormone replacement therapy and the risk of invasive epithelial ovarian cancer in Swedish women. J Natl Cancer Inst. 2002;94(7):497–504.
148. Weiss NS, Lyon JL, Krishnamurthy S, Dietert SE, Liff JM, Daling JR. Noncontraceptive estrogen use and the occurrence of ovarian cancer. J Natl Cancer Inst. 1982;68(1):95–8.
149. Braem MG, Onland-Moret NC, van den Brandt PA, et al. Reproductive and hormonal factors in association with ovarian cancer in the Netherlands cohort study. Am J Epidemiol. 2010;172(10):1181–9.
150. Coughlin SS, Giustozzi A, Smith SJ, Lee NC. A meta-analysis of estrogen replacement therapy and risk of epithelial ovarian cancer. J Clin Epidemiol. 2000;53(4):367–75.
151. Garg PP, Kerlikowske K, Subak L, Grady D. Hormone replacement therapy and the risk of epithelial ovarian carcinoma: a meta-analysis. Obstet Gynecol. 1998;92(3):472–9.
152. Kaufman DW, Kelly JP, Welch WR, et al. Noncontraceptive estrogen use and epithelial ovarian cancer. Am J Epidemiol. 1989;130(6): 1142–51.
153. Beral V, Bull D, Green J, Reeves G. Ovarian cancer and hormone replacement therapy in the Million Women Study. Lancet. 2007;369(9574):1703–10.
154. Pearce CL, Chung K, Pike MC, Wu AH. Increased ovarian cancer risk associated with menopausal estrogen therapy is reduced by adding a progestin. Cancer. 2009;115(3):531–9.
155. Greiser CM, Greiser EM, Dören M. Menopausal hormone therapy and risk of ovarian cancer: systematic review and meta-analysis. Hum Reprod Update. 2007;13(5):453–63.
156. Zhou B, Sun Q, Cong R, et al. Hormone replacement therapy and ovarian cancer risk: a meta-analysis. Gynecol Oncol. 2008;108(3):641–51.
157. Folsom AR, Anderson JP, Ross JA. Estrogen replacement therapy and ovarian cancer. Epidemiology. 2004;15(1):100–4.
158. Lacey Jr JV, Brinton LA, Leitzmann MF, et al. Menopausal hormone therapy and ovarian cancer risk in the National Institutes of Health-AARP Diet and Health Study Cohort. J Natl Cancer Inst. 2006;98(19):1397–405.
159. Lacey Jr JV, Mink PJ, Lubin JH, et al. Menopausal hormone replacement therapy and risk of ovarian cancer. JAMA. 2002;288(3):334–41.
160. Rodriguez C, Patel AV, Calle EE, Jacob EJ, Thun MJ. Estrogen replacement therapy and ovarian cancer mortality in a large prospective study of US women. JAMA. 2001;285(11):1460–5.
161. Danforth KN, Tworoger SS, Hecht JL, Rosner BA, Colditz GA, Hankinson SE. A prospective study of postmenopausal hormone use and ovarian cancer risk. Br J Cancer. 2007;96(1):151–6.
162. Hildebrand JS, Gapstur SM, Feigelson HS, Teras LR, Thun MJ, Patel AV. Postmenopausal hormone use and incident ovarian cancer: associations differ by regimen. Int J Cancer. 2010;127(12):2928–35.
163. Rossing MA, Cushing-Haugen KL, Wicklund KG, Doherty JA, Weiss NS. Menopausal hormone therapy and risk of epithelial ovarian cancer. Cancer Epidemiol Biomarkers Prev. 2007;16(12):2548–56.
164. Tsilidis KK, Allen NE, Key TJ, et al. Menopausal hormone therapy and risk of ovarian cancer in the European prospective investigation into cancer and nutrition. Cancer Causes Control. 2011;22(8):1075–84.
165. Morch LS, Lokkegaard E, Andreasen AH, Kruger-Kjaer S, Lidegaard O. Hormone therapy and ovarian cancer. JAMA. 2009;302(3):298–305.
166. Canchola AJ, Chang ET, Bernstein L, et al. Body size and the risk of ovarian cancer by hormone therapy use in the California Teachers Study cohort. Cancer Causes Control. 2010;21(12):2241–8.
167. Risch HA. Estrogen replacement therapy and risk of epithelial ovarian cancer. Gynecol Oncol. 1996; 63(2):254–7.
168. Kumar V, Robbins SL. Robbins basic pathology. 8th ed. Philadelphia: Saunders/Elsevier; 2007.
169. Rodriguez C, Calle EE, Fakhrabadi-Shokoohi D, Jacobs EJ, Thun MJ. Body mass index, height, and the risk of ovarian cancer mortality in a prospective cohort of postmenopausal women. Cancer Epidemiol Biomarkers Prev. 2002;11(9):822–8.
170. Renehan AG, Tyson M, Egger M, Heller RF, Zwahlen M. Body-mass index and incidence of cancer: a systematic review and meta-analysis of prospective observational studies. Lancet. 2008; 371(9612):569–78.
171. Olsen CM, Green AC, Whiteman DC, Sadeghi S, Kolahdooz F, Webb PM. Obesity and the risk of epithelial ovarian cancer: a systematic review and meta-analysis. Eur J Cancer. 2007;43(4):690–709.
172. Lahmann PH, Cust AE, Friedenreich CM, et al. Anthropometric measures and epithelial ovarian cancer risk in the European Prospective Investigation into Cancer and Nutrition. Int J Cancer. 2010; 126(10):2404–15.
173. Schouten LJ, Rivera C, Hunter DJ, et al. Height, body mass index, and ovarian cancer: a pooled analysis of 12 cohort studies. Cancer Epidemiol Biomarkers Prev. 2008;17(4):902–12.
174. Leitzmann MF, Koebnick C, Danforth KN, et al. Body mass index and risk of ovarian cancer. Cancer. 2009;115(4):812–22.
175. Kotsopoulos J, Baer HJ, Tworoger SS. Anthropometric measures and risk of epithelial

ovarian cancer: results from the nurses' health study. Obesity. 2009;18(8):1625–31.
176. Yang HP, Trabert B, Murphy MA, et al. Ovarian cancer risk factors by histologic subtypes in the NIH-AARP diet and health study. Int J Cancer. 2012;131(4):938–48.
177. Schulz M, Lahmann PH, Riboli E, Boeing H. Dietary determinants of epithelial ovarian cancer: a review of the epidemiologic literature. Nutr Cancer. 2004; 50(2):120–40.
178. Kolahdooz F, van der Pols JC, Bain CJ, et al. Meat, fish, and ovarian cancer risk: results from 2 Australian case-control studies, a systematic review, and meta-analysis. Am J Clin Nutr. 2010;91(6): 1752.
179. Wallin A, Orsini N, Wolk A. Red and processed meat consumption and risk of ovarian cancer: a dose-response meta-analysis of prospective studies. Br J Cancer. 2011;104(7):1196–201.
180. Gilsing AMJ, Weijenberg MP, Goldbohm RA, van den Brandt PA, Schouten LJ. Consumption of dietary fat and meat and risk of ovarian cancer in the Netherlands Cohort Study. Am J Clin Nutr. 2011; 93(1):118–26.
181. Oppeneer SJ, Robien K. Tea consumption and epithelial ovarian cancer risk: a systematic review of observational studies. Nutr Cancer. 2011;63(6): 817–26.
182. Larsson SC, Wolk A. Coffee consumption is not associated with ovarian cancer incidence. Cancer Epidemiol Biomarkers Prev. 2005;14(9):2273–4.
183. Riman T, Dickman PW, Nilsson S, Nordlinder H, Magnusson CM, Persson IR. Some life-style factors and the risk of invasive epithelial ovarian cancer in Swedish women. Eur J Epidemiol. 2004;19(11): 1011–9.
184. Whittemore AS, Wu ML, Paffenbarger Jr RS, et al. Personal and environmental characteristics related to epithelial ovarian cancer. II. Exposures to talcum powder, tobacco, alcohol, and coffee. Am J Epidemiol. 1988;128(6):1228–40.
185. Arab L. Epidemiologic evidence on coffee and cancer. Nutr Cancer. 2010;62(3):271–83.
186. Baker JA, Boakye K, McCann SE, et al. Consumption of black tea or coffee and risk of ovarian cancer. Int J Gynecol Cancer. 2007;17(1):50–4.
187. Nagle CM, Olsen CM, Bain CJ, Whiteman DC, Green AC, Webb PM. Tea consumption and risk of ovarian cancer. Cancer Causes Control. 2010;21(9): 1485–91.
188. Holick MF. Vitamin D, deficiency. N Engl J Med. 2007;357(3):266–81.
189. Zheng W, Danforth KN, Tworoger SS, et al. Circulating 25-hydroxyvitamin D and risk of epithelial ovarian cancer. Am J Epidemiol. 2010; 172(1):70.
190. Cook LS, Neilson HK, Lorenzetti DL, Lee RC. A systematic literature review of vitamin D and ovarian cancer. Am J Obstet Gynecol. 2010;203(1): 70.e1–8.
191. Yin L, Grandi N, Raum E, Haug U, Arndt V, Brenner H. Meta-analysis: circulating vitamin D and ovarian cancer risk. Gynecol Oncol. 2011;121:369–75.
192. Tworoger SS, Lee IM, Buring JE, Rosner B, Hollis BW, Hankinson SE. Plasma 25-hydroxyvitamin D and 1, 25-dihydroxyvitamin D and risk of incident ovarian cancer. Cancer Epidemiol Biomarkers Prev. 2007;16(4):783–8.
193. McTiernan A. Mechanisms linking physical activity with cancer. Nat Rev Cancer. 2008;8(3):205–11.
194. Chionh F, Baglietto L, Krishnan K, et al. Physical activity, body size and composition, and risk of ovarian cancer. Cancer Causes Control. 2010;21(12):2183–94.
195. Bertone ER, Willett WC, Rosner BA, et al. Prospective study of recreational physical activity and ovarian cancer. J Natl Cancer Inst. 2001; 93(12):942–8.
196. Anderson JP, Ross JA, Folsom AR. Anthropometric variables, physical activity, and incidence of ovarian cancer: the Iowa Women's Health Study. Cancer. 2004;100(7):1515–21.
197. Hannan LM, Leitzmann MF, Lacey Jr JV, et al. Physical activity and risk of ovarian cancer: a prospective cohort study in the United States. Cancer Epidemiol Biomarkers Prev. 2004;13(5):765–70.
198. Schnohr P, Grønbæk M, Petersen L, Ole Hein H, Ia Sørensen T. Physical activity in leisure-time and risk of cancer: 14-year follow-up of 28,000 Danish men and women. Scand J Public Health. 2005;33(4): 244–9.
199. Biesma RG, Schouten LJ, Dirx MJ, Goldbohm RA, van den Brandt PA. Physical activity and risk of ovarian cancer: results from the Netherlands Cohort Study (The Netherlands). Cancer Causes Control. 2006;17(1):109–15.
200. Patel AV, Rodriguez C, Pavluck AL, Thun MJ, Calle EE. Recreational physical activity and sedentary behavior in relation to ovarian cancer risk in a large cohort of US women. Am J Epidemiol. 2006;163(8):709.
201. Weiderpass E, Margolis KL, Sandin S, et al. Prospective study of physical activity in different periods of life and the risk of ovarian cancer. Int J Cancer. 2006;118(12):3153–60.
202. Lahmann PH, Friedenreich C, Schulz M, et al. Physical activity and ovarian cancer risk: the European Prospective Investigation into Cancer and Nutrition. Cancer Epidemiol Biomarkers Prev. 2009;18(1):351–4.
203. Leitzmann MF, Koebnick C, Moore SC, et al. Prospective study of physical activity and the risk of ovarian cancer. Cancer Causes Control. 2009;20(5): 765–73.
204. Pukkala E, Poskiparta M, Apter D, Vihko V. Life-long physical activity and cancer risk among Finnish female teachers. Eur J Cancer Prev. 1993;2(5):369.
205. Zheng W, Shu XO, Gao YT, McLaughlin JK, Chow WH, Blot WJ. Occupational physical activity and the incidence of cancer of the breast, corpus uteri,

and ovary in Shanghai. Cancer. 1993;71(11): 3620–4.
206. Moorman PG, Jones LW, Akushevich L, Schildkraut JM. Recreational physical activity and ovarian cancer risk and survival. Ann Epidemiol. 2011;21(3): 178–87.
207. Cottreau CM, Ness RB, Kriska AM. Physical activity and reduced risk of ovarian cancer. Obstet Gynecol. 2000;96(4):609.
208. Bertone ER, Newcomb PA, Willett WC, Stampfer MJ, Egan KM. Recreational physical activity and ovarian cancer in a population-based case-control study. Int J Cancer. 2002;99(3):431–6.
209. Pan SY, Ugnat AM, Mao Y. Physical activity and the risk of ovarian cancer: a case-control study in Canada. Int J Cancer. 2005;117(2):300–7.
210. Olsen CM, Bain CJ, Jordan SJ, et al. Recreational physical activity and epithelial ovarian cancer: a case-control study, systematic review, and meta-analysis. Cancer Epidemiol Biomarkers Prev. 2007; 16(11):2321–30.
211. Carnide N, Kreiger N, Cotterchio M. Association between frequency and intensity of recreational physical activity and epithelial ovarian cancer risk by age period. Eur J Cancer Prev. 2009;18(4):322.
212. Rossing MA, Cushing-Haugen KL, Wicklund KG, Doherty JA, Weiss NS. Recreational physical activity and risk of epithelial ovarian cancer. Cancer Causes Control. 2010;21(4):485–91.
213. Tavani A, Gallus S, La Vecchia C, et al. Physical activity and risk of ovarian cancer: an Italian case-control study. Int J Cancer. 2001;91(3):407–11.
214. Dosemeci M, Hayes RB, Vetter R, et al. Occupational physical activity, socioeconomic status, and risks of 15 cancer sites in Turkey. Cancer Causes Control. 1993;4(4):313–21.
215. Zhang M, Lee AH, Binns CW. Physical activity and epithelial ovarian cancer risk: a case-control study in China. Int J Cancer. 2003;105(6):838–43.
216. Zhang M, Xie X, Lee AH, Binns CW. Sedentary behaviours and epithelial ovarian cancer risk. Cancer Causes Control. 2004;15(1):83–9.
217. Franks AL, Lee NC, Kendrick JS, Rubin GL, Layde PM. Cigarette smoking and the risk of epithelial ovarian cancer. Am J Epidemiol. 1987;126(1):112–7.
218. Smith EM, Sowers MF, Burns TL. Effects of smoking on the development of female reproductive cancers. J Natl Cancer Inst. 1984;73(2):371–6.
219. Modugno F, Ness RB, Cottreau CM. Cigarette smoking and the risk of mucinous and nonmucinous epithelial ovarian cancer. Epidemiology. 2002;13(4): 467–71.
220. Jordan SJ, Whiteman DC, Purdie DM, Green AC, Webb PM. Does smoking increase risk of ovarian cancer? A systematic review. Gynecol Oncol. 2006; 103(3):1122–9.
221. Rossing MA, Cushing-Haugen KL, Wicklund KG, Weiss NS. Cigarette smoking and risk of epithelial ovarian cancer. Cancer Causes Control. 2008;19(4): 413–20.
222. Gwinn ML, Webster LA, Lee NC, Layde PM, Rubin GL. Alcohol consumption and ovarian cancer risk. Am J Epidemiol. 1986;123(5):759–66.
223. Adami HO, McLaughlin JK, Hsing AW, et al. Alcoholism and cancer risk: a population-based cohort study. Cancer Causes Control. 1992;3(5): 419–25.
224. Larsson SC, Wolk A. Wine consumption and epithelial ovarian cancer. Cancer Epidemiol Biomarkers Prev. 2004;13(11 Pt 1):1823; author reply 1823–4.
225. Modugno F, Ness RB, Allen GO. Alcohol consumption and the risk of mucinous and nonmucinous epithelial ovarian cancer. Obstet Gynecol. 2003;102(6): 1336–43.
226. Goodman MT, Tung KH. Alcohol consumption and the risk of borderline and invasive ovarian cancer. Obstet Gynecol. 2003;101(6):1221–8.
227. Kelemen LE, Sellers TA, Vierkant RA, Harnack L, Cerhan JR. Association of folate and alcohol with risk of ovarian cancer in a prospective study of postmenopausal women. Cancer Causes Control. 2004; 15(10):1085–93.
228. Webb PM, Purdie DM, Bain CJ, Green AC. Alcohol, wine, and risk of epithelial ovarian cancer. Cancer Epidemiol Biomarkers Prev. 2004;13(4): 592–9.
229. Peterson NB, Trentham-Dietz A, Newcomb PA, et al. Alcohol consumption and ovarian cancer risk in a population-based case-control study. Int J Cancer. 2006;119(10):2423–7.
230. Schouten LJ, Zeegers MP, Goldbohm RA, van den Brandt PA. Alcohol and ovarian cancer risk: results from the Netherlands Cohort Study. Cancer Causes Control. 2004;15(2):201–9.
231. Genkinger JM, Hunter DJ, Spiegelman D, et al. Alcohol intake and ovarian cancer risk: a pooled analysis of 10 cohort studies. Br J Cancer. 2006; 94(5):757–62.
232. Kim HS, Kim JW, Shouten LJ, et al. Wine drinking and epithelial ovarian cancer risk: a meta-analysis. J Gynecol Oncol. 2010;21(2):112–8.
233. Shen N, Weiderpass E, Antilla A, et al. Epidemiology of occupational and environmental risk factors related to ovarian cancer. Scand J Work Environ Health. 1998;24(3):175–82.
234. Shields T, Gridley G, Moradi T, Adami J, Plato N, Dosemeci M. Occupational exposures and the risk of ovarian cancer in Sweden. Am J Ind Med. 2002;42(3):200–13.
235. Heller DS, Gordon RE, Westhoff C, Gerber S. Asbestos exposure and ovarian fiber burden. Am J Ind Med. 1996;29(5):435–9.
236. Langseth H, Johansen BV, Nesland JM, Kjaerheim K. Asbestos fibers in ovarian tissue from Norwegian pulp and paper workers. Int J Gynecol Cancer. 2007;17(1):44–9.
237. Roggli VL. Experimental models of asbestos-related diseases. In: Rogglie VL, Greenberg SD, Pratt PC, editors. Pathology of asbestos-associated diseases. Boston: Little Brown & Company; 1992.

238. Reid A, de Klerk N, Musk AW. Does exposure to asbestos cause ovarian cancer? A systematic literature review and meta-analysis. Cancer Epidemiol Biomarkers Prev. 2011;20(7):1287–95.
239. IARC Monographs on the Evaluation of Carcinogenic Risks to Humans. Overall evaluations of carcinogenicity: an updating of IARC monographs supplement 7. International Agency for Research on Cancer, Lyon; 1987.
240. Huncharek M, Geschwind JF, Kupelnick B. Perineal application of cosmetic talc and risk of invasive epithelial ovarian cancer: a meta-analysis of 11,933 subjects from sixteen observational studies. Anticancer Res. 2003;23(2C):1955–60.
241. Gates MA, Tworoger SS, Terry KL, et al. Talc use, variants of the GSTM1, GSTT1, and NAT2 genes, and risk of epithelial ovarian cancer. Cancer Epidemiol Biomarkers Prev. 2008;17(9): 2436–44.
242. Muscat JE, Huncharek MS. Perineal talc use and ovarian cancer: a critical review. Eur J Cancer Prev. 2008;17(2):139–46.
243. Turner MC, Chen Y, Krewski D, Ghadirian P. An overview of the association between allergy and cancer. Int J Cancer. 2006;118(12):3124–32.
244. Elmasri WM, Tran TH, Mulla ZD. A case-control study of asthma and ovarian cancer. Arch Environ Occup Health. 2010;65(2):101–5.
245. Pinheiro SP, Tworoger SS, Cramer DW, Rosner BA, Hankinson SE. Use of nonsteroidal antiinflammatory agents and incidence of ovarian cancer in 2 large prospective cohorts. Am J Epidemiol. 2009;169(11):1378–87.
246. Prizment AE, Folsom AR, Anderson KE. Nonsteroidal anti-inflammatory drugs and risk for ovarian and endometrial cancers in the Iowa Women's Health Study. Cancer Epidemiol Biomarkers Prev. 2010;19(2):435–42.
247. Li D. Metformin as an antitumor agent in cancer prevention and treatment. J Diabetes. 2011;3(4):320–7.
248. Bodmer M, Becker C, Meier C, Jick SS, Meier CR. Use of metformin and the risk of ovarian cancer: a case-control analysis. Gynecol Oncol. 2011;123: 200–4.

2 Genetic Risks of Ovarian Cancer

Christopher A. Friedrich

Introduction

Most cases of ovarian cancer occur sporadically, but the presence of germline mutations in some genes can increase the risk for developing ovarian cancer well above that of the general population. It is essential for the practitioner to recognize characteristics of an individual patient or a family to identify those who are more likely to carry one of these mutations and who might benefit from genetic testing. There is not a known gene that increases the risk only for ovarian cancer. Mutations in two well-established genes, *BRCA1* and *BRCA2*, increase the risk substantially for both breast cancer and ovarian cancer. Mutations in other more recently discovered and less common cancer susceptibility syndrome genes increase the risk for ovarian cancer, along with increasing the risk for several other cancers specific to each syndrome. Identifying members of these families involves taking an appropriate family medical history in order to identify relatives whose medical history may be related to the current patient's situation. It is also necessary to understand the strategies to follow in identifying which family member is most informative for initial testing, how to interpret the test results, and what to recommend regarding testing for relatives. While the majority of investigations have been performed on families carrying mutations in the *BRCA1* and *BRCA2* breast/ovarian cancer susceptibility genes, recent discoveries in a number of other tumor susceptibility syndrome genes have increased the number of syndromes for which germline mutation testing is available commercially, and practitioners must be aware of manifestations of these syndromes in relatives that may identify an at-risk family. For patients at increased risk of developing ovarian cancer due to germline mutations, guidelines have been published with the goal of reducing morbidity and mortality among those at highest risk.

Background

Ovarian cancer carries a lifetime risk for women of about 1 in 71 (1.4 %) and is the fifth most deadly cancer affecting women [1, 2]. In 2013, the National Cancer Institute estimates that about 22,240 cases will be diagnosed and there will be about 14,230 deaths from ovarian cancer [3]. It is the most lethal gynecologic malignancy, primarily due to the lack of symptoms that occur early in the disease and the lack of effective screening programs for the general population. It has been estimated that among white women in the USA, about 10–15 % of cases of ovarian cancer occur in patients with a germline mutation in *BRCA1* or *BRCA2* [4]. Because of this high prevalence, evaluation for genetic risk for any woman with

C.A. Friedrich, MD, PhD
Division of Oncology, Department of Medicine,
University of Mississippi Medical Center,
2500 North State Street, Jackson, MS 39216-4505, USA
e-mail: cfriedrich@umc.edu

S.A. Farghaly (ed.), *Advances in Diagnosis and Management of Ovarian Cancer*,
DOI 10.1007/978-1-4614-8271-0_2, © Springer Science+Business Media New York 2014

ovarian, fallopian tube, or primary peritoneal cancer is recommended in guidelines published by the National Comprehensive Cancer Network (NCCN) and other organizations [5]. Estimates of the risk of developing ovarian cancer among women with mutations in *BRCA1* or *BRCA2* range from 11 to 39 % [6, 7]. Identifying individuals at increased risk, followed by applying surveillance guidelines, may allow early detection and intervention when the disease is more likely to be curable.

Hereditary Breast and Ovarian Cancer (HBOC) Due to *BRCA1* or *BRCA2* Mutations

Taking a Family History

Families in which a germline mutation in *BRCA1* or *BRCA2* is being transmitted may show some characteristic features. These include multiple generations containing members with breast cancer (either invasive or ductal carcinoma in situ (DCIS)), ovarian cancer (or fallopian tube or primary peritoneal cancer), or both. Breast cancer may occur at a younger age (i.e., <50 years old). The affected relatives must be on the same side of the family. Males may be affected with breast cancer. The family may contain individuals who have had multiple primary cancers, including bilateral breast cancers or both breast and ovarian cancers. The family may come from an ethnic group with an increased risk due to particular mutations prevalent within that group (e.g., Ashkenazi Jews). A member of the family may be known to have a *BRCA1* or *BRCA2* mutation already. Pancreatic cancer may be present in the family.

Since this is an autosomal dominant condition, it is important to obtain information about both the maternal and paternal family histories, as men may have a germline mutation although they are much less likely to express it, but can pass it on to their daughters. Any mutation carrier, of either sex, has a 50 % chance of transmitting the mutation to any child of either sex.

Information about all adult relatives, including siblings, parents, grandparents, aunts, uncles, and cousins, or younger relatives with any kind of malignancy may be useful to identify patterns suggesting an autosomal dominant condition in the family.

Even if a mutation is present in a family, it may be difficult to appreciate its presence if the family is small or if there are few females living past age 45 in either side of the family. If a patient is adopted and nothing is known about the birth parents, then the family history is not available. If a woman has had an oophorectomy for a reason not related to malignancy (e.g., benign ovarian cysts), then the risk of breast cancer is reduced, and the risk for ovarian cancer is greatly reduced; therefore the expression of the mutated gene is less likely to be evident.

Although some families may show an obvious pattern of breast or ovarian cancer at young ages in first- or second-degree relatives in multiple generations, in other families the pattern is less clear-cut, and quantitative estimates of the likelihood of a *BRCA1* or *BRCA2* mutation being present may help guide the decision to recommend germline genetic testing or not. The BRCAPRO computer program is a Bayesian probability model that uses information about a family history of breast cancer, ovarian cancer, or both in first- and second-degree relatives to estimate the likelihood that a *BRCA1* or *BRCA2* mutation is present in the family [8]. The software has been updated regularly since its original publication to incorporate the revised population prevalence of mutations, and it also factors in variables including age-specific penetrance values as well as Ashkenazi Jewish heritage.

Another software package to estimate the likelihood of the presence of a *BRCA1* or *BRCA2* mutation is available from Myriad Genetics Laboratories on their web site and does not require a license [9, 10]. The program is updated with mutation prevalence results from the clinical test results obtained by Myriad Genetic Laboratories. The program takes into account a personal history of breast or ovarian cancer, a history of breast cancer in a relative, the age of onset for breast cancer in the patient or a relative(s) (<50 years or >50 years), the number of relatives with breast cancer, the presence or absence of Ashkenazi Jewish ancestry, and the presence or absence of ovarian cancer in the patient or in first- or second-degree relatives.

Other probability models exist but are not used as widely in clinical situations in the USA. It should be noted that the American Society of Clinical Oncology guidelines [11] do not recommend relying solely on quantitative estimates in deciding whether or not to recommend testing:

> Given the known limitations and wide variations inherent in models for estimating mutation probability in a given family or individual, and the lack of such models for many cancer predisposition syndromes, it is neither feasible nor practical to set numerical thresholds for recommending genetic risk assessment services. The American Society of Clinical Oncology therefore recommends that evaluation by a health care professional experienced in cancer genetics should be relied on in making interpretations of pedigree information and determinations of the appropriateness of genetic testing.

Germline Genetic Testing

Pretest Counseling

Before testing is offered, the patient should receive genetic counseling that includes a discussion of the risks and benefits of testing. Issues that may be present can vary widely among patients. The privacy of the patient must be respected, and it must be ascertained that the patient is requesting testing of his or her own volition, and not under duress from a relative, employer, insurer, or other party. The patient must understand that germline testing cannot determine the presence or absence of cancer. The patient's support systems must be explored, as the patient may receive results that cause anxiety, guilt, or depression. It must be determined whether or not the patient is willing to share her or his test results with other family members, and the patient must be assured that her or his test results will not be provided to anyone without her or his consent. The patient should be aware that test results may indicate an increased risk of developing cancer, or they may indicate the risk may be no different than that of the general population; in some cases the results may be ambiguous. Possible potential changes in cancer screening recommendations should be discussed before testing is performed. The possible risk to other family members (e.g., the patient's children), if a mutation is detected, should be discussed. The patient should understand that testing children for adult-onset genetic syndromes is not recommended under guidelines issued by several organizations [12]. For adult-onset conditions the consensus is that testing should not be offered until the child becomes an adult and can make his or her own decision regarding whether or not to undergo testing. Since the passage of the Genetic Information Nondiscrimination Act in 2008, it is illegal for health insurance companies to discriminate against individuals based on the results of genetic tests, but some patients are still concerned about the effects of adverse test results on their insurability and their employability if their health insurance is provided by their employer [13].

Molecular Testing

Three main types of tests are available: sequence analysis of entire genes, deletion/duplication analysis, and targeted mutation analysis of a specific mutation known to be in the family. In almost all cases anticoagulated whole blood is sent for DNA extraction and analysis. Buccal swabs do not provide enough DNA for comprehensive testing. In patients who have undergone an allogeneic bone marrow transplant, another tissue must be analyzed, usually fibroblasts from a skin biopsy.

In sequence analysis the precise sequence of nucleotides in the *BRCA1* and *BRCA2* genes is determined and compared to the consensus sequence in the general population and against a data base of known deleterious mutations from families affected by HBOC. This test is usually the most appropriate test for the first person to be tested from a family (see below for exceptions).

In a small number of families, large-scale rearrangements are present and deletion/duplication analysis can detect large or multiexon deletions, duplications, or rearrangements in *BRCA1* or *BRCA2*.

In some circumstances, more limited testing is appropriate as the initial test for a family. There are three common mutations found in Ashkenazi Jews (c.68_69delAG in *BRCA1*, c.5266dupC in *BRCA1*, and c.5946delT in *BRCA2*), and testing for the presence or absence of these three mutations first is recommended for members of this group [14–16]. If none of these three mutations are present and the family has a high likelihood of harboring a *BRCA1* or *BRCA2* mutation, then sequence analysis and deletion/duplication studies should be performed next.

Similarly, in a member of a family in which a deleterious mutation in *BRCA1* or *BRCA2* is known to be present, targeted mutation analysis for the familial mutation is most appropriate. An exception to this recommendation would exist if breast or ovarian cancer was present in both the paternal and maternal lineages and the familial mutation was only known for one side of the family. Then sequence analysis and deletion/duplication analysis would be indicated [17].

Determining the Most Appropriate Family Member for Initial Testing

It is essential to perform the initial testing on the person in the family who is most likely to have a detectable mutation. This is usually someone in the family who has unusual clinical features, including (1) early onset, (2) multiple primary cancers, or (3) male breast cancer. This will reduce the chance of genotyping someone whose cancer has occurred sporadically. If a mutation cannot be detected in a family member with features suspicious for an inherited cancer susceptibility syndrome, then there is no point in testing other relatives [17].

Interpreting Results

Three main types of results may be reported: (1) known deleterious mutation present; (2) a result of unknown clinical significance; or (3) no mutation is detected. These results must be interpreted in light of what is known about the patient and the family in order to avoid providing false reassurance to a patient. It should also be emphasized that if a mutation in a cancer susceptibility gene is known to be in a family and a family member is tested and found not to have inherited the mutation, their risk for the associated cancer is not zero but is the same as for anyone in the general population with similar nongenetic risk factors for the disease.

In a study of another autosomal dominant cancer susceptibility syndrome, familial adenomatous polyposis (FAP), Giardiello et al. found that in 31.6 % of the cases physicians misinterpreted genetic test results [18]. This syndrome, characterized by the development of numerous colon polyps and early onset of colon cancer, is caused by mutations in the *APC* gene. They analyzed 177 patients from 125 families tested for *APC* mutations. Among the subjects, 83 % had clinical features of FAP or were at risk for FAP due to their family history. Only 79.4 % of those seeking presymptomatic testing had an affected relative tested first.

The main mistake was lack of understanding that failure to identify a mutation ("no mutation found") could represent a false-negative unless an *APC* gene mutation had previously been identified in a relative. They also learned that only 18.6 % of the subjects received pretest genetic counseling and only 16.9 % of patients provided written informed consent prior to undergoing testing.

Hereditary Ovarian Cancer Due to Mutations in Other Genes

An increased risk for ovarian cancer has been known to exist in a small number of other genetic syndromes (Table 2.1). Recent technological advances have identified mutations in the associated genes and allowed the introduction of clinical testing for mutations in many of these genes. Recognition of the presence of particular cancers in the family may allow tentative diagnosis of a cancer susceptibility syndrome and guide molecular testing. The principles discussed previously regarding

Table 2.1 Hereditary ovarian cancer due to mutations in other genes

Syndrome	Manifestations	Inheritance	Gene(s)	Reference
Hereditary breast and ovarian cancer	Early-onset breast or ovarian cancer, multiple primary cancers, cancer in several generations, male breast cancer	AD	*BRCA1* *BRCA2*	[19] [20]
Hereditary nonpolyposis Colon cancer (HNPCC; aka Lynch syndrome)	Colon cancer, uterine cancer, ovarian cancer, stomach cancer, cancer in several generations	AD	*MLH1* *MSH2* *MSH6* *PMS2* *EPCAM*	[21] [22] [23] [24] [25]
Familial pancreatic cancer	Pancreatic cancer, breast cancer, ovarian cancer, cancer in several generations	AD	*PALB2*	[26]
Fanconi anemia	Skeletal defects, anemia, bone marrow failure, eye or ear defects, congenital heart defects, renal defects	AR	*BARD1* *BRIP1* *MRE11A* *NBN* *RAD50* *RAD51C*	[27] [28] [29] [30] [31] [32]
Li-Fraumeni syndrome	Breast, brain, adrenal, sarcomas, leukemia	AD	*TP53*	[33]
Peutz-Jeghers syndrome	Multiple gastrointestinal hamartomatous polyps; melanocytic macules of the lips, buccal mucosa, and digits; GI cancers; breast, lung, thyroid, pancreatic, uterine, ovarian sex cord tumors	AD	*STK11*	[34]
CHEK2	Breast cancer; may resemble Li-Fraumeni syndrome phenotype	AD	*CHEK2*	[27]
Cowden syndrome	Gastrointestinal hamartomatous polyps; breast, ovarian, uterine, cervical, thyroid, bladder cancers; mucocutaneous lesions	AD	*PTEN*	[35]
Bannayan-Ruvalcaba-Riley syndrome	Macrocephaly, angiomatosis, lipomatosis, childhood onset (cf. Cowden)	AD	*PTEN*	[36]
Although clinical testing is available for these genes, there seems to be no significantly increased risk for ovarian cancer associated with them, although there is for other gynecologic malignancies:				
Ataxia-telangiectasia	Cerebellar ataxia, telangiectases, immune system defects, breast cancer in heterozygous relatives of probands (not ovarian cancer)	AR	*ATM*	[37]
Hereditary diffuse gastric cancer	Gastric cancer	AD	*CDH1*	[38]
Familial adenomatous polyposis, Type 2	Multiple colorectal adenomas	AD	*MUTYH*	[39]

taking a family history, pretest counseling, identifying the most appropriate person in a family for initial testing, and interpreting test results also apply to patients with an increased risk due to mutations in these other genes.

Massively parallel sequencing (also called next-generation sequencing) is a high-throughput group of technologies that allows rapid simultaneous determination of single-base substitutions, small deletions and insertions, and large gene rearrangements in several genes. Recent studies of inherited mutations in breast and ovarian cancer [40] and ovarian, fallopian tube, and peritoneal carcinoma [41] have demonstrated the utility of the technique and identified several genes not previously suspected of being involved in ovarian cancer. In the latter study, 360 women undergoing primary surgery (273 with ovarian carcinomas, 48 with peritoneal carcinomas, 31 with fallopian tube carcinomas, and 8 with synchronous ovarian and endometrial carcinomas) had their germline DNA analyzed for several genes. Deleterious mutations were found in 24 % of the subjects, 18 % in *BRCA1* and *BRCA2*, and 6 % in several other genes (*BARD1, BRIP1, CHEK2, MRE11A, MSH6, NBN, PALB2, RAD50, RAD51C, or TP53*). In the women with inherited mutations, over 30 % had no family history of breast or ovarian cancer, and more than 35 % were over 60 years old at the time of diagnosis. The authors stated that massively parallel sequencing of several genes simultaneously, as compared to sequential sequencing of individual genes, could lower the cost while increasing the identification of patients and families with germline mutations.

Recently, testing for several genes using next-generation sequencing has become available on a clinical basis. Since mutations in each of these genes are much less prevalent than mutations in *BRCA1* or *BRCA2*, testing these genes should usually be considered a second-tier option for most patients, reserved for patients who do not have a detectable mutation in *BRCA1* or *BRCA2*. One commercially available panel offers testing for *ATM, BARD1, BRIP1, MRE11A, NBN, RAD50, RAD51C, CHEK2, CDH1, EPCAM, MLH1, MSH2, MSH6, PMS2, MUTYH, PALB2, PTEN, STK11*, and *TP53*. It should be noted that some of these genes are associated with an increased risk of breast or uterine cancer, not ovarian cancer, but testing for individual genes in this panel is also available.

Management of High-Risk Patients

Identification of a *BRCA1* or *BRCA2* mutation warrants more intensive surveillance and more aggressive management due to the increased risk for a cancer that typically causes few symptoms in the early stages. There is evidence that risk-reducing oophorectomy reduces the incidence of ovarian cancer substantially in mutation carriers [42–44], although the risk of peritoneal cancer remains at about 2 % after surgery [45, 46].

For women with a mutation, the NCCN has specific recommendations [47]. For prevention or early detection of breast or ovarian cancer, these recommendations include: (1) breast self-exam and education starting at age 18; (2) clinical breast exam every 6–12 months starting at age 25; (3) annual mammogram and breast magnetic resonance imaging screening starting at age 25 or earlier based on the earliest age of onset of breast cancer in the family; (4) a discussion of prophylactic mastectomy; (5) risk-reducing salpingo-oophorectomy, ideally between ages 35 and 40 and after childbearing is complete or earlier based on the earliest age of onset of ovarian cancer in the family; (6) for those not electing risk-reducing salpingo-oophorectomy, the recommendation is transvaginal ultrasound, preferably during days 1–10 of menstrual cycle in premenopausal women, plus cancer antigen 125 (CA-125) measurements (preferably after day 5 of the menstrual cycle in premenopausal woman) every 6 months starting at age 35 or 5–10 years before the earliest age of first diagnosis of ovarian cancer in the family; (7) consideration of chemoprevention (e.g., tamoxifen, raloxifene, exemestane); and (8) considering investigational imaging and screening studies when available in the context of a clinical trial. Regarding the salpingo-oophorectomy recommendation, NCCN Guidelines state: "Counseling includes a discussion of reproductive desires, extent of cancer risk, degree of protection for breast and ovarian cancer, management of menopausal symptoms, possible short term hormone replacement therapy (HRT) to a recommended maximum age of natural menopause, and related medical issues" [5]. There is no evidence that transvaginal ultrasound and serum CA-125 measurements reduce ovarian cancer mortality [48, 49].

Research studies have shown that oral contraceptive use is associated with a decreased risk for ovarian cancer among women with a germline *BRCA1* or *BRCA2* mutation [50]. Longer use of oral contraceptives was associated with a greater reduction in ovarian cancer incidence [51].

Family Planning

If a mutation is identified in any man or woman, there is a 50 % chance of passing on that mutation to any child they have. If the potential parent does not want to pass on the mutation to the next generation, prenatal diagnosis and preimplantation genetic diagnosis are technically possibly but rarely requested in clinical practice and beyond the scope of this chapter.

Conclusion

Ovarian cancer remains a diagnosis with a grim prognosis, mainly due to the late stage at which is it usually diagnosed. For a group of patients, however, there is hope for an improved outcome due to the recognition of some germline mutations that can identify those with an increased risk for developing the disease. There is some evidence that earlier and more frequent surveillance of these patients may result in (1) prevention of the disease, mainly through prophylactic oophorectomies and (2) decreased morbidity and mortality due to earlier diagnosis and treatment.

Recognition of the characteristics of patients likely to have such a mutation, as well as features that are typically found in families affected by these mutations, is critical to identifying those who are most likely to benefit from genetic testing. Understanding the ethical, legal, and social implications of identifying persons with a high risk for a potentially fatal disease is a difficult area that may benefit from referral to a geneticist or genetic counselor with expertise in inherited cancer susceptibility syndromes.

Families with a very high incidence of breast and ovarian cancer have been known for over a century [52], but the discovery of the *BRCA1* and *BRCA2* genes allowed the definite determination of those within the families who had the increased risk for malignancy. It also allowed the definite identification of those who did not inherit their family's mutation and whose risk for these cancers was no more than that of the general population. Subsequent study of those with deleterious germline mutations has allowed the identification of some interventions that reduce morbidity and mortality [53]. More recently, mutations in other genes have been found that increase the risk of ovarian cancer, although each of these genes seems to contribute much less to the burden of disease than *BRCA1* or *BRCA2*. It remains to be determined how effective interventions will be in improving outcomes for persons with mutations in these genes.

In June, 2013, the United States Supreme Court ruled the patents on the BrCa1 and BrCa2 gene sequences that had been awarded to Myriad Laboratories were invalid. Since that time several other laboratories have announced they will be offering BrCa1 and BrCa1 testing on a clinical basis. Because of numerous lawsuits that were filed after these announcements it is unclear how many other laboratories will be offering this testing, or what effect this will have on the cost of testing.

References

1. Statistics. Ovarian Cancer National Alliance. Available at: https://www.ovariancancer.org/about-ovarian-cancer/statistics/. Accessed 22 May 2013.
2. PDQ® Cancer Information Summary. National Cancer Institute; Bethesda, MD. Genetics of breast and ovarian cancer (PDQ®) – health professional. Date last modified 31 May 2012. Available at: http://www.cancer.gov/cancertopics/pdq/genetics/breast-and-ovarian/health-professional. Accessed 25 June 2012.
3. Ovarian cancer. American Cancer Society. Last updated 21 Mar 2013. Available at: http://www.cancer.org/cancer/ovariancancer/detailedguide/ovarian-cancer-key-statistics. Accessed 22 May 2013.
4. Campeau PM, Foulkes WD, Tischkowitz MD. Hereditary breast cancer: new genetic developments, new therapeutic avenues. Hum Genet. 2008;124(1):31–42.
5. NCCN Guidelines™ Version 1.2011. Breast and/or Ovarian Cancer Genetic Assessment. National Comprehensive Cancer Network. Last updated 7 April 2011. Available at: http://www.nccn.org/professionals/physician_gls/pdf/genetics_screening.pdf. Accessed 25 June 2012.
6. Antoniou A, Pharoah PD, Narod S, et al. Average risks of breast and ovarian cancer associated with BRCA1 or BRCA2 mutations detected in case Series unselected for family history: a combined analysis of 22 studies. Am J Hum Genet. 2003;72(5):1117–30.
7. Chen S, Parmigiani G. Meta-analysis of BRCA1 and BRCA2 penetrance. J Clin Oncol. 2007;25(11):1329–33.
8. Parmigiani G, Berry D, Aguilar O. Determining carrier probabilities for breast cancer-susceptibility

genes BRCA1 and BRCA2. Am J Hum Genet. 1998;62:145–58.
9. Frank TS, Deffenbaugh AM, Reid JE, Hulick M, Ward BE, Lingenfelter B, Gumpper KL, Scholl T, Tavtigian SV, Pruss DR, Critchfield GC. Clinical characteristics of individuals with germline mutations in BRCA1 and BRCA2: analysis of 10,000 individuals. J Clin Oncol. 2002;20:1480–90.
10. Myriad®: BRCA risk calculator. Available at https://www.myriadpro.com/brca-risk-calculator. Accessed 29 June 2012.
11. American Society of Clinical Oncology. American Society of Clinical Oncology policy statement update: genetic testing for cancer susceptibility (pdf). 2003. Available at http://www.asco.org/asco/downloads/GeneticTesting.pdf. Accessed 26 June 2010.
12. American Society of Human Genetics and American College of Medical Genetics. Points to consider: ethical, legal, and psychosocial implications of genetic testing in children and adolescents. Am J Hum Genet. 1995;57(5):1233–41. Available at http://www.ncbi.nlm.nih.gov/pmc/articles/PMC1801355/. Accessed 23 June 2012.
13. The National Human Genome Research Institute. GINA: The Genetic Information Nondiscrimination Act of 2008: Information for Researchers and Health Care Professionals. Retrieved 23 June 2012, from: http://www.genome.gov/Pages/PolicyEthics/GeneticDiscrimination/GINAInfoDoc.pdf.
14. Struewing JP, Abeliovich D, Peretz T, Avishai N, Kaback MM, Collins FS, Brody LC. The carrier frequency of the BRCA1 185delAG mutation is approximately 1 percent in Ashkenazi Jewish individuals. Nat Genet. 1995;11:198–200.
15. Spence CW, Judkins T, Schoenberger J, Balzotti M, Rajamani S, Colvin C, Burbidge A, Chen S, Frost M, Trost J, Wenstrup R, Roa B. Clinical testing experience for large genomic rearrangements in the BRCA1 and BRCA2 genes for hereditary breast and ovarian cancer. Poster. San Diego: 57th Annual Meeting of the American Society of Human Genetics; 2007
16. Stadler ZK, Saloustros E, Hansen NAL, Schluger AE, Kauff ND, Offit K, Robson ME. Absence of genomic BRCA1 and BRCA2 rearrangements in Ashkenazi breast and ovarian cancer families. Breast Cancer Res Treat. 2010;123:581–5.
17. Petrucelli N, Daly MB, Feldman GL. BRCA1 and BRCA2 hereditary breast and ovarian cancer. 1998 [Updated 20 Jan 2011]. In: Pagon RA, Bird TD, Dolan CR, et al., editors. GeneReviews™ [Internet]. Seattle (WA): University of Washington, Seattle; 1993-. Available from: http://www.ncbi.nlm.nih.gov/books/NBK1247/. Accessed 23 June 2012.
18. Giardiello FM, Brensinger JD, Petersen GM, Luce MC, Hylind LM, Bacon JA, Booker SV, Parker RD, Hamilton SR. The use and interpretation of commercial *APC* gene testing for familial adenomatous polyposis. N Engl J Med. 1997;336:823–7.
19. Breast-ovarian cancer, familial, susceptibility to, 1; BROVCA1. Online mendelian inheritance in man. Available at: http://omim.org/entry/604370. Accessed 25 June 2012.
20. Breast-ovarian cancer, familial, susceptibility to, 2; BROVCA2. Online mendelian inheritance in man. Available at: http://omim.org/entry/612555. Accessed 25 June 2012.
21. Colorectal cancer, hereditary nonpolyposis, type 2; HNPCC2. Online mendelian inheritance in man. Available at: http://omim.org/entry/609310. Accessed 25 June 2012.
22. Colorectal cancer, hereditary nonpolyposis, type 1; HNPCC1. Online mendelian inheritance in man. Available at: http://omim.org/entry/120435. Accessed 25 June 2012.
23. Colorectal cancer, hereditary nonpolyposis, type 5; HNPCC5. Online mendelian inheritance in man. Available at: http://omim.org/entry/614350. Accessed 25 June 2012.
24. Colorectal cancer, hereditary nonpolyposis, type 4; HNPCC4. Online mendelian inheritance in man. Available at: http://omim.org/entry/614337. Accessed 25 June 2012.
25. Colorectal cancer, hereditary nonpolyposis, type 8; HNPCC8. Online mendelian inheritance in man. Available at: http://omim.org/entry/613244. Accessed 25 June 2012.
26. Pancreatic cancer, susceptibility to, 3; online mendelian inheritance in man. Available at: http://omim.org/entry/613348. Accessed 25 June 2012.
27. Breast cancer. Online mendelian inheritance in man. Available at: http://omim.org/entry/114480. Accessed 25 June 2012.
28. Fanconi Anemia, Complementation Group J; FANCJ. Online mendelian inheritance in man. Available at: http://omim.org/entry/609054. Accessed 25 June 2012.
29. Meiotic recombination 11, S. Cerevisiae, Homolog of, A; MRE11A. Online mendelian inheritance in man. Available at: http://omim.org/entry/600814. Accessed 25 June 2012.
30. Porhanova NV, Sokolenko AP, Sherina NY, Ponomariova DN, Tkachenko NN, Matsko DE, Imyanitov EN. Ovarian cancer patient with germline mutations in both BRCA1 and NBN genes. (Letter). Cancer Genet Cytogenet. 2008;186:122–4.
31. RAD50, S. Cerevisiae, Homolog of; RAD50. Online mendelian inheritance in man. Available at: http://omim.org/entry/600814. Accessed 25 June 2012.
32. Fanconi Anemia, Complementation Group O; FANCO. Online mendelian inheritance in man. Available at: http://omim.org/entry/604040. Accessed 25 June 2012.
33. Li-Fraumeni Syndrome 1; LFS1. Online mendelian inheritance in man. Available at: http://omim.org/entry/151623. Accessed 25 June 2012.
34. Peutz-Jeghers Syndrome; PJS. Online mendelian inheritance in man. Available at: http://omim.org/entry/175200. Accessed 25 June 2012.
35. Cowden Disease; CD. Online mendelian inheritance in man. Available at: http://omim.org/entry/158350. Accessed 25 June 2012.

36. Bannayan-Riley-Ruvalcaba Syndrome; BRRS. Online mendelian inheritance in man. Available at: http://omim.org/entry/153480. Accessed 25 June 2012.
37. Ataxia-Telangiectasia; AT. Online mendelian inheritance in man. Available at: http://omim.org/entry/208900. Accessed 25 June 2012.
38. Gastric Cancer, Hereditary Diffuse; HDGC. Online mendelian inheritance in man. Available at: http://omim.org/entry/137215. Accessed June 25, 2012.
39. Familial Adenomatous Polyposis, 2; FAP2. Online mendelian inheritance in man. Available at: http://omim.org/entry/608456. Accessed 25 June 2012.
40. Walsh T, Lee MK, Casadei S, Thornton AM, Stray SM, Pennil C, Nord AS, Mandell JB, Swisker EM, King M-C. Detection of inherited mutations for breast and ovarian cancer using genomic capture and massively parallel sequencing. Proc Natl Acad Sci U S A. 2010;107:12629–33.
41. Walsh T, Casadei S, Lee MK, Pennil CC, Nord AS, Thornton AM, Roeb W, Agnew KJ, Stray SM, Wickramanayake A, Norquist B, Pennington KP, Garcia RL, King M-C, Swisher EM. Mutations in 12 genes for inherited ovarian, fallopian tube, and peritoneal carcinoma identified by massively parallel sequencing. Proc Natl Acad Sci U S A. 2011;108: 18032–7.
42. Kauff ND, et al. Risk-reducing salpingo-oophorectomy for the prevention of *BRCA1*- and *BRCA2*-associated breast and gynecologic cancer: a multicenter, prospective study. J Clin Oncol. 2008;26:1331–7.
43. Rebbeck TR, Kauff ND, Domchek SM. Meta-analysis of risk reduction estimates associated with risk-reducing salpingo-oophorectomy in *BRCA1* or *BRCA2* mutation carriers. J Natl Cancer Inst. 2009; 101:80–7.
44. Rutter JL, Wacholder S, Chetrit A, Lubin F, Menczer J, Ebbers S, Tucker MA, Struewing JP, Hartge P. Gynecologic surgeries and risk of ovarian cancer in women with BRCA1 and BRCA2 Ashkenazi founder mutations: an Israeli population-based case–control study. J Natl Cancer Inst. 2003;95:1072–8.
45. Piver MS, Jishi MF, Tsukada Y, Nava G. Primary peritoneal carcinoma after prophylactic oophorectomy in women with a family history of ovarian cancer. A Report of the Gilda Radner Familial Ovarian Cancer Registry. Cancer. 1993;71:2751–5.
46. Casey MJ, Synder C, Bewtra C, Narod SA, Watson P, Lynch HT. Intra-abdominal carcinomatosis after prophylactic oophorectomy in women of hereditary breast ovarian cancer syndrome kindreds associated with BRCA1 and BRCA2 mutations. Gynecol Oncol. 2005;97:457–67.
47. Daly MB, Axilbund JE, Buys S, Crawford B, Farrell CD, Friedman S, Garber JE, Goorha S, Gruber SB, Hampel H, Kaklamani V, Kohlmann W, Kurian W, Litton J, Marcom PK, Nussbaum R, Offit K, Pal Y, Pasche B, Pilarski R, Reiser W, Shannon KM, Smith JR, Swisher E, Weitzel JN. Genetic/familial high-risk assessment: breast and ovarian. J Natl Compr Canc Netw. 2010;8(5):562–94.
48. Clarke-Pearson DL. Screening for ovarian cancer. N Engl J Med. 2009;361:170–7.
49. Goozner M. Personalizing ovarian cancer screening. JNCI J Natl Cancer Inst. 2010;102(15):1112–3.
50. Narod SA, Ford D, Devilee P, Barkardottir RB, Lynch HT, Smith SA, Ponder BA, Weber BL, Garber JE, Birch JM, et al. An evaluation of genetic heterogeneity in 145 breast-ovarian cancer families. Breast Cancer Linkage Consortium. Am J Hum Genet. 1995;56:254–64.
51. Whittemore AS, Balise RR, Pharoah PD, Dicioccio RA, Oakley-Girvan I, Ramus SJ, Daly M, Usinowicz MB, Garlinghouse Jones K, Ponder BA, Buys S, Senie R, Andrulis I, John E, Hopper JL, Piver MS. Oral contraceptive use and ovarian cancer risk among carriers of BRCA1 or BRCA2 mutations. Br J Cancer. 2004;91:1911–5.
52. Broca P. Traité des Tumeurs. Paris: Asselin; 1866.
53. Friedrich CA. The role of DNA testing in breast, ovarian, and colon cancers. Am J Med Sci. 2003; 325(3):120–4.

Ovarian Cancer Screening and Early Detection

3

Brian M. Nolen and Anna E. Lokshin

Early Detection of Ovarian Cancer: Requirements and Reality [1]

Ovarian cancer represents the eighth most common cancer among women and the second most frequently diagnosed gynecological malignancy in the USA and Europe [2]. The overall mortality attributed to ovarian cancer exceeds that of any other gynecological cancer with over 50 % of the more than 200,000 women newly diagnosed each year worldwide expected to perish from the disease [3]. A critical factor in the elevated mortality associated with ovarian cancer is the lack of disease-specific symptoms. This difficulty is underscored in a joint recommendation recently issued by a high-profile consortium of public health organizations termed the Ovarian Cancer Symptom Index (OCSI), which listed bloating, pelvic or abdominal pain, difficulty eating/fullness, and urinary symptoms as those more likely to occur in ovarian cancer patients than healthy women [4]. Compounding the problem of ubiquitous clinical presentation is the observation that the majority of early-stage cancers are asymptomatic resulting in over three-quarters of all diagnoses being made at a time when the disease has already established regional or distant metastases [5]. Despite aggressive cytoreductive surgery and platinum-based chemotherapy, the 5-year survival rate for patients with clinically advanced ovarian cancer is only 15–20 %, although the cure rate for stage I disease is usually greater than 90 % [5, 6]. This strongly suggests that finding and removing tumors that remain confined to the ovary should confer a substantial improvement in survival. A stochastic model developed for annual screening indicated that shifting diagnosis from late (stage III) to early (stage I) stages could result in 3.4 years of life saved per patient [7]. Therefore, biomarker-based screening methodologies aimed at detecting ovarian cancer at its earliest stages have the potential to result in substantial improvements in overall survival for this disease.

Considering the low prevalence of ovarian cancer, any proposed screening strategy must demonstrate a minimum specificity (SP) of 99.6 % and a sensitivity (SN) of >75 % to achieve a positive predictive value (PPV) of 10 % and avoid an unacceptable level of false-positive results [8, 9]. Present methods for detecting ovarian cancer include physical examination, assessment of symptoms, imaging by several modalities (transvaginal ultrasound [TVU], Doppler ultrasound,

B.M. Nolen, PhD (✉)
University of Pittsburgh Cancer Institute,
Hillman Cancer Center 1.18, 5117 Centre Avenue,
Pittsburgh, PA 15213, USA
e-mail: nolanb@upmc.edu

A.E. Lokshin, PhD
University of Pittsburgh Cancer Institute,
Hillman Cancer Center 1.19d, 5117 Centre Avenue,
Pittsburgh, PA 15213, USA

Departments of Medicine, Pathology, and Ob/Gyn,
School of Medicine, University of Pittsburgh,
Pittsburgh, PA, USA
e-mail: lokshin@upmc.edu

S.A. Farghaly (ed.), *Advances in Diagnosis and Management of Ovarian Cancer*,
DOI 10.1007/978-1-4614-8271-0_3, © Springer Science+Business Media New York 2014

computed tomography [CT], magnetic resonance imaging [MRI], positron emission tomography [PET]), and serum levels of the cancer antigen 125 (CA-125) biomarker of ovarian cancer (reviewed in [10]) [11, 12]. CA-125 is the most robust and well-known serum biomarker for detection of ovarian cancer. The initial finding of CA-125 levels greater than 35 U/mL in approximately 83 % of patients with advanced epithelial ovarian cancer and in only 1–2 % of the normal population led to investigations into its use as a biomarker for ovarian cancer [13, 14]. Furthermore, elevated levels of CA-125 are most strongly associated with serous tumors, which represent the most aggressive histological type of ovarian cancer [15]. Subsequent analyses of CA-125 have revealed a number of limitations for the test. Although CA-125 is frequently elevated in advanced-stage ovarian cancer, the protein is elevated in less than 50 % of stage I disease and is often normal in mucinous, endometrioid, and clear cell carcinomas [16–22]. Moreover, a number of benign and malignant conditions may result in falsely elevated CA-125 values [23, 24]. Additional factors may influence the CA-125 level, such as race/ethnicity, age, hysterectomy, smoking history, and obesity [25]. Despite these well-recognized limitations, CA-125 remains the most widely studied serum biomarker for ovarian cancer. The best currently available protocol for early detection of ovarian cancer, a combination of screening for elevated CA-125 and transvaginal ultrasound in the presence of elevated CA-125 [26, 27], does not meet the stringent criteria for cost-effectiveness espoused by the US Preventive Services Task Force [28]. As a result, no professional group currently recommends screening for ovarian cancer in the general population [29–31]. Thus, there is a critical need to develop additional informative biomarkers capable of complementing CA-125 in order to achieve the requisite diagnostic performance necessary for clinical advancement.

Two large, randomized trials designed to determine whether ovarian cancer screening improves survival have recently reported their findings. In the Prostate, Lung, Colon, and Ovarian (PLCO) Cancer Screening Trial, 34,261 healthy women between the ages of 55 and 74 years were randomly assigned to undergo either annual CA-125 testing plus TVU or to receive "usual care." [32] A positive finding was defined as a CA-125 level of more than 35 U/mL or TVU evidence of an abnormal ovarian volume or an ovarian cyst with papillary projections or solid components. Diagnostic follow-up of positive screens was performed at the discretion of participants' physicians. The PPV of a positive screening test was 1.0–1.3 % during the 4 years of screening. The overall ratio of surgeries to screen-detected cancers was 19.5:1. Importantly, 72 % of screen-detected cases were stage III or IV, indicating that screening has not resulted in stage shift [32]. The PLCO project team recently released its final report on survival in which they conclude that the CA-125/TVU screening approach does not reduce disease-specific mortality in comparison to usual care, but does result in an increase in invasive medical procedures and associated harms [33]. In the United Kingdom Collaborative Trial of Ovarian Cancer Screening (UKCTOCS), 202,638 postmenopausal women between the ages of 50 and 74 years who were deemed to be at average risk for ovarian cancer were randomly assigned to undergo annual pelvic examination (control group), annual TVU (ultrasonography or USS group), or annual measurement of CA-125 (evaluated over time with the use of Risk of Ovarian Cancer Algorithm [ROCA] [34]) plus TVU in cases in which the CA-125 level was elevated (multimodality or MMS group) [35]. Women with persistent abnormality on repeat screens underwent evaluation by a clinical oncologist and, where appropriate, surgery. As compared with ultrasonography alone, multimodality screening had a significantly greater SP (99.8 % vs. 98.2 %) and a higher PPV (35.1 % vs. 2.8 %) ($P<0.001$); SN did not differ significantly between the two groups. The proportion of primary invasive ovarian and fallopian tube cancers diagnosed with stage I/II disease (48 %) was encouraging compared with the 26 % rate in the clinical series [36] and 22 % in the prevalence screen of the PLCO screening trial in the USA [37]. Both the USS and MMS arms demonstrated a higher proportion of stage I–II cancers. The apparent difference between PLCO and UKCTOCS in proportion of screen-detected early cases could possibly be explained by the mode of diagnostic follow-up utilized in each trial wherein the suspicious cases identified in the PLCO trial were cared for by their physicians and in the UKCTOCS trial the majority were referred to a gynecological oncologist.

The World Health Organization (WHO) has specified prerequisite criteria that must be met for a screening test to be effective [38]. Notably, a sufficient interval must exist between onset of early-stage disease and development of advanced disease to allow for screening and intervention. Although ovarian cancer satisfies many of the WHO requirements, several particular aspects of the etiology and epidemiology of ovarian cancer complicate the question of screening:

1. Due to the lack of knowledge of a precursor lesion, screening must focus on early detection of invasive cancer.
2. The transition time from stage I to stage III is unclear, since it is not known whether there is an evolution from an early to an advanced stage or whether the disease may initially arise as a diffuse process in the peritoneal cavity.
3. Clinical evidence indicates that methods in common use today are not able to identify cancers at early enough stages to improve upon the natural history of the disease.
4. Approximately 90 % of ovarian cancers appear to be sporadic directing screening algorithms toward a general population of women.
5. Given a low prevalence of ovarian cancer (40 per 100,000 per year) among postmenopausal women, screening tests must achieve an SN of at least 75 % and an SP of greater than 99.6 % to attain a PPV of 10 %, which would translate into ten surgeries for every one case of cancer detected.

Biomarker Development

Biomarker Discovery

A number of cell-surface antigens and serum proteins are produced by ovarian tumors and can be assayed using monoclonal antibodies. Some of these assays have been applied clinically as markers of disease status and are useful in the detection of subclinical disease and in the diagnosis of recurrent ovarian cancer [39, 40]. As mentioned above, of all the serum biomarkers of ovarian cancer, CA-125 has been the most extensively studied; however, a growing number of additional biomarkers elevated in patients with ovarian cancer have been identified and evaluated in preclinical studies (Table 3.1) including the following: CA 15-3, CA 54/61, CA 19-9, TAG-72, OVX1, M-CSF, carcinoembriogenic antigen (CEA), cancer-associated serum antigen (CASA), lipid-associated sialic acid (LASA), urinary gonadotropin fragment (UGF), HER2/neu (ErbB2), EGFR, sICAM-1, VEGF, and lysophosphatidic acid [17, 41–49]. In addition, several members of the kallikrein family of proteins have been identified as potential serum markers of ovarian cancer [50–56]. The use of gene expression array analysis has identified a number of novel markers, including HE4 [57], prostasin [58], and osteopontin [59]. HE4, or human epididymis protein 4, is a secreted glycoprotein product of the *WFDC2* gene which has shown great promise as a diagnostic biomarker for ovarian cancer and has also recently been approved by the US Food and Drug Administration for disease monitoring [60]. With the exception of HE4, the identification of additional biomarkers associated with ovarian cancer has not translated into widespread clinical implementation. Although several of these biomarkers are currently utilized clinically in other disease settings, most notably CA 15-3 and CA 19-9 for disease monitoring in breast and pancreatic cancer, respectively, none have shown significant diagnostic capabilities.

Phases of Cancer Biomarker Development

Biomarker development efforts to date clearly indicate that no individual biomarker, including CA-125, can provide sufficient SN at high SP for the early detection of ovarian cancer. Therefore, the bulk of research efforts are now focused on the development of robust multimarker algorithms incorporating additional informative biomarkers which complement CA-125. According

Table 3.1 Alternative biomarkers of ovarian cancer

Biomarker	Description	Method	Reference
CA 15-3	Tumor antigen	Serum ELISA	Woolas et al. [41]
CA 19-9	Tumor antigen	Serum ELISA	Woolas et al. [41]
TAG-72	Tumor antigen	Serum ELISA	Woolas et al. [41].
CA 54/61	Tumor antigen	IHC	Suzuki et al. [42].
OVX1	Tumor antigen	Serum RIA	Woolas et al. [17]
M-CSF	Growth factor	Serum RIA	Woolas et al. [17].
CEA	Tumor antigen	Luminex® (serum)	Yurkovetsky et al. [43].
CASA	Tumor antigen	Serum ELISA	Sehouli et al. [44].
LASA	Tumor antigen	Serum ELISA	Crump et al. [45]
UGF	Tumor antigen	Serum ELISA	Crump et al. [45]
HER2/neu	Growth factor receptor	Serum ELISA	Crump et al. [45]
EGFR	Growth factor receptor	MS/serum ELISA	Baron et al. [46].
sICAM1	Adhesion molecule	Serum ELISA	Callet et al. [47].
VEGF	Angiogenesis factor	Serum ELISA	Oehler et al. [48].
Lysophosphatidic acid	Mitogenic factor	Plasma ELISA	Xu et al. [49].
Kallikreins 4–8,11,15	Proteases	Various methods	Diamandis and colleagues [50–56]
HE4	Tumor antigen	Microarray	Schummer et al. [57].
Prostasin	Protease	Microarray	Mok et al. [58].
Osteopontin	Bone factor	Microarray	Kim et al. [59].

to the requirements of the Early Detection Research Network/NIH, biomarker development should include five phases: preclinical exploratory Phase 1, clinical development and validation in Phase 2, validation in a retrospective longitudinal study in Phase 3, prospective screening in Phase 4, and randomized clinical trials in Phase 5 [61].

Methodological Approaches to Protein Biomarkers Development

Noninvasive biomarker testing is essential for practical general population monitoring. Therefore, biomarkers that can be detected in bodily fluids such as blood, urine, saliva, or cervical mucus could be considered. The candidate marker must be both stable in these body fluids and present in quantities that can quantitatively differentiate individuals with ovarian cancer from individuals without disease. In the arena of Phase 1 protein biomarker development, a number of conceptual and methodological approaches have been utilized for biomarker discovery in bodily fluids. Early efforts, including those responsible for the identification of CA-125, described the analysis of murine antibodies capable of reacting with tumor cells from ovarian cancer patients [62–64]. Later, biomarker discovery was achieved primarily by means of high-throughput screening methodologies, such as genomic, transcriptional, and proteomic profiling [2, 65–75]. Proteomic profiling provides direct information about proteins differentially expressed in cancer patients and control individuals. Such profiling has been performed by mass spectrometry (reviewed in [66]) and, lately, through the use of antibody arrays, such as multiplex bead-based arrays or reverse antigen arrays [43, 76]. Both approaches have limitations. To date, mass spectrometry (MS)-based methods have demonstrated limited analytical sensitivity, and consequently most of the biomarkers discovered by proteomics represent high-abundance, predominantly acute-phase proteins [4]. Recently developed methods aimed at the depletion of abundant serum proteins may overcome this limitation and lead to the enhanced discovery of lower-abundance biomarkers [77, 78]. Immunoassays permit the analysis of proteins present in bodily fluids at much lower concentrations, as low as fg/mL, but this approach is limited by the availability of suitable

Table 3.2 Ovarian cancer-associated proteins

Biological function	Biomarkers	Role in cancer
Cytokines/ chemokines	IL-1,IL- 6, IL-7, IL-8, IL-10, IL-11, IL-12, IL-16, IL-18, IL-21, IL-23, IL-28A, IL-33, LIF, TNFR1-2, HVEM (TNFRSF14), IL-1Rα,b, IL-2R, M-CSF, MIP-1α, TNF-α, CD40, RANTES, CD40L, MIF, IFN-β, MCP-4 (CCL13), MIG (CXCL9), MIP-1delta (CCL15), MIP-3α (CCL20), MIP-4 (CCL18), MPIF-1, SDF-1a+b (CXCL12), CD137/4-1BB, lymphotactin (XCL1), eotaxin-1 (CCL11), eotaxin-2 (CCL24), 6Ckine (CCL21), BLC (CXCL13), CTACK (CCL27), BCA-1 (CXCL13), HCC4 (CCL16), CTAP-3 (CXCL7)	Tumor growth, angiogenesis, immune functions, inflammation, invasion
Growth/angiogenic factors	IGF-I, VEGF, VEGFR3, EGFR, ErbB2, CTGF, PDGF AA, BB, PDGFRb, bFGF, TGFbRIII, betacellulin, IGFBP-1–4, 6, BDNF, PEDF, angiopoietin-2, renin, lysophosphatidic acid (LPA), b2-microglobulin, sialyl TN, ACE	Tumor growth, angiogenesis
Adhesion molecules/ proteases/related molecules	CA-125, CA 19-9, CEA, CA 15-3, CA-50, CA 72-4, OVX1, mesothelin, sialyl TN [80], MMP-2,3,7,9, VAP-1, TIMP1-2, tenascin C, VCAM-1, osteopontin, KIM-1, NCAM, tetranectin, nidogen-2, cathepsin L, prostasin, matriptase, kallikreins 2,6,10, cystatin C, claudin, spondin-2, SLPI	Invasion/metastases
Hormones/related molecules	bHCG, urinary gonadotropin peptide, inhibin, leptin, adiponectin, GH, TSH, ACTH, PRL, FSH, LH, cortisol, TTR, osteocalcin, insulin, ghrelin, GIP, GLP-1, amylin, glucagon, peptide YY (PYY), follistatin, hepcidin	Tumor growth, transformation
Acute phase reactants/coagulation factors	CRP, ApoA1, CIII, H, transthyretin (TTR), SAA, SAP, complement C3,4, complement factor H, albumin, ceruloplasmin, haptoglobin, beta-hemoglobin, transferrin, ferritin, fibrinogen, thrombin, von Willebrand factor, myoglobin, immunosuppressive acidic protein, lipid-associated sialic acid (LASA), S100A12 (EN-RAGE), fetuin A, clusterin, alpha1-antitrypsin, a2-macroglobulin, serpin1 (human plasminogen activator inhibitor-1, tPAI-1), Cox-1, Hsp27, Hsp60, Hsp80, Hsp90, lectin-type oxidized LDL receptor 1 (LOX-1), CD14, lipocalin 2, ITIH4	Inflammation, tumor growth, angiogenesis
Apoptosis factors	sFasL, Cyfra 21-1, TPA, perforin, DcR3	Tumor growth, immune functions
Energy homeostasis	AGRP, creatine kinase-MB	Tumor growth
Proteins with undefined or other functions	HE4, human milk fat globule (HMFG 1–2), NT-Pro-BNP, neuron-specific enolase (NSE), CASA, NB/70 K, AFP, afamin (AFM), collagen, prohibitin, keratin-6, PARC, B7-H4, YK-L40	

Based on findings reported in [66, 76, 77, 79, 81–124]

immunoassays. However, the menu of candidate biomarker immunoassays continues to expand as the popularity of multiplex bead-based platforms grows. For instance, three large screening exercises aimed at the identification of ovarian cancer biomarkers using multiplex bead-based immunoassays evaluated over 300 candidate biomarkers in serum obtained from large groups of ovarian cancer patients and controls [43, 76, 79].

A comprehensive review of the relevant literature identified over 160 proteins reported to be differentially expressed in early ovarian cancer in comparison to healthy controls (Table 3.2). The ongoing analysis of these proteins and the biological and pathological pathways they regulate could provide powerful tools for determining the mechanisms of ovarian cancer initiation and progression that could eventually lead to individualized molecular medicine. However, as mentioned above, further validation steps are necessary to determine the diagnostic value of these proteins, and relatively few have been evaluated in studies

Table 3.3 Trends in serum biomarker alteration in three large studies

Biological function	Trend in OC	Biomarkers
Cytokines/chemokines	Elevated	IL-10[a], IL-6[a], TNF-α[a], TNFR2[a], 6Ckine, BCA-1, BLC/CXCL, CCL20/MIP-3α, CD40, CXCL9/MIG, IL-1Rα, IL-11, IL-16, IL-1β, IL-21, IL-28A, IL-2R, IL-33, IL-7, IL-8, LIF, MIF, MIP-1δ, RANTES, sCD137/4, TNFR1
	Decreased	Eotaxin-1, eotaxin-2, IL-18, macrophage-derived chemokine, XCL1/lymphotactin
Growth/angiogenic factors	Elevated	IGFBP-1[a], angiopoietin-2, β2-microglobulin, betacellulin, CTGF, bFGF, heparin-binding EGF-like growth factor, IGFBP-2, IGFBP-4, PDGF, VEGF
	Decreased	EGFR[b], BDNF[a], ErbB2[a], IGFBP-3, IGFBP-6, IGF-I, PEDF, stem cell factor
Adhesion molecules/proteases	Elevated	CA-125[a], CA 19-9[a], OPN[a], TIMP-1[a], CA 15-3, CA 72-4, cathepsin D, MMP-9, tenascin C
	Decreased	VCAM-1[a], MMP-2, MMP-3, NCAM
Hormones	Elevated	ACTH, GH, GLP-1, prolactin, TSH
	Decreased	Adiponectin, estrogen receptor α, FSH, ghrelin, GIP, insulin, leptin, LH, osteocalcin, thrombopoietin
Acute phase reactants/coagulation factors	Elevated	α1-Antitrypsin[a], CRP[a], EN-RAGE, ferritin, fibrinogen, haptoglobin, HSA, PAI-1, protein S100-A12 (EN-RAGE), SAP, von Willebrand factor
	Decreased	a2-Macroglobulin[a], ApoA1[a], apolipoprotein CIII, apolipoprotein H, clusterin, complement C3, complement C4, Factor VII, fetuin A, prealbumin[a]
Apoptosis factors	Elevated	Cyfra 21-1
	Decreased	Fas, perforin
Energy homeostasis	Elevated	AGRP
	Decreased	Creatine kinase-MB
Undefined or other functions	Elevated	Anti-TFF-3, FABP, HE4, NSE, NT-Pro-BNP
	Decreased	none

Biomarker results compiled from [43, 76] and unpublished observations
[a]trend agreement in two studies
[b]trend agreement in three studies

which meet the criteria for Phase 2 and/or 3 biomarker development [43, 76, 125–129].

The complex and multifaceted process of ovarian epithelial tumorigenesis necessitates the development of an equally complex tumor microenvironment. Within this microenvironment, tumor cells, stromal fibroblasts, and infiltrating leukocytes produce a multitude of autocrine and paracrine factors, including but not limited to cytokines, chemokines, growth factors, hormones, inflammatory mediators, and acute-phase reaction molecules. It is this complex signaling network which mediates tumor/stroma interactions and facilitates tumor proliferation, invasion, neoangiogenesis, and metastasis. As illustrated in Table 3.2, concentrations of numerous proteins involved in the above listed tumorigenic biological functions are altered in the circulation of ovarian cancer patients [130]. Mediators of inflammation, including cytokines and acute-phase reactants, were the most numerous among the various biological groups followed by adhesion molecules/proteases, growth/angiogenic factors, and hormones. Contrary to the commonly held notion that useful biomarkers represent proteins which are significantly elevated in the circulation of cancer patients, many of the identified proteins were observed to be significantly decreased in the ovarian cancer group in a number of studies (Table 3.3). These findings represent the complexity of signaling mechanisms at work in ovarian cancer development and a potential paradigm shift in biomarker research.

Advances in Population-Based Screening for Ovarian Cancer

The development of multimarker panels for the diagnosis of ovarian cancer is currently advancing on two fronts. The first of these fronts includes investigators seeking improved tools for use in screening strategies for ovarian cancer in the general population. Given the limited performance of currently used imaging techniques and CA-125 testing as well as the overall rarity of ovarian cancer, routine population-based screening is not recommended by any of the major relevant professional societies [24]. It also remains unlikely that any stand-alone biomarker-based screening test will be capable of overcoming the 10 % PPV level required for implementation. However, work has persisted based on the notion that biomarker testing may prove effective in sufficiently defined high-risk groups or as part of a multimodal screening strategy involving TVU or an equivalent imaging method as a second-line test. The second front in the clinical use of ovarian cancer biomarkers pertains to the use of multimarker panels in the triage of women presenting with a pelvic mass. This aspect of early detection is discussed in depth in the next section.

Current State of Ovarian Cancer Screening: Clinical Trials

In addition to the PLCO and UKCTOCS screening trials, a number of additional clinical trials have examined the efficacy of imaging and CA-125. Imaging of the ovary has been proposed as a strategy to detect changes in size and architecture that might precede the development of symptoms and detection by pelvic examination. Studies involving healthy women have established the upper limit of ovarian size as greater than 5 cm and a set of morphologic characteristics of ovarian masses in order to identify malignant neoplasms [131, 132]. Therefore, considering the above model, these trials could be expected to preferentially diagnose cancer at invasive late stages, thus limiting their efficacy as screening tools [133]. In fact, several prospective studies of transvaginal ultrasonography that involved more than 136,000 women had mixed results, with some but not others showing a nonsignificant trend toward the diagnosis of ovarian cancer at an early stage [12, 32, 134–139]. The PPV of ultrasonography in these studies ranged from 1.0 to 27 % [137]. The interpretation of these results is complicated by differences with respect to inclusion criteria, with some studies enrolling only women at high risk (on the basis of a family history) [12, 135], some enrolling only women at average risk [32, 134, 138, 139], and others enrolling both women at high risk and those at average risk [136, 137].

An alternative strategy is to evaluate serum tumor markers for the early detection of ovarian cancer. This strategy is potentially attractive in that measurement of markers is broadly available, can be repeated at appropriate intervals, and is minimally invasive. In addition, biomarker testing does not depend on operator interpretation and is less costly than ultrasonography. As of yet, the most robust serum biomarker for detection of ovarian cancer is CA-125. In clinical trials, CA-125 as a single screening biomarker demonstrated limited utility when examined in a retrospective analysis of serum samples from 5,550 women enrolled in a population-based registry in Sweden [140]. Later it was suggested that measurement of CA-125 values in an individual patient over time could improve the estimation of a patient's risk of ovarian cancer [141]. To evaluate CA-125 dynamics, the ROCA was developed based on the slope of serial CA-125 measurements drawn at regular intervals [34]. This algorithm was based on the observation that irrespective of the initial level, CA-125 measurements are stable in non-cases for periods of more than 5 years, indicating that each woman has her own baseline level of CA-125 [34]. In contrast, exponentially increasing serial values readily identify cases. When the ROCA score exceeds a 1 % risk of having ovarian cancer, patients undergo TVU to determine whether additional intervention is warranted. In a retrospective examination of 33,621 serum samples from 9,233 women, ROCA provided an SN of 86 % at a fixed SP of 98 % for the preclinical detection of ovarian cancer, as compared with an SN of 62 % for a single CA-125 value [34]. This algorithm was confirmed to have a reasonably high PPV (19 %) in a subsequent prospective pilot study involving more than 13,000 postmenopausal women [142]. This strategy is currently being prospectively studied among more than 2,600 high-risk women by the Gynecologic Oncology Group (protocol #199) as well as in a parallel trial being conducted by the National Cancer Institute-Cancer Genetics Network [143]. Another algorithm used in screening of high-risk women is the Parametric Empirical Bayes (PEB) algorithm [45, 144]. In the PEB model, each woman's complete screening history, not only her most recent index value, acts as her own control, and the slightest deviation from that person-specific norm is used to detect elevated values at a fixed SP. The PEB model will assign the great majority of subjects lower thresholds, allowing their cancers to be detected earlier. Additionally, PEB allows for assessment of multiple markers.

Selection of Multimarker Panels Based on Postdiagnostic Samples

A number of studies have utilized different criteria for biomarker prioritization and selection (Table 3.4). In the study by Mor et al., 169 proteins were analyzed in serum samples obtained from ovarian cancer patients by means of RCA immunoassay microarray, and 35 of these proteins were found to be differentially expressed between cases and controls [79]. Biomarkers were further prioritized for independent ELISA testing if (1) similar levels of expression were observed in newly diagnosed patients and patients with recurrent disease; (2) ELISA tests were available commercially for these analytes; and

Table 3.4 Multimarker panels which discriminate ovarian cancer cases from healthy controls

Panel	Cases/ controls	SN/SP	Analytical platform	Bioinformatics method	Biomarker prioritization	Year/reference
CA-125, ApoA1, TTR	200/142[b]	74/97	MS	SVM	No	2004 [129]
CA-125, CA 72-4, M-CSF	123/224[b]	70/98	ELISA	CT, MDA, LR	Yes	2004 [127]
CA-125, IL-6, IL-8, VEGF, EGF	44/45	85/95	BBIA	CT	No	2005 [145]
CA-125, TTR, ApoA1	20/82	89/92	MS	LR	No	2007 [146]
CA-125, leptin, PRL, OPN, IGF-II, MIF	156/362[b]	95.3/99.4	BBIA	LR	No	2008 [128]
CA-125, HE4, glycodelin, Plau-R, MUC1, PAI1	200/396	80–89/87	BBIA	LR	Yes	2008 [147]
CA-125, HE4, CEA, VCAM-1	456/2,000[b]	86–93/98	BBIA	MMC	No	2010 [43]
CA-125, CA 19-9, EGFR, CRP, myoglobin, ApoA1, CIII, MIP-1α, IL-6, IL-18, tenascin C	176/187[b]	91.3/88.5	BBIA	Knowledge Discovery Engine-VS	No	2008–2009 [76, 125]
CA-125, CRP, SAA, IL-6, IL-8	150/212[b]	94.1/91.3	BBIA	LR	Yes	2010 [126]
CA-125, HE4, SI[a]	74/137	84/98.5	ELISA	N/A	Yes	2010 [148]

BBIA bead-based immunoassay, *CT* classification trees
[a]Symptom Index
[b]Includes independent validation set

(3) they had compelling biological reasons for their evaluation. These analytes were EGF, MIF-1, TNF-α, leptin, prolactin, IL-17, OPN, and IGF-II. Leptin, prolactin, OPN, and IGF-II showed perfect correlation between the RCA microarray immunoassays and the ELISA assays and were able, when used together, to discriminate the control and cancer training group samples with 95 % SN at 95 % SP. Adding CA-125 and MIF to this panel provided a classification power of 92 % SN at 99 % SP. This panel was equally sensitive to different histological subtypes of primary epithelial ovarian cancers: papillary serous, clear cell, endometrioid, and mixed [128]. Unfortunately, following a high level of initial enthusiasm and the subsequent marketing of this panel under the trade name OvaSure, deficiencies in study design have been identified which illustrate the challenges facing biomarker development efforts in general. The most prominent among these deficiencies was the inaccurate calculation of PPV based on improper estimates of ovarian cancer prevalence [143, 149]. This observation coupled with the lack of evaluation in a large prospective study led to performance revisions and the withdrawal of the commercial kit.

In the recent study by Havrilevsky et al. [147], a literature review was conducted for investigations describing transcriptional profiling of epithelial ovarian cancer. Candidate biomarkers meeting the following inclusion criteria were selected: (1) overexpression of candidate gene in epithelial ovarian cancer relative to normal ovarian epithelium; (2) overexpression of encoded protein in ovarian tissue; (3) localization of encoded proteins to extracellular compartment as membrane-bound or secreted protein; and (4) discrimination of ovarian cancer from normal sera utilizing prototype immunological assays. Correlation with CA-125 was not evaluated. Based on these criteria, eight genes, HE4, glycodelin (PAEP), MMP-7, MUC-1, PAI-1, and SLPI, Plau-R, and inhibin A, were selected as candidate markers for inclusion. Several combinations of these proteins were evaluated, and a combination of CA-125, HE4, glycodelin, Plau-R, and MMP7 was selected that offered 79 % SN at 93 % SP for early-stage ovarian cancer [147].

Yurkovetsky et al. utilized a subject cohort which included more than 2,000 healthy women in an unbiased analysis of serum biomarker candidates [43]. Feature selection was performed based on both bioinformatics and the following biological considerations: high accuracy in early-stage disease, equal classification of all ovarian cancer histologies, and selectivity for ovarian cancer versus benign disease and other epithelial cancers [43]. The identified panel of CA-125, HE4, CEA, and vascular cell adhesion molecule-1 (VCAM-1) was found to discriminate early-stage ovarian cancer from the control group with 86 % SN at 98 % SP.

In a multicenter case-control study, Zhang et al. utilized surface-enhanced laser desorption/ionization (SELDI) to analyze sera obtained from 195 patients with invasive epithelial or other types of ovarian cancer along with patients diagnosed with benign pelvic masses and healthy control women [129]. The investigators employed subsets of five separate centers for sequential components of their analysis. Two centers were designated for biomarker discovery, and candidate peaks from the proteomic analysis were identified by cross-validation. These candidate biomarker peaks were then validated in sera collected at two additional sites. Validated biomarker peaks were then identified and the corresponding proteins purified. Candidate biomarkers for which suitable immunoassays were available were then chosen for validation in sera collected at the fifth site. Analysis of immunoassay results led to the identification of a four-biomarker panel consisting of CA-125, ApoA1, transthyretin (TTR), and H418. In the validation set, this panel provided an SN of 74 % at an SP of 97 % for the discrimination of early-stage ovarian cancer from healthy women.

In a separate study, Skates et al. evaluated serum levels of four biomarkers by immunoassay in patients enrolled at 3 independent collection centers [127]. Sera collected at the first center constituted the training set, and biomarker data was analyzed using three statistical models: logistic regression, classification tree, and mixture discriminant analysis (MDA). The MDA model is unique in that it emulates the heterogeneity of ovarian cancer with respect to histological subtype and utilizes the distribution of biomarker levels within each subtype to estimate the histological type of each sample analyzed. The authors conclude that logistic regression and MDA modeling perform similarly and both outperform classification tree in the discrimination of ovarian cancer cases from controls. The combination of CA-125, CA 15-3, CA 72-4, and M-CSF, identified using the MDA model, performed best in the independent validation set, providing an SN of 70 % at 98 % SP for early-stage ovarian cancer.

Recently, Edgell et al. reported on a retrospective case-control study (Phase 2 biomarker study) in which the authors utilized a multiplexed bead-based immunoassay platform to evaluate five ovarian cancer biomarkers (CA-125, CRP, SAA, IL-6, IL-8) in 362 plasma samples obtained from ovarian cancer patients and healthy controls split into independent training and validation sets [126]. Through multivariate modeling the authors demonstrated SN/SP of 94.1/91.3 for the five-biomarker panel in the validation set and an SN/SP of 92.3/91.3 for all early-stage ovarian cancers.

In another recent study, Amonkar et al. demonstrated the value of multiplexed analysis in their evaluation of 104 candidate biomarkers in a cohort of over 350 ovarian cancer patients and controls [125]. The cohort represented various stages of disease and each of the most common histological subtypes of epithelial ovarian cancer and most prevalent benign ovarian conditions. Their training analysis led to the identification of an 11-analyte profile consisting of CA-125, CA 19-9, EGFR, CRP, myoglobin, ApoA1, ApoCIII, MIP-1α, IL-6, IL-18, and tenascin C. In an independent validation set, this panel provided an SN of 91.3 % at an SP of 88.5 %.

Multimarker Panels in Prediagnostic Samples

While many of the reports represented in Table 3.4 are initially encouraging, several hurdles remain before any of the identified models can be implemented clinically on a widespread basis. Foremost is the need to evaluate the most promising panels in prospective randomized clinical trials. Additional preclinical validation will be required to fully characterize the efficacy of selected panels before this significant next step is warranted. A key component of this validation process is the evaluation of panels in samples obtained from prediagnostic ovarian cancer patients. Progress toward this type of validation is greatly hindered by the rarity of this sample type; however, several significant findings have been reported by a group under the direction of Nicole Urban. In a pair of reports, this group first describes elevated levels of CA-125, HE4, and mesothelin in the sera of symptomatic ovarian cancer patients and then in the sera of patients 0–3 years prior to diagnosis, noting an optimal lead time of 1 year [150, 151]. In a separate study, the investigators utilize a combinatorial approach including CA-125 and HE4 measurements in addition to the Symptom Index (SI) to prospectively classify benign from malignant pelvic masses with an SN of 84 % at an SP of 98.5 % (Table 3.4) [148].

Recently, a collaborative study was performed to assess the prediagnostic performance of candidate biomarkers in the PLCO trial [152, 153]. Forty-one biomarkers selected by five leading ovarian cancer biomarker laboratories from Harvard University, Fred Hutchinson Medical Center, MD Anderson Cancer Center, University of Pittsburgh, and Yale University were utilized in the analysis of 118 cases and 473 matched healthy controls [153, 154]. The selection of these markers proceeded from a Phase 2 validation study using a common reference set of 160 ovarian cancer cases (approximately 50 % stage I/II) and 480 general population controls based solely on individual performance (SN at 95 % SP, AUC). The study demonstrated that none of these biomarkers or multimarker panels added any appreciable improvement in SN over that of CA-125 alone. In addition, levels of CA-125 began to increase, on average, less than 1 year prior to diagnosis with ovarian cancer (Fig. 3.1). Subsequent analyses revealed that 10 of the selected biomarkers, HE4, mesothelin, CA 15-3,

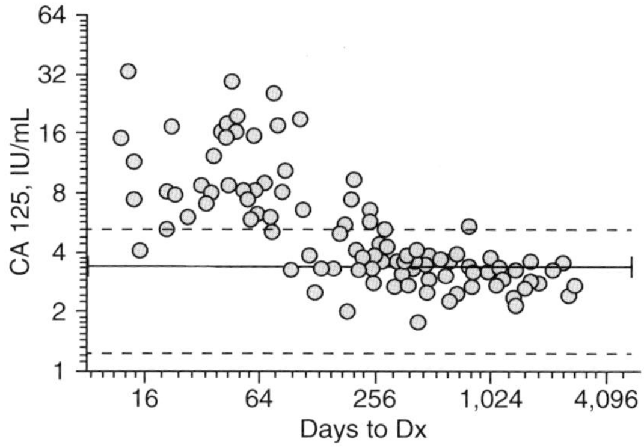

Fig. 3.1 Distribution of CA-125 concentrations in case samples from PLCO trial in relation to time of blood draw to diagnosis. *Solid line* mean for healthy controls, *hatched line* SD (minus outliers)

CA 72-4, KLK6, spondin-2, TTR, Cyfra 21-1, IGFBP-2, and YKL-40, were strongly (r>0.35) correlated with CA-125. This lack of feature independence could be credited as a limiting factor in the ability of these additional biomarkers to complement the diagnostic performance of CA-125. Similarly, Anderson et al. [151] measured several biomarkers over time in prediagnostic samples obtained from ovarian cancer patients and matched controls and observed that CA-125 (along with HE4 and mesothelin, but not of B7-H4, DcR3, and spondin-2) demonstrated appreciable increases in patients approximately 3 years before diagnosis. However, this CA-125 velocity reached detectable elevations only within the final year before diagnosis implying that a more sensitive assay could possibly detect early individual changes.

In nearly all reports, efforts aimed at novel biomarker development have relied upon the use of biological fluid samples collected at the time of first diagnosis. It would appear from the disappointing results of the PLCO study and others that this approach is not optimized for the development of prediagnostic tests offering a potential window of early successful intervention. Ongoing efforts of this type are unlikely to be productive, and the incorporation of new strategies focused on the characterization and detection of preclinical disease will be necessary for true advancement. Recent work suggests that a precursor lesion for serous carcinomas, termed serous tubal intraepithelial carcinoma (STIC), does indeed exist [155]. STICs originate from the fimbriated end of the fallopian tube, indicating a tubal, rather than ovarian epithelial, origin for serous carcinomas. The identification of the potential STIC precursor of serous carcinomas represents an important finding that may lead to advances in detecting these tumors at an earlier stage. Perhaps, analysis of blood samples from patients who had undergone prophylactic oophorectomy where preneoplastic lesions were discovered could prove useful although substantial effort would be needed to collect a statistically meaningful set of such samples. In fact, a recent publication based on mathematical modeling of ovarian cancer development using pathological findings from prophylactic bilateral salpingo-oophorectomies (PBSOs) suggested that ovarian cancers spend more than 4.3 years as in situ or stage I–II disease and that serous ovarian cancers have already progressed to a late stage by approximately 1 year prior to their discovery [133]. Therefore, if, as suggested above, changes in CA-125 levels are detectable within 3–12 months before clinical diagnosis, then current strategies are doomed to identify lower-volume high-grade disease, at best. Indeed, the authors conclude that in order to achieve 50 % SN in detecting tumors before they advance to stage III, an annual screen would need to detect tumors of less than 1.3 cm in diameter, whereas 80 % SN would require detecting tumors of less than 0.4 cm in diameter. No imaging modality could presently detect such small lesions, and therefore improved biomarker testing including the use of additional biomarkers and assays capable of detecting CA-125 with greater SN represents the most promising tools for early detection.

Advances in the Diagnosis and Triage of Malignant Pelvic Masses

The use of biomarker panels for the differential diagnosis of pelvic masses represents a clinical setting within the management of ovarian cancer where significant improvements could be achieved in the near future. According to current estimates, 1.4 % of women born today, or 1 in 72, will be diagnosed with ovarian cancer at some point in their lifetime. This year in the USA, there will be over 21,000 new cases of ovarian cancer along with nearly 14,000 deaths [156]. These cases arise from a much larger group of women presenting with pelvic masses. The overall prevalence of pelvic abnormalities is estimated at 7 %, and it is expected that 5–10 % of American women will receive prophylactic surgery for suspected ovarian cancer at some point in their lives [157]. Effective preoperative risk assessment of the pelvic mass is currently an area of great unmet need. At present, a patient's age and menopausal status are the most important factors to consider upon the identification of an pelvic abnormality as the associated risk of malignancy increases from 13 % in premenopausal women to 45 % in postmenopausal women [158].

Although the vast majority of women diagnosed with ovarian carcinoma will initially present with a pelvic mass, only a small proportion of all masses detected will prove to be malignant. The expeditious triage of these patients often represents the most important component of their clinical management. The burden of early identification of potential ovarian cancer falls predominantly upon the obstetrician/gynecologist whose training in the management of cancer patients is usually limited. While these practitioners can effectively manage the high percentage of patients diagnosed with functional cysts and benign neoplasms through observation and surgery, respectively, the clinical outcome for a patient presenting with a malignant mass can be drastically worsened if she is not immediately referred to a gynecological oncologist [159–161]. A series of diverse studies have demonstrated a decrease in the relative risk of reoperation and increases in disease-free interval and overall survival for women operated on by gynecological oncologists compared with gynecologists and general surgeons [162–164]. The overall prognosis for patients diagnosed with ovarian cancer has improved significantly over the past 30 years, demonstrated by an increase in 5-year survival from 20 to 50 % [165, 166]. This improvement can be largely attributed to the development and application of cytoreductive surgical techniques and the optimization of chemotherapeutic regimens. Despite these findings and advancements, referral rates remain disappointingly low for patients diagnosed with a pelvic mass [167]. Improvements upon current screening methodologies and the emergence of new techniques should aid gynecologists and general practitioners in making appropriate referral decisions leading to improvements in the overall clinical management of ovarian cancer.

A pelvic examination is the method most widely utilized in the identification of a pelvic mass; however, a physical exam alone cannot discriminate between benign and malignant lesions. TVU has proven useful as a secondary diagnostic tool; however, its utility as a first-line screening tool remains questionable given its demonstrated low PPV (3–5 %) and clinically insufficient levels of SN (75 %) [35]. Advanced imaging techniques such as CT or MRI have proven too expensive for widespread use given their limited SN and SP. Positron emission tomography (PET)/CT has proven useful in the evaluation of a pelvic mass [168] (SN/SP of 100 %/92.5 %; $n=97$); however, the high cost of this technique also limits its routine use. In addition to family history, pelvic examination, ascites, and evidence of local or distant metastases, the CA-125 blood test is included in the standard criteria espoused by the Society of Gynecologic Oncology and the American College of Obstetricians and Gynecologists regarding referral of a patient with a pelvic mass to a gynecological oncologist. This set of criteria has produced disappointing results in prospective studies, particularly those evaluating premenopausal women with early-stage disease, with SN/SP levels as low as 47 %/77 % [169]. This disappointing performance reflects the well-noted limitations of CA-125, including poor SN for early-stage disease, frequent elevation in a number of benign peritoneal conditions, and poor performance in premenopausal women. Much of the research into improved diagnostic tools is now focused on the identification of additional biomarkers capable of complementing the performance of CA-125. The potential clinical impact of a biomarker-based diagnostic test is considerable, given the reduced performance requirements necessary for implementation in comparison to general screening. In this setting, a diagnostic test would be used as a risk assessment tool to aid physicians in the decision to refer a patient presenting with a suspicious pelvic mass for evaluation by a gynecological oncologist and/or laparoscopy. Sensitivity is paramount within this strategy and should meet or approach 100 % in order to ensure proper referral of all malignant cases. Specificity should be sufficient to produce a meaningful reduction in unnecessary laparoscopies in order to be cost-effective and beneficial to the target population.

Recent Progress in Risk Assessment Tool Development

The Risk of Malignancy Index (RMI), first described by Jacobs et al. in 1990 [170], is the most widely used and accepted diagnostic index for the assessment of a pelvic mass. The RMI combines ultrasound findings with the measurement of CA-125 and menopausal status. Risk assessment using the RMI is achieved through direct multiplication of scores representing each parameter, rendering this model relatively simple to use and cost-effective. In an initial analysis, the RMI achieved an SN of 85 % at an SP of 97 % for the prediction of malignancy in women diagnosed with a pelvic mass. The model has been modified in several subsequent studies, and its performance has been validated in multiple trials with SN and SP values ranging between 71 and 88.5 % and 74.3 and 97 %, respectively [171–174]. The RMI is used routinely in the UK and several other European countries. A recent evaluation of the use of the RMI in a tertiary care setting in Denmark which included 1,159 women diagnosed with a pelvic mass, reported SN and SP values of 92 and 82 %, respectively, with a PPV of 62 % and a negative predictive value (NPV) of 97 % [175].

In light of the well-described limitations exhibited by CA-125, investigators have adopted a number of distinct approaches aimed at improved risk of malignancy assessment for women presenting with a pelvic mass. Several models of this type are compared systematically in a recent review by Geomini et al. [176]. In that review, the authors concluded that the RMI performed optimally with respect to all other models for the preoperative assessment of a pelvic mass with a pooled SN of 78 % at an SP of 87 %. Timmerman et al. [177]. recently described a diagnostic index composed of over 50 discrete clinical variables evaluated in over 1,000 patients enrolled by the International Ovarian Tumor Analysis (IOTA) group. A subset of 12 of these variables incorporated into a logistic regression model provided an SN of 93 % and an SP of 77 % in the IOTA cohort. The descriptive factors comprising this model included age, personal history of ovarian cancer, maximum diameter of the lesion, maximum diameter of the solid component, presence of ascites, Doppler blood flow, presence of a purely solid lesion, irregular cyst wall, increased color score, hormone therapy, and pain with ultrasound. This model and several related IOTA models were found to outperform the RMI in an external prospective validation study [178]. The performance of these models does appear encouraging and may represent a cost-effective method of risk assessment; however, the complex nature of the algorithms involved may present a barrier to broad clinical implementation.

A number of groups have reported encouraging results through the use of multimarker panels which attempt to improve upon the performance of CA-125 by combining it with various additional biomarkers found to be associated with ovarian cancer (Table 3.5). The most recent findings related to this endeavor are discussed here. Hogdall et al. recently described the development of [a pelvic mass risk index, termed the DK index, comprising CA-125, age, and three additional serum biomarkers identified through SELDI-TOF-MS proteomic analysis (beta-2-microglobulin (B2M), transthyretin (TT), transferrin (TF)) [179]. In a large group of women diagnosed with pelvic masses, the DK index provided an SN of 95 % at an SP of 81 %. Additional work by this group suggests that the

Table 3.5 Multimarker panels which discriminate benign from malignant pelvic masses

Panel	Cases	Controls	SN	SP	Reference
CA-125, β2-microglobulin, transthyretin, transferrin	144	509	95	81	Hogdall et al. [179]
CA-125, midkine, anterior gradient 2 protein	46	61	95.2	97.7	Rice et al. [180].
CA-125, G-CSF, IL-6, EGF, VEGF	44	37	86.5	93	Gorelik et al. [145]
CA-125, IL-7	187	45	69	100	Lambeck et al. [181]
CA-125, HE4, IL-2Rα, α1-antitrypsin, CRP, YKL-40, cellular fibronectin, CA 72-4, prostasin	149	350	90	89.9	Yip et al. [182]

incorporation of urine biomarkers identified through proteomic techniques into biomarker-based tools may result in improved diagnostic performance [183]. In a separate study, a panel of CA-125, midkine (MDK), and anterior gradient 2 protein (AGR2) performed very well in the discrimination of benign and malignant pelvic masses with an SN/SP of 95.2 %/97.7 % [180]. This study was limited by a relatively small sample size and a lack of validation; however, further analysis of this panel appears warranted. Elsewhere, several groups have examined the role of cytokines in ovarian cancer diagnosis in an attempt to utilize the network of local and systemic signaling involved in ovarian tumorigenesis. A panel consisting of CA-125, G-CSF, IL-6, EGF, and VEGF provided an SN/SP of 86.5 %/93 % in a small preliminary study [145], while the combination of CA-125 and IL-7 provided an SN of 69 % at 100 % SP in a somewhat larger patient group [181]. While the high level of SP achieved by the latter study is certainly meritorious, this model should be further examined to determine if it is capable of providing the high SN required of a diagnostic test in this setting. Yip et al. conducted an analysis of 175 circulating biomarkers in 499 women scheduled for surgery for pelvic abnormalities, including 149 cases of ovarian cancer [182]. A nine-biomarker combination was identified through logistic regression that provided an SN of 90 % at an SP of 88.9 % for the discrimination of benign versus malignant patients. Notably, this combination outperformed the five-biomarker panel comprising the OVA1 diagnostic test (discussed below); however, the performance of this panel has not been independently validated.

The CA-125/HE4 Combination and ROMA

Gene expression profiling indicates that HE4 is expressed in several tissues outside of the male reproductive system and is highly overexpressed in epithelial ovarian cancers [184]. Studies focusing on the potential use of HE4 as a biomarker of ovarian cancer suggest that it is elevated in over 50 % of ovarian cancer patients whose tumors do not express CA-125 [185]. HE4 has also demonstrated greater SN than CA-125 among early-stage ovarian cancer patients and greater SP in comparison with benign ovarian lesions [185, 186]. A diagnostic assay for HE4 has been developed and commercialized by Fujirebio Diagnostics, Inc. (Malvern, PA), and the use of HE4 for ovarian cancer monitoring has recently been approved by the US Food and Drug Administration (FDA) [60]. Investigations into the use of HE4 as an ovarian cancer biomarker have proceeded both in the area of population-based screening and in the differential diagnosis of a pelvic mass. Despite a number of promising reports, it has become apparent that HE4 is not sufficiently sensitive or specific to function effectively as a stand-alone test. However, the combined use of CA-125 and HE4 in the differential diagnosis of pelvic masses has received a considerable amount of attention (Table 3.6).

The diagnostic potential of the CA-125/HE4 combination was first recognized by Moore et al. in an investigation of circulating levels of nine biomarkers (CA-125, SMRP, HE4, CA 72-4, activin, inhibin, osteopontin, EGFR, ErbB2) in sera obtained from 233 women diagnosed with a pelvic mass [185]. HE4 was identified as the most

Table 3.6 The CA-125/HE4 combination in the differential diagnosis of a pelvic mass

Panel	Cases	Controls	SN	SP	Reference
CA-125, HE4	129	352	92.3	75	Moore et al. [186]
CA-125, HE4	14	129[a]	92.9	95	Huhtinen et al. [187]
CA-125, HE4	491[b]	299[b]	83	85	Nolen et al. [188]
CA-125, HE4	34	195	91.2	55.4	Holcomb et al. [189]
ROMA[c]	89	383	93.8	74.9	Moore et al. [190]

[a]Ovarian endometriotic cysts
[b]Includes independent validation set
[c]Negative predictive value: 98 %

sensitive marker in that study, and this was especially true among early-stage ovarian cancer patients. The combination of CA-125 and HE4 provided a greater overall classification accuracy than either biomarker used alone and provided an SN of 76.4 % at an SP of 95 %. Moore et al. then utilized this combination in a prospective multicenter study involving 531 patients [186]. Measurements of CA-125 and HE4 were used to categorize patients into high or low risk of ovarian cancer with 93.8 % of ovarian cancer patients correctly classified into the high-risk group [186]. Elsewhere, Huhtinen et al. demonstrated the efficacy of this combination in the discrimination of malignant ovarian masses from benign ovarian endometriotic cysts with an SN of 92.9 % at 95 % SP [187]. In a separate and independent study involving 790 patients separated into distinct training and validation sets, Nolen et al. evaluated circulating levels of 65 biomarkers and determined that the combination of CA-125 and HE4 performed optimally with respect to all other possible panels, resulting in an SN of 83 % at an SP of 85 % [188]. In that study, HE4 was the most highly elevated biomarker among cancer patients, followed by Cyfra 21-1, CA-125, and CA 19-9 (Fig. 3.2a). In the vast majority of cases, the magnitude of biomarker level changes, both upregulated and downregulated, was significantly more pronounced in late-stage disease, and for many biomarkers, the observed differences were significant in only the late-stage patients (Fig. 3.2b). Another recent study by Holcomb et al. reported that the combination of CA-125 and HE4 provided an SN of 91.2 % at an SP of 55.4 % with a PPV of 26.3 % and a NPV of 97.3 % [189]. Although SP is this study is somewhat diminished, the high NPV is encouraging given the paucity of ovarian cancers 16/229 (8 %) included in the cohort of premenopausal women.

Recently, Steven Skates and colleagues developed a scoring model termed the Risk of Ovarian Malignancy Algorithm (ROMA) which incorporates measurements of CA-125 and HE4 along with menopausal status in order to assign high or low risk of malignancy to a woman presenting with a pelvic mass. In a comparison of ROMA and RMI in 467 patients, the ROMA provided a higher SN (94.3 % vs. 84.6 %) at an SP of 75 % [191]. This was particularly evident among stage I and II cancer, where ROMA detected 85 % and RMI 65 %. The comparative performance of ROMA versus RMI remains in question, however, as a subsequent evaluation by a separate group found that RMI outperformed ROMA among both pre- and postmenopausal women diagnosed with a pelvic mass (n=432) [192]. In the latter study, both ROMA and RMI were outperformed by subjective assessment by ultrasound. Most recently, ROMA was evaluated in a prospective, multicenter, blinded clinical trial involving 472 patients diagnosed with a pelvic mass, 89 of which were found to have ovarian cancer [190]. In that trial, ROMA provided an overall SN of 93.8 % at an SP of 74.9 % with a NPV of 98 %. ROMA performed particularly well in the premenopausal patient subset, achieving an SN of 100 % at an SP of 74.2 %. Based upon the results of this clinical trial, ROMA was recently approved by the FDA for use in determining the risk of ovarian cancer in pre- and postmenopausal women with a pelvic mass.

Recent evaluations of HE4 and ROMA have produced mixed results. A number of studies have reported results which reaffirm the complementary performance of HE4 to CA-125 and the superior diagnostic abilities of the HE4/CA-125 combination or ROMA over CA-125 alone [187, 189, 193–197]. However, several groups have reported contrary results. Van Gorp et al. [198]. concluded that the addition of HE4 or the use of ROMA does not offer improvement upon CA-125 based on a large prospective study of women diagnosed with a pelvic mass. Several notable differences in the composition of the patient cohorts exist between this study and the previous study by Moore et al. [186]. These differences include an increased proportion in the number of overall cancers, mucinous tumors, borderline tumors, metastatic tumors, and postmenopausal women in the later study. Montagnana et al. [199]. found that ROMA was effective in ovarian cancer diagnosis in postmenopausal women but not in premenopausal women; however, HE4 alone outperformed ROMA in either group. The study design here also differed from Moore et al. regarding the incidence of ovarian cancer in the pre- and postmenopausal groups. A third study, which included a large proportion of borderline and extra-ovarian tumors found that HE4 offered several advantages over CA-125 for ovarian cancer diagnosis; however, no diagnostic benefit was derived from combining them [200]. Thus, variability in the composition of the target population appears to impact the performance of the CA-125/HE4 combination. Going forward, this issue may be addressed through a reevaluation of the specific threshold values employed in the test to better respond to this variability or through the incorporation of additional useful biomarkers which make the test more robust.

The OVA1 Test

A biomarker-based diagnostic test for the evaluation of patients with a pelvic mass was approved by the FDA in September of 2009 and is currently available under the trade name OVA1 (Vermillion, Inc.) [201]. The test utilizes a five-biomarker combination (CA-125, transthyretin, ApoA1, β2-microglobulin, transferrin) identified through serum proteomics using SELDI [202]. Following validation of SELDI-derived markers in retrospective samples, the final combination was assembled based on the successful

a

	All cancer	Stage I–II	Stage III–IV
HE4	1095.9	316.8	2775.6
Cyfra 21-1	380.8	158.4	857.4
CA-125	314.2	100.5	744.0
CA 19-9	300.0	376.7	135.9
IL-1Ra	*201.9*	*60.0*	483.7
CA72-4	129.0	183.0	*14.8*
IL-10	93.3	82.2	116.8
DRS	83.1	*30.5*	181.0
DA-153	78.0	44.1	152.8
IL-6	69.3	42.9	125.7
IL-2R	67.9	32.4	151.1
IL-8	66.2	75.5	46.4
TNF-RI	51.5	18.5	127.6
IL-7	35.9	31.6	45.2
MMP-9	35.8	38.2	31.2
TNF-RII	31.6	17.0	61.1
IGFBP-1	27.9	72.6	−66.7
tPAI 1	22.8	15.6	37.9
MPO	20.0	*16.1*	28.3
ErbB2	16.5	5.1	40.9
IP-10	13.6	−6.2	64.2
Fas	12.0	2.6	32.1
TNF-a	11.5	−2.4	41.2
Kallikrein 10	9.1	7.4	12.6
EOTAXIN	5.7	−6.8	32.2
sVCAM-1	−7.2	−6.5	−8.6
Apolipoprotein AI	−7.7	−5.6	−14.0
MMP-2	−10.3	−6.8	−17.8
RGFR	−13.1	−7.4	−25.3
sFasl	−17.2	−13.7	−24.8
TTR	−19.6	−11.7	−43.8
ACTH	−26.9	−17.3	−47.3

Fig. 3.2 Summary of biomarker changes observed in the sera of women diagnosed with benign and malignant adnexal masses. (**a**) Biomarker heat map. Values represent the percentage change over observed biomarker levels in the benign group for the training set: 141 women with benign masses and 264 women diagnosed with ovarian cancer. *Red* indicates an increase in cancer levels over benign, while *green* indicates a decrease. The minimum level of significance in differences was $P<0.05$ by Mann-Whitney U test (values in *italics* were nonsignificant). (**b**) Biological trends. Trends in biomarker level changes observed in malignant versus benign masses are organized according to each biological category of biomarkers evaluated

Fig. 3.2 (continued)

b

Biomarker group	Elevated throughout	Elevated early	Elevated late	Decreased
Inflammatory mediators	IL-10 IL-1Ra IL-2R IL-6 IL-7 TNFR-1 TNFR-2	IL-8	IP-10 eotaxin-1 MPO TNFa	
Growth/angiogenic factors		IGFBP-1	Her2/neu	EGFR IGFBP-1
Tumor-associated antigens	CA 125 CA 15-3 HE4	CA 19-9 CA 72-4		
Apoptotic proteins	Cyfra 21-1 DRS		sFas	sFasL
Proteases/inhibitors		MMP-9	Kallikrein 10 tPAI-1	MMP-2
Adhesion molecules				sVCAM-1
Hormones				ACTH
Other markers				ApoA1

development of immunoassays. The test is currently approved for use as an adjunct to physical examination and imaging and produces a risk assessment score within the range of 0 to 10. Separate cutoff values are employed for premenopausal (5.0) and postmenopausal women (4.4). Although the full impact of clinical implementation of the OVA1 test remains to be evaluated, the advancement of the test thus far is testament to the beneficial use of systemic biomarkers and a marked divergence from other efforts which rely heavily on tumor-derived factors such as CA-125 and HE4.

The panel was evaluated in a clinical trial which utilized immunoassays targeting each of the five markers in a set of 524 women diagnosed with a pelvic mass and recommended for surgery [203, 204]. At the time of surgery, there were 363 benign tumors and 161 malignancies of which 151 were ovarian cancers. In a pair of reports, the developers of the kit evaluate its efficacy in several clinical settings (Table 3.7). When the OVA1 panel was substituted for CA-125 within the American College of Obstetricians and Gynecologists (ACOG) ovarian tumor referral guidelines, it provided an SN of 94 % at an SP of 35 % with a PPV of 40 % and a NPV of 93 %. This represented an increase in SN and NPV in comparison to CA-125, but also a decrease in SP and PPV. When the OVA1 test was added to a normal physician assessment, it provided an SN of 96 % at an SP of 35 % with a PPV of 40 % and a NPV of 95 %. Among gynecological oncologists, SN and NPV were higher at 99 and 98 %, respectively; however, SP was lower at 26 %. In comparison to physician assessment alone, the incorporation of the OVA1 test again resulted in improvements in SN and NPV along with decreased levels of SP and PPV. When the OVA1 test was directly compared to CA-125, similar

Table 3.7 Clinical evaluation of the OVA1 test

	SN	SP	PPV	NPV
ACOG + CA-125	77	68	52	87
ACOG + OVA1	94	35	40	93
PA alone	75	79	62	88
PA + OVA1	96	35	40	95
CA-125 alone	69–77	73–84	56–65	86–88
OVA1 alone	93	43	42	93

Reported in [203, 204]
ACOG American College of Obstetricians and Gynecologists' ovarian tumor referral guidelines, *PA* physician assessment

trends in performance were observed. A recent evaluation of the OVA1 markers, which included all seven proteins originally identified by SELDI-TOF-MS, suggested that these markers do not improve upon the performance of CA-125 in prediagnostic samples [205]. A similar finding by Cramer et al. in prediagnostic samples collected as part of the large PLCO trial may indicate a potential limitation in the usefulness of the OVA1 test [153].

The ROMA and OVA1 test have not been compared directly in a single trial, and such an evaluation would be eagerly anticipated. Based on the separate results of the clinical trials involving each test, the two are likely to perform with similar levels of SN and NPV. The most notable difference between the two tests is SP, wherein ROMA appears to be substantially more specific (75 % vs. 43 %). While such a difference in SP should not affect patient outcomes, it could produce an impact on cost-effectiveness and the distribution of medical resources. Some comparative information may also be gleaned from several studies which evaluate the biomarkers included in each panel individually. In the report by Yip et al., CA-125, HE4, and each of the OVA1 markers were evaluated in 499 women scheduled for pelvic mass surgery [182]. HE4 was the highest-performing individual marker in that study, while none of the OVA1 markers were among the top nine analytes selected for panel development. Similarly, when each of the markers were evaluated in prediagnostic samples collected during the PLCO trial, HE4 was found to outperform all other biomarkers with the exception of CA-125 [153]. Although transthyretin ranked third among all markers evaluated in that study, its performance in samples drawn ≤6 months prior to ovarian cancer diagnosis was significantly less than HE4 (SN of 2 % vs. 73 % at 95 % SP).

In conclusion, the successful development of the ROMA and OVA1 test represents a significant milestone in the clinical management of women diagnosed with a pelvic mass. The limited amount of clinical data available suggests that ROMA may be advantageous to OVA1 in terms of SP and this advantage may stem from the inclusion of HE4, a marker which has demonstrated superior performance on an individual basis. However, additional clinical validation will be necessary to fully evaluate the impact of either test on the overall burden of ovarian cancer.

Conclusion

The search for biomarker-based screening tools for the early detection of ovarian cancer has yielded a number of promising findings. Biomarker panels offering levels of SN and SP exceeding 90 % have been identified by a number of groups utilizing a variety of analysis techniques and statistical models. Each of the panels identified demonstrates a clear performance advantage over the individual performance of CA-125. Clinical implementation of biomarker tools has been delayed, and sometimes reversed, in large part due to the stringent performance requirements associated with the detection of a rare disease and the lack of a demonstrated survival benefit.

Despite intense preclinical and clinical effort aimed at the development of screening strategies for ovarian cancer, a truly effective method of early detection remains elusive. Factors contributing to our inability to achieve a screening breakthrough include the low prevalence of ovarian cancer, the lack of well-defined high-risk populations, and significant deficiencies in our understanding of the early events of ovarian tumorigenesis and the transition from early to advanced disease. The high degree of disease heterogeneity is an additional complicating factor wherein less prevalent histological subtypes of ovarian epithelial cancer such as mucinous, endometrioid, clear cell, and low-grade serous carcinomas represent tumors which are amenable to screening while the more prevalent high-grade serous subtype remains undetectable throughout early, treatable stages.

The limited performance of serum biomarkers in the testing of prediagnostic samples indicates the need to identify additional useful biomarkers which may display alterations earlier in disease development. Further investigation into the tumorigenic pathways associated with each subtype of epithelial ovarian cancer is likely to provide a basis for additional biomarker discovery and development. The identification of the potential STIC precursor of serous carcinomas represents an important finding that may lead to advances in detecting these tumors at an earlier stage. Currently, findings related to the subtype specific production of ovarian cancer biomarkers are sporadic and incomplete. The ongoing paradigm shift regarding the tissue of origin and pathogenesis of disease subtypes should give rise to additional investigations of this type. A greater appreciation of the natural history of each subtype of ovarian cancer, including the involvement or absence of precursor lesions, should further refine the search for useful prediagnostic biomarkers.

Recent reports describing the clinical performance of several multianalyte and multimodal models for pelvic mass triage indicate that the widespread implementation of this type of testing into clinical practice is near at hand. The FDA-approved ROMA and OVA1 tests are the clearest examples of advancement within the field. Both developments represent variations upon a common theme, which is the inclusion of biomarker alternatives to CA-125 which complement its diagnostic performance. The underlying goal of such a strategy is to detect a wider range of ovarian cancers, including early-stage disease and disease among premenopausal women, while providing a beneficial level of SP with respect to benign masses. Ongoing efforts must now focus on determining whether or not the improvements noted for these multianalyte tests are of sufficient magnitude to produce a meaningful impact on the clinical management of the pelvic mass and a measurable reduction in ovarian cancer-related disease burden. Measurements of success in this clinical setting include a reduction in morbidity and cost resulting from unnecessary surgical procedures and improved outcome for ovarian cancer patients achieved by efficient referral to clinical centers of excellence.

References

1. Nolen BM, Lokshin AE. Screening for ovarian cancer: old tools, new lessons. Cancer Biomark. 2010;8(4–5):177–86.
2. Badgwell D, Bast Jr RC. Early detection of ovarian cancer. Dis Markers. 2007;23(5–6):397–410.
3. Altekruse SF, Kosary CL, Krapcho M, Neyman N, Aminou R, Waldron W, et al. SEER Cancer Statistics Review, 1975–2007. Bethesda, MD: National Cancer Institute; 2010.
4. Moshkovskii SA, Serebryakova MV, Kuteykin-Teplyakov KB, Tikhonova OV, Goufman EI, Zgoda VG, et al. Ovarian cancer marker of 11.7 kDa detected by proteomics is a serum amyloid A1. Proteomics. 2005;5(14):3790–7.
5. Holschneider CH, Berek JS. Ovarian cancer: epidemiology, biology, and prognostic factors. Semin Surg Oncol. 2000;19(1):3–10.
6. Baker TR, Piver MS. Etiology, biology, and epidemiology of ovarian cancer. Semin Surg Oncol. 1994;10(4):242–8.
7. Skates SJ, Singer DE. Quantifying the potential benefit of CA 125 screening for ovarian cancer. J Clin Epidemiol. 1991;44(4–5):365–80.
8. Jacobs IJ, Menon U. Progress and challenges in screening for early detection of ovarian cancer. Mol Cell Proteomics. 2004;3(4):355–66.
9. Menon U, Jacobs IJ. Ovarian cancer screening in the general population: current status. Int J Gynecol Cancer. 2001;11 Suppl 1:3–6.
10. Bast Jr RC, Xu FJ, Yu YH, Barnhill S, Zhang Z, Mills GB. CA 125: the past and the future. Int J Biol Markers. 1998;13(4):179–87.
11. Kinkel K, Hricak H, Lu Y, Tsuda K, Filly RA. US characterization of ovarian masses: a meta-analysis. Radiology. 2000;217(3):803–11.
12. Fishman DA, Cohen L, Blank SV, Shulman L, Singh D, Bozorgi K, et al. The role of ultrasound evaluation in the detection of early-stage epithelial ovarian cancer. Am J Obstet Gynecol. 2005;192(4):1214–21; discussion 1221–2.

13. Zurawski Jr VR, Orjaseter H, Andersen A, Jellum E. Elevated serum CA 125 levels prior to diagnosis of ovarian neoplasia: relevance for early detection of ovarian cancer. Int J Cancer. 1988;42(5):677–80.
14. Bast Jr RC, Klug TL, St John E, Jenison E, Niloff JM, Lazarus H, et al. A radioimmunoassay using a monoclonal antibody to monitor the course of epithelial ovarian cancer. N Engl J Med. 1983;309(15): 883–7.
15. Tseng PC, Sprance HE, Carcangiu ML, Chambers JT, Schwartz PE. CA 125, NB/70K, and lipid-associated sialic acid in monitoring uterine papillary serous carcinoma. Obstet Gynecol. 1989;74(3 Pt 1):384–7.
16. Jacobs I, Bast Jr RC. The CA 125 tumour-associated antigen: a review of the literature. Hum Reprod. 1989;4(1):1–12.
17. Woolas RP, Xu FJ, Jacobs IJ, Yu YH, Daly L, Berchuck A, et al. Elevation of multiple serum markers in patients with stage I ovarian cancer. J Natl Cancer Inst. 1993;85(21):1748–51.
18. Slotman BJ, Rao BR. Ovarian cancer (review). Etiology, diagnosis, prognosis, surgery, radiotherapy, chemotherapy and endocrine therapy. Anticancer Res. 1988;8(3):417–34.
19. Yancik R. Ovarian cancer. Age contrasts in incidence, histology, disease stage at diagnosis, and mortality. Cancer. 1993;71(2 Suppl):517–23.
20. Gocze P, Vahrson H. [Ovarian carcinoma antigen (CA 125) and ovarian cancer (clinical follow-up and prognostic studies)]. Orv Hetil. 1993;134(17):915–8.
21. Molina R, Filella X, Jo J, Agusti C, Ballesta AM. CA 125 in biological fluids. Int J Biol Markers. 1998;13(4):224–30.
22. Kaku T, Ogawa S, Kawano Y, Ohishi Y, Kobayashi H, Hirakawa T, Nakano H. Histological classification of ovarian cancer. Med Electron Microsc. 2003; 36(1):9–17.
23. Neesham D. Ovarian cancer screening. Aust Fam Physician. 2007;36(3):126–8.
24. Clarke-Pearson DL. Clinical practice. Screening for ovarian cancer. N Engl J Med. 2009;361(2):170–7.
25. Johnson CC, Kessel B, Riley TL, Ragard LR, Williams CR, Xu JL, et al. The epidemiology of CA-125 in women without evidence of ovarian cancer in the Prostate, Lung, Colorectal and Ovarian Cancer (PLCO) Screening Trial. Gynecol Oncol. 2008;110(3): 383–9.
26. Menon U. Ovarian cancer screening. CMAJ. 2004; 171(4):323–4.
27. Urban N, McIntosh MW, Andersen M, Karlan BY. Ovarian cancer screening. Hematol Oncol Clin North Am. 2003;17(4):989–1005, ix.
28. Calogne N. Screening for ovarian cancer: recommendation statement. Ann Fam Med. 2004;2(3):260–2.
29. U.S. Preventive Services Task Force. Screening for ovarian cancer: recommendation statement. Am Fam Physician. 2005;71(4):759–62.
30. ACOG committee opinion. Role of loop electrosurgical excision procedure in the evaluation of abnormal Pap test results. Number 195, November 1997. Committee on Gynecologic Practice. American College of Obstetricians and Gynecologists. Int J Gynaecol Obstet. 1998;61(2):203–4.
31. Brown DL, Andreotti RF, Lee SI, Dejesus Allison SO, Bennett GL, Dubinsky T, et al. ACR appropriateness criteria(c) ovarian cancer screening. Ultrasound Q. 2010;26(4):219–23.
32. Partridge E, Kreimer AR, Greenlee RT, Williams C, Xu JL, Church TR, et al. Results from four rounds of ovarian cancer screening in a randomized trial. Obstet Gynecol. 2009;113(4):775–82.
33. Buys SS, Partridge E, Black A, Johnson CC, Lamerato L, Isaacs C, et al. Effect of screening on ovarian cancer mortality: the Prostate, Lung, Colorectal and Ovarian (PLCO) Cancer Screening Randomized Controlled Trial. JAMA. 2011;305(22):2295–303.
34. Skates SJ, Menon U, MacDonald N, Rosenthal AN, Oram DH, Knapp RC, Jacobs IJ, et al. Calculation of the risk of ovarian cancer from serial CA-125 values for preclinical detection in postmenopausal women. J Clin Oncol. 2003;21(10 Suppl):206s–10.
35. Menon U, Gentry-Maharaj A, Hallett R, Ryan A, Burnell M, Sharma A, et al. Sensitivity and specificity of multimodal and ultrasound screening for ovarian cancer, and stage distribution of detected cancers: results of the prevalence screen of the UK Collaborative Trial of Ovarian Cancer Screening (UKCTOCS). Lancet Oncol. 2009;10(4):327–40.
36. Ueland FR, DePriest PD, Pavlik EJ, Kryscio RJ, van Nagell Jr JR. Preoperative differentiation of malignant from benign ovarian tumors: the efficacy of morphology indexing and Doppler flow sonography. Gynecol Oncol. 2003;91(1):46–50.
37. Buys SS, Partridge E, Greene MH, Prorok PC, Reding D, Riley TL, et al. Ovarian cancer screening in the Prostate, Lung, Colorectal and Ovarian (PLCO) cancer screening trial: findings from the initial screen of a randomized trial. Am J Obstet Gynecol. 2005; 193(5):1630–9.
38. Wilson JM, Jungner YG. [Principles and practice of mass screening for disease]. Bol Oficina Sanit Panam. 1968;65(4):281–393.
39. Herbst AL. The epidemiology of ovarian carcinoma and the current status of tumor markers to detect disease. Am J Obstet Gynecol. 1994;170(4):1099–105; discussion 1105–7.
40. Niloff JM. Ovarian malignancy. Curr Opin Obstet Gynecol. 1991;3(1):66–72.
41. Woolas RP, Oram DH, Jeyarajah AR, Bast RC, Jacobs IJ. Ovarian cancer identified through screening with serum markers but not by pelvic imaging. Int J Gynecol Cancer. 1999;9(6):497–501.
42. Suzuki M, Sekiguchi I, Tamada T. Clinical evaluation of tumor-associated mucin-type glycoprotein CA 54/61 in ovarian cancers: comparison with CA 125. Obstet Gynecol. 1990;76(3 Pt 1):422–7.
43. Yurkovetsky Z, Skates S, Lomakin A, Nolen B, Pulsipher T, Modugno F, et al. Development of a multimarker assay for early detection of ovarian cancer. J Clin Oncol. 2010;28(13):2159–66.

44. Sehouli J, Akdogan Z, Heinze T, Könsgen D, Stengel D, Mustea A, Lichtenegger W, et al. Preoperative determination of CASA (Cancer Associated Serum Antigen) and CA-125 for the discrimination between benign and malignant pelvic tumor mass: a prospective study. Anticancer Res. 2003;23(2A):1115–8.
45. Crump C, McIntosh MW, Urban N, Anderson G, Karlan BY. Ovarian cancer tumor marker behavior in asymptomatic healthy women: implications for screening. Cancer Epidemiol Biomarkers Prev. 2000;9(10):1107–11.
46. Baron AT, Cora EM, Lafky JM, et al. Soluble epidermal growth factor receptor (sEGFR/sErbB1) as a potential risk, screening, and diagnostic serum biomarker of epithelial ovarian cancer. Cancer Epidemiol Biomarkers Prev. 2003;12(2):103–13.
47. Callet N, Delaunay J, Pichon MF. Serum sICAM-1 (soluble intercellular adhesion molecule-1) and M-CSF (macrophage colony-stimulating growth factor) throughout monitoring of 34 non-serous ovarian cancers. Eur J Gynaecol Oncol. 2000;21(2):135–40.
48. Oehler MK, Caffier H. Diagnostic value of serum VEGF in women with ovarian tumors. Anticancer Res. 1999;19(4A):2519–22.
49. Xu Y, Shen Z, Wiper DW, Wu M, Morton RE, Elson P, et al. Lysophosphatidic acid as a potential biomarker for ovarian and other gynecologic cancers. JAMA. 1998;280(8):719–23.
50. Borgono CA, Fracchioli S, Yousef GM. Rigault de la Longrais IA, Luo LY, Soosaipillai A, et al. Favorable prognostic value of tissue human kallikrein 11 (hK11) in patients with ovarian carcinoma. Int J Cancer. 2003;106(4):605–10.
51. Diamandis EP, Scorilas A, Fracchioli S, Van Gramberen M, De Bruijn H, Henrik A, et al. Human kallikrein 6 (hK6): a new potential serum biomarker for diagnosis and prognosis of ovarian carcinoma. J Clin Oncol. 2003;21(6):1035–43.
52. Kishi T, Grass L, Soosaipillai A, Scorilas A, Harbeck N, Schmalfeldt B, et al. Human kallikrein 8, a novel biomarker for ovarian carcinoma. Cancer Res. 2003;63(11):2771–4.
53. Kyriakopoulou LG, Yousef GM, Scorilas A, Katsaros D, Massobrio M, Fracchioli S, Diamandis EP, et al. Prognostic value of quantitatively assessed KLK7 expression in ovarian cancer. Clin Biochem. 2003;36(2):135–43.
54. Obiezu CV, Scorilas A, Katsaros D, Massobrio M, Yousef GM, Fracchioli S, et al. Higher human kallikrein gene 4 (KLK4) expression indicates poor prognosis of ovarian cancer patients. Clin Cancer Res. 2001;7(8):2380–6.
55. Yousef GM, Scorilas A, Katsaros D, Fracchioli S, Iskander L, Borgono C, et al. Prognostic value of the human kallikrein gene 15 expression in ovarian cancer. J Clin Oncol. 2003;21(16):3119–26.
56. Yousef GM, Polymeris ME, Grass L, Soosaipillai A, Chan PC, Scorilas A, et al. Human kallikrein 5: a potential novel serum biomarker for breast and ovarian cancer. Cancer Res. 2003;63(14):3958–65.
57. Schummer M, Ng WV, Bumgarner RE, Nelson PS, Schummer B, Bednarski DW, et al. Comparative hybridization of an array of 21,500 ovarian cDNAs for the discovery of genes overexpressed in ovarian carcinomas. Gene. 1999;238(2):375–85.
58. Mok SC, Chao J, Skates S, Wong K, Yiu GK, Muto MG, et al. Prostasin, a potential serum marker for ovarian cancer: identification through microarray technology. J Natl Cancer Inst. 2001;93(19):1458–64.
59. Kim JH, Skates SJ, Uede T, Wong KK, Schorge JO, Feltmate CM, et al. Osteopontin as a potential diagnostic biomarker for ovarian cancer. JAMA. 2002;287(13):1671–9.
60. Drapkin R, von Horsten HH, Lin Y, Mok SC, Crum CP, Welch WR, Hecht JL. Human epididymis protein 4 (HE4) is a secreted glycoprotein that is overexpressed by serous and endometrioid ovarian carcinomas. Cancer Res. 2005;65(6):2162–9.
61. Pepe MS, Etzioni R, Feng Z, Potter JD, Thompson ML, Thornquist M, et al. Phases of biomarker development for early detection of cancer. J Natl Cancer Inst. 2001;93(14):1054–61.
62. Koprowski H, Herlyn M, Steplewski Z, Sears HF. Specific antigen in serum of patients with colon carcinoma. Science. 1981;212(4490):53–5.
63. Gold P, Freedman SO. Demonstration of tumor-specific antigens in human colonic carcinomata by immunological tolerance and absorption techniques. J Exp Med. 1965;121:439–62.
64. Bast Jr RC, Feeney M, Lazarus H, Nadler LM, Colvin RB, Knapp RC. Reactivity of a monoclonal antibody with human ovarian carcinoma. J Clin Invest. 1981;68(5):1331–7.
65. Husseinzadeh N. Status of tumor markers in epithelial ovarian cancer has there been any progress? A review. Gynecol Oncol. 2011;120(1):152–7.
66. Zhang B, Barekati Z, Kohler C, Radpour R, Asadollahi R, Holzgreve W, Zhong XY. Proteomics and biomarkers for ovarian cancer diagnosis. Ann Clin Lab Sci. Summer 2010;40(3):218–25.
67. Makridakis M, Vlahou A. Secretome proteomics for discovery of cancer biomarkers. J Proteomics. 2010;73(12):2291–305.
68. Dutta S, Wang FQ, Phalen A, Fishman DA. Biomarkers for ovarian cancer detection and therapy. Cancer Biol Ther. 2010;9(9):668–77.
69. Tung CS, Wong KK, Mok SC. Biomarker discovery in ovarian cancer. Womens Health (Lond Engl). 2008;4:27–40.
70. Coticchia CM, Yang J, Moses MA. Ovarian cancer biomarkers: current options and future promise. J Natl Compr Canc Netw. 2008;6(8):795–802.
71. McLemore MR, Miaskowski C, Aouizerat BE, Chen LM, Dodd M. Rules of tumor cell development and their application to biomarkers for ovarian cancer. Oncol Nurs Forum. 2008;35(3):403–9.
72. Merritt WM, Sood AK. Markers of angiogenesis in ovarian cancer. Dis Markers. 2007;23(5–6):419–31.

73. Munkarah A, Chatterjee M, Tainsky MA. Update on ovarian cancer screening. Curr Opin Obstet Gynecol. 2007;19(1):22–6.
74. Bast Jr RC, Badgwell D, Lu Z, Marquez R, Rosen D, Liu J, et al. New tumor markers: CA125 and beyond. Int J Gynecol Cancer. 2005;15 Suppl 3:274–81.
75. Nossov V, Amneus M, Su F, Lang J, Janco JM, Reddy ST, Farias-Eisner R. The early detection of ovarian cancer: from traditional methods to proteomics. Can we really do better than serum CA-125? Am J Obstet Gynecol. 2008;199(3):215–23.
76. Bertenshaw GP, Yip P, Seshaiah P, Zhao J, Chen TH, Wiggins WS, et al. Multianalyte profiling of serum antigens and autoimmune and infectious disease molecules to identify biomarkers dysregulated in epithelial ovarian cancer. Cancer Epidemiol Biomarkers Prev. 2008;17(10):2872–81.
77. Lin B, White JT, Wu J, Lele S, Old LJ, Hood L, Odunsi K, et al. Deep depletion of abundant serum proteins reveals low-abundant proteins as potential biomarkers for human ovarian cancer. Proteomics Clin Appl. 2009;3(7):853–61.
78. Qian WJ, Kaleta DT, Petritis BO, Jiang H, Liu T, Zhang X, et al. Enhanced detection of low abundance human plasma proteins using a tandem IgY12-SuperMix immunoaffinity separation strategy. Mol Cell Proteomics. 2008;7(10):1963–73.
79. Mor G, Visintin I, Lai Y, Zhao H, Schwartz P, Rutherford T, et al. Serum protein markers for early detection of ovarian cancer. Proc Natl Acad Sci U S A. 2005;102(21):7677–82.
80. Pinho S, Marcos NT, Ferreira B, Carvalho AS, Oliveira MJ, Santos-Silva F, et al. Biological significance of cancer-associated sialyl-Tn antigen: modulation of malignant phenotype in gastric carcinoma cells. Cancer Lett. 2007;249(2):157–70.
81. Bast Jr RC. Status of tumor markers in ovarian cancer screening. J Clin Oncol. 2003;21(10 Suppl):200s–5.
82. Moore RG, Maclaughlan S. Current clinical use of biomarkers for epithelial ovarian cancer. Curr Opin Oncol. 2010;22(5):492–7.
83. Pitteri SJ, JeBailey L, Faca VM, Thorpe JD, Silva MA, Ireton RC, et al. Integrated proteomic analysis of human cancer cells and plasma from tumor bearing mice for ovarian cancer biomarker discovery. PLoS One. 2009;4(11):e7916.
84. Gadducci A, Ferdeghini M, Castellani C, Annicchiarico C, Gagetti O, Prontera C, et al. Serum levels of tumor necrosis factor (TNF), soluble receptors for TNF (55- and 75-kDa sTNFr), and soluble CD14 (sCD14) in epithelial ovarian cancer. Gynecol Oncol. 1995;58(2):184–8.
85. Naldini A, Morena E, Belotti D, Carraro F, Allavena P, Giavazzi R. Identification of thrombin-like activity in ovarian cancer associated ascites and modulation of multiple cytokine networks. Thromb Haemost. 2011;106(4):705–11.
86. Morin PJ. Claudin proteins in ovarian cancer. Dis Markers. 2007;23(5–6):453–7.
87. Pyle-Chenault RA, Stolk JA, Molesh DA, Boyle-Harlan D, McNeill PD, Repasky EA, et al. VSGP/F--spondin: a new ovarian cancer marker. Tumour Biol. 2005;26(5):245–57.
88. Simon I, Liu Y, Krall KL, Urban N, Wolfert RL, Kim NW, McIntosh MW. Evaluation of the novel serum markers B7-H4, Spondin 2, and DcR3 for diagnosis and early detection of ovarian cancer. Gynecol Oncol. 2007;106(1):112–8.
89. Dupont J, Tanwar MK, Thaler HT, Fleisher M, Kauff N, Hensley ML, et al. Early detection and prognosis of ovarian cancer using serum YKL-40. J Clin Oncol. 2004;22(16):3330–9.
90. Hogdall E, Fung ET, Christensen IJ, Yip C, Nedergaard L, Engelholm SA, et al. Proteomic biomarkers for overall and progression-free survival in ovarian cancer patients. Proteomics Clin Appl. 2010;4(12):940–52.
91. Cho H, Kim JH. Lipocalin2 expressions correlate significantly with tumor differentiation in epithelial ovarian cancer. J Histochem Cytochem. 2009;57(5): 513–21.
92. Tsukishiro S, Suzumori N, Nishikawa H, Arakawa A, Suzumori K. Use of serum secretory leukocyte protease inhibitor levels in patients to improve specificity of ovarian cancer diagnosis. Gynecol Oncol. 2005;96(2):516–9.
93. Strieter RM, Burdick MD, Mestas J, Gomperts B, Keane MP, Belperio JA. Cancer CXC chemokine networks and tumour angiogenesis. Eur J Cancer. 2006;42(6):768–78.
94. Barton DP, Blanchard DK, Michelini-Norris B, Nicosia SV, Cavanagh D, Djeu JY. High serum and ascitic soluble interleukin-2 receptor alpha levels in advanced epithelial ovarian cancer. Blood. 1993;81(2):424–9.
95. Bast Jr RC. Early detection of ovarian cancer: new technologies in pursuit of a disease that is neither common nor rare. Trans Am Clin Climatol Assoc. 2004;115:233–47; discussion 247–8.
96. Bast Jr RC, Brewer M, Zou C, Daley M, Ozols R, Lu K, et al. Prevention and early detection of ovarian cancer: mission impossible? Recent Results Cancer Res. 2007;174:91–100.
97. Bast Jr RC, Urban N, Shridhar V, Smith D, Zhang Z, Skates S, et al. Early detection of ovarian cancer: promise and reality. Cancer Treat Res. 2002;107:61–97.
98. Clarke CH, Yip C, Badgwell D, Fung ET, Coombes KR, Zhang Z, et al. Proteomic biomarkers apolipoprotein A1, truncated transthyretin and connective tissue activating protein III enhance the sensitivity of CA125 for detecting early stage epithelial ovarian cancer. Gynecol Oncol. 2011;122(3):548–53.
99. Cole LA, Nam JH. Urinary gonadotropin fragment (UGF) measurements in the diagnosis and management of ovarian cancer. Yale J Biol Med. 1989;62(4):367–78.
100. Cooke I, O'Brien M, Charnock FM, Groome N, Ganesan TS. Inhibin as a marker for ovarian cancer. Br J Cancer. 1995;71(5):1046–50.

101. Dieplinger H, Ankerst DP, Burges A, Lenhard M, Lingenhel A, Fineder L, et al. Afamin and apolipoprotein A-IV: novel protein markers for ovarian cancer. Cancer Epidemiol Biomarkers Prev. 2009;18(4):1127–33.
102. Dobrzycka B, Terlikowski SJ, Garbowicz M, Niklińska W, Bernaczyk PS, Nikliński J, et al. Tumor necrosis factor-alpha and its receptors in epithelial ovarian cancer. Folia Histochem Cytobiol. 2009;47(4):609–13.
103. Gadducci A, Cosio S, Tana R, Genazzani AR. Serum and tissue biomarkers as predictive and prognostic variables in epithelial ovarian cancer. Crit Rev Oncol Hematol. 2009;69(1):12–27.
104. Gagnon A, Ye B. Discovery and application of protein biomarkers for ovarian cancer. Curr Opin Obstet Gynecol. 2008;20(1):9–13.
105. Hata K, Dhar DK, Kanasaki H, Nakayama K, Fujiwaki R, Katabuchi H, et al. Serum endostatin levels in patients with epithelial ovarian cancer. Anticancer Res. 2003;23(2C):1907–12.
106. Hogdall CK, Hogdall EV, Hording U, Toftager-Larsen K, Arends J, Nørgaard-Pedersen B, Clemmensen I. Use of tetranectin, CA-125 and CASA to predict residual tumor and survival at second- and third-look operations for ovarian cancer. Acta Oncol. 1996;35(1):63–9.
107. Johnson MD, Oberst MD, Lin CY, Dickson RB. Possible role of matriptase in the diagnosis of ovarian cancer. Expert Rev Mol Diagn. 2003;3(3):331–8.
108. Kocbl H, Tatra G, Bieglmayer C. A comparative study of immunosuppressive acidic protein (IAP), CA 125 and acute-phase proteins as parameters for ovarian cancer monitoring. Neoplasma. 1988;35(2):215–20.
109. Koh SH, Cauchi MN. Prognostic significance of oncofetal antigens in patients with ovarian cancer. Aust N Z J Obstet Gynaecol. 1983;23(2):69–72.
110. Kuk C, Gunawardana CG, Soosaipillai A, Kobayashi H, Li L, Zheng Y, Diamandis EP. Nidogen-2: a new serum biomarker for ovarian cancer. Clin Biochem. 2010;43(4–5):355–61.
111. Lim R, Lappas M, Ahmed N, Permezel M, Quinn MA, Rice GE. 2D-PAGE of ovarian cancer: analysis of soluble and insoluble fractions using medium-range immobilized pH gradients. Biochem Biophys Res Commun. 2011;406(3):408–13.
112. Maccio A, Lai P, Santona MC, Pagliara L, Melis GB, Mantovani G. High serum levels of soluble IL-2 receptor, cytokines, and C reactive protein correlate with impairment of T cell response in patients with advanced epithelial ovarian cancer. Gynecol Oncol. 1998;69(3):248–52.
113. Moradi MM, Carson LF, Weinberg B, Haney AF, Twiggs LB, Ramakrishnan S. Serum and ascitic fluid levels of interleukin-1, interleukin-6, and tumor necrosis factor-alpha in patients with ovarian epithelial cancer. Cancer. 1993;72(8):2433–40.
114. Moshkovskii SA, Vlasova MA, Pyatnitskiy MA, Tikhonova OV, Safarova MR, Makarov OV, Archakov AI. Acute phase serum amyloid A in ovarian cancer as an important component of proteome diagnostic profiling. Proteomics Clin Appl. 2007;1(1):107–17.
115. Nayak SB, Bhat VR, Mayya SS. Serum copper, ceruloplasmin and thiobarbituric acid reactive substance status in patients with ovarian cancer. Indian J Physiol Pharmacol. 2004;48(4):486–8.
116. Pledger DR, Belfield A, Kennedy JH, Kaye SB. Onco-developmental protein concentrations in the sera of patients with ovarian cancer prior to treatment. Eur J Cancer Clin Oncol. 1988;24(2):219–22.
117. Polterauer S, Grimm C, Seebacher V, Concin N, Marth C, Tomovski C, Concin N, Marth C, Tomovski C, et al. Plasma fibrinogen levels and prognosis in patients with ovarian cancer: a multicenter study. Oncologist. 2009;14(10):979–85.
118. Tempfer C, Zeisler H, Sliutz G, Haeusler G, Hanzal E, Kainz C. Serum evaluation of interleukin 6 in ovarian cancer patients. Gynecol Oncol. 1997;66(1):27–30.
119. Wang X, Wang E, Kavanagh JJ, Freedman RS. Ovarian cancer, the coagulation pathway, and inflammation. J Transl Med. 2005;3:25.
120. Ward BG, McGuckin MA, Ramm LE, Coglan M, Sanderson B, Tripcony L, Free KE. The management of ovarian carcinoma is improved by the use of cancer-associated serum antigen and CA 125 assays. Cancer. 1993;71(2):430–8.
121. Yabushita H, Masuda T, Ogawa A, Noguchi M, Ishihara M. Combination assay of CA125, TPA, IAP, CEA, and ferritin in serum for ovarian cancer. Gynecol Oncol. 1988;29(1):66–75.
122. Ye B, Cramer DW, Skates SJ, Gygi SP, Pratomo V, Fu L, Gygi SP, Pratomo V, Fu L, et al. Haptoglobin-alpha subunit as potential serum biomarker in ovarian cancer: identification and characterization using proteomic profiling and mass spectrometry. Clin Cancer Res. 2003;9(8):2904–11.
123. Yousef GM, Diamandis EP. The human kallikrein gene family: new biomarkers for ovarian cancer. Cancer Treat Res. 2009;149:165–87.
124. Zeisler H, Tempfer C, Joura EA, Sliutz G, Koelbl H, Wagner O, Kainz C. Serum interleukin 1 in ovarian cancer patients. Eur J Cancer. 1998;34(6):931–3.
125. Amonkar SD, Bertenshaw GP, Chen TH, Bergstrom KJ, Zhao J, Seshaiah P, et al. Development and preliminary evaluation of a multivariate index assay for ovarian cancer. PLoS One. 2009;4(2):e4599.
126. Edgell T, Martin-Roussety G, Barker G, Autelitano DJ, Allen D, Grant P, Rice GE. Phase II biomarker trial of a multimarker diagnostic for ovarian cancer. J Cancer Res Clin Oncol. 2010;136(7):1079–88.
127. Skates SJ, Horick N, Yu Y, Xu FJ, Berchuck A, Havrilesky LJ, et al. Preoperative sensitivity and specificity for early-stage ovarian cancer when combining cancer antigen CA-125II, CA 15-3, CA 72-4, and macrophage colony-stimulating factor using mixtures of multivariate normal distributions. J Clin Oncol. 2004;22(20):4059–66.

128. Visintin I, Feng Z, Longton G, Ward DC, Alvero AB, Lai Y, et al. Diagnostic markers for early detection of ovarian cancer. Clin Cancer Res. 2008;14(4):1065–72.
129. Zhang Z, Bast Jr RC, Yu Y, Li J, Sokoll LJ, Rai AJ, et al. Three biomarkers identified from serum proteomic analysis for the detection of early stage ovarian cancer. Cancer Res. 2004;64(16):5882–90.
130. Nolen BM, Lokshin AE. Protein biomarkers of ovarian cancer: the forest and the trees. Future Oncol. 2012;8(1):55–71.
131. DePriest PD, Varner E, Powell J, Fried A, Puls L, Higgins R, et al. The efficacy of a sonographic morphology index in identifying ovarian cancer: a multi-institutional investigation. Gynecol Oncol. 1994; 55(2):174–8.
132. Schulman H, Conway C, Zalud I, Farmakides G, Haley J, Cassata M. Prevalence in a volunteer population of pelvic cancer detected with transvaginal ultrasound and color flow Doppler. Ultrasound Obstet Gynecol. 1994;4(5):414–20.
133. Brown PO, Palmer C. The preclinical natural history of serous ovarian cancer: defining the target for early detection. PLoS Med. 2009;6(7):e1000114.
134. Sato S, Yokoyama Y, Sakamoto T, Futagami M, Saito Y. Usefulness of mass screening for ovarian carcinoma using transvaginal ultrasonography. Cancer. 2000;89(3):582–8.
135. Bourne TH, Campbell S, Reynolds KM, Whitehead MI, Hampson J, Royston P, et al. Screening for early familial ovarian cancer with transvaginal ultrasonography and colour blood flow imaging. BMJ. 1993;306(6884):1025–9.
136. van Nagell Jr JR, DePriest PD, Reedy MB, Gallion HH, Ueland FR, Pavlik EJ, Kryscio RJ. The efficacy of transvaginal sonographic screening in asymptomatic women at risk for ovarian cancer. Gynecol Oncol. 2000;77(3):350–6.
137. van Nagell Jr JR, DePriest PD, Ueland FR, DeSimone CP, Cooper AL, McDonald JM, et al. Ovarian cancer screening with annual transvaginal sonography: findings of 25,000 women screened. Cancer. 2007;109(9):1887–96.
138. Hayashi H, Yaginuma Y, Kitamura S, Saitou Y, Miyamoto T, Komori H, et al. Bilateral oophorectomy in asymptomatic women over 50 years old selected by ovarian cancer screening. Gynecol Obstet Invest. 1999;47(1):58–64.
139. Tabor A, Jensen FR, Bock JE, Hogdall CK. Feasibility study of a randomised trial of ovarian cancer screening. J Med Screen. 1994;1(4):215–9.
140. Einhorn N, Sjovall K, Knapp RC, Hall P, Scully RE, Bast Jr RC, Zurawski Jr VR, et al. Prospective evaluation of serum CA 125 levels for early detection of ovarian cancer. Obstet Gynecol. 1992;80(1):14–8.
141. Skates SJ, Xu FJ, Yu YH, Sjövall K, Einhorn N, Chang Y, et al. Toward an optimal algorithm for ovarian cancer screening with longitudinal tumor markers. Cancer. 1995;76(10 Suppl):2004–10.
142. Menon U, Skates SJ, Lewis S, Rosenthal AN, Rufford B, Sibley K, et al. Prospective study using the risk of ovarian cancer algorithm to screen for ovarian cancer. J Clin Oncol. 2005;23(31):7919–26.
143. Greene MH, Piedmonte M, Alberts D, Gail M, Hensley M, Miner Z, et al. A prospective study of risk-reducing salpingo-oophorectomy and longitudinal CA-125 screening among women at increased genetic risk of ovarian cancer: design and baseline characteristics: a Gynecologic Oncology Group study. Cancer Epidemiol Biomarkers Prev. 2008; 17(3):594–604.
144. McIntosh MW, Urban N, Karlan B. Generating longitudinal screening algorithms using novel biomarkers for disease. Cancer Epidemiol Biomarkers Prev. 2002;11(2):159–66.
145. Gorelik E, Landsittel DP, Marrangoni AM, Modugno F, Velikokhatnaya L, Winans MT, et al. Multiplexed immunobead-based cytokine profiling for early detection of ovarian cancer. Cancer Epidemiol Biomarkers Prev. 2005;14(4):981–7.
146. Su F, Lang J, Kumar A, Ng C, Hsieh B, Suchard MA, Ng C, Hsieh B, Suchard MA, et al. Validation of candidate serum ovarian cancer biomarkers for early detection. Biomark Insights. 2007;2:369–75.
147. Havrilesky LJ, Whitehead CM, Rubatt JM, Cheek RL, Groelke J, He Q, et al. Evaluation of biomarker panels for early stage ovarian cancer detection and monitoring for disease recurrence. Gynecol Oncol. 2008;110(3):374–82.
148. Andersen MR, Goff BA, Lowe KA, Scholler N, Bergan L, Drescher CW, et al. Use of a Symptom Index, CA125, and HE4 to predict ovarian cancer. Gynecol Oncol. 2010;116(3):378–83.
149. McIntosh M, Anderson G, Drescher C, Hanash S, Urban N, Brown P, et al. Ovarian cancer early detection claims are biased. Clin Cancer Res. 2008;14(22):7574; author reply 7577–9.
150. Palmer C, Duan X, Hawley S, Scholler N, Thorpe JD, Sahota RA, et al. Systematic evaluation of candidate blood markers for detecting ovarian cancer. PLoS One. 2008;3(7):e2633.
151. Anderson GL, McIntosh M, Wu L, Barnett M, Goodman G, Thorpe JD, et al. Assessing lead time of selected ovarian cancer biomarkers: a nested case-control study. J Natl Cancer Inst. 2010;102(1):26–38.
152. Gohagan JK, Prorok PC, Hayes RB, Kramer BS. The Prostate, Lung, Colorectal and Ovarian (PLCO) Cancer Screening Trial of the National Cancer Institute: history, organization, and status. Control Clin Trials. 2000;21(6 Suppl):251S–72.
153. Cramer DW, Bast Jr RC, Berg CD, Diamandis EP, Godwin AK, Hartge P, et al. Ovarian cancer biomarker performance in prostate, lung, colorectal, and ovarian cancer screening trial specimens. Cancer Prev Res (Phila). 2011;4(3):365–74.
154. Zhu CS, Pinsky PF, Cramer DW, Ransohoff DF, Hartge P, Pfeiffer RM, et al. A framework for evaluating biomarkers for early detection: validation of

biomarker panels for ovarian cancer. Cancer Prev Res (Phila). 2011;4(3):375–83.
155. Folkins AK, Jarboe EA, Roh MH, Crum CP. Precursors to pelvic serous carcinoma and their clinical implications. Gynecol Oncol. 2009;113(3):391–6.
156. Ries LAG, Melbert D, Krapcho M, Stinchcomg DG, Howlader N, Horner MJ, Mariotto A, et al. SEER cancer statistics review, 1975-2005. Bethesda: National Cancer Institute; 2008.
157. Disaia PJ, Creasman WT. The adnexal mass and early ovarian cancer. In: Clinical gynecological oncology. 5th ed. St. Louis: Mosby-Year Book; 1997. p. 253–81.
158. Drake J. Diagnosis and management of the adnexal mass. Am Fam Physician. 1998;57(10):2471–6, 2479–80.
159. Droegenmueller W. Benign gynecological lesions. In: Mishell Jr DR, editor. Comprehensive gynecology. 4th ed. St. Louis: Mosby; 2001. p. 479–525.
160. Stany MP, Hamilton CA. Benign disorders of the ovary. Obstet Gynecol Clin North Am. 2008;35(2): 271–84, ix.
161. Earle CC, Schrag D, Neville BA, Yabroff KR, Topor M, Fahey A, et al. Effect of surgeon specialty on processes of care and outcomes for ovarian cancer patients. J Natl Cancer Inst. 2006;98(3):172–80.
162. Tingulstad S, Skjeldestad FE, Hagen B. The effect of centralization of primary surgery on survival in ovarian cancer patients. Obstet Gynecol. 2003;102(3): 499–505.
163. Bristow RE, Tomacruz RS, Armstrong DK, Trimble EL, Montz FJ. Survival effect of maximal cytoreductive surgery for advanced ovarian carcinoma during the platinum era: a meta-analysis. J Clin Oncol. 2002;20(5):1248–59.
164. Eisenkop SM, Spirtos NM, Montag TW, Nalick RH, Wang HJ. The impact of subspecialty training on the management of advanced ovarian cancer. Gynecol Oncol. 1992;47(2):203–9.
165. Chan JK, Cheung MK, Husain A, Teng NN, West D, Whittemore AS, et al. Patterns and progress in ovarian cancer over 14 years. Obstet Gynecol. 2006;108(3 Pt 1):521–8.
166. Goodman MT, Howe HL. Descriptive epidemiology of ovarian cancer in the United States, 1992-1997. Cancer. 2003;97(10 Suppl):2615–30.
167. Gostout BS, Brewer MA. Guidelines for referral of the patient with an adnexal mass. Clin Obstet Gynecol. 2006;49(3):448–58.
168. Risum S, Høgdall C, Loft A, Berthelsen AK, Høgdall E, Nedergaard L, et al. The diagnostic value of PET/CT for primary ovarian cancer–a prospective study. Gynecol Oncol. 2007;105(1):145–9.
169. Dearking AC, Aletti GD, McGree ME, Weaver AL, Sommerfield MK, Cliby WA. How relevant are ACOG and SGO guidelines for referral of adnexal mass? Obstet Gynecol. 2007;110(4):841–8.
170. Jacobs I, Oram D, Fairbanks J, Turner J, Frost C, Grudzinskas JG. A risk of malignancy index incorporating CA 125, ultrasound and menopausal status for the accurate preoperative diagnosis of ovarian cancer. Br J Obstet Gynaecol. 1990;97(10):922–9.
171. Tingulstad S, Hagen B, Skjeldestad FE, Onsrud M, Kiserud T, Halvorsen T, Nustad K. Evaluation of a risk of malignancy index based on serum CA125, ultrasound findings and menopausal status in the pre-operative diagnosis of pelvic masses. Br J Obstet Gynaecol. 1996;103(8):826–31.
172. Tingulstad S, Hagen B, Skjeldestad FE, Halvorsen T, Nustad K, Onsrud M. The risk-of-malignancy index to evaluate potential ovarian cancers in local hospitals. Obstet Gynecol. 1999;93(3):448–52.
173. Bailey J, Tailor A, Naik R, Lopes A, Godfrey K, Hatem HM, et al. Risk of malignancy index for referral of ovarian cancer cases to a tertiary center: does it identify the correct cases? Int J Gynecol Cancer. 2006;16 Suppl 1:30–4.
174. Enakpene CA, Omigbodun AO, Goecke TW, Odukogbe AT, Beckmann MW. Preoperative evaluation and triage of women with suspicious adnexal masses using risk of malignancy index. J Obstet Gynaecol Res. 2009;35(1):131–8.
175. Håkansson F, Høgdall EV, Nedergaard L, Lundvall L, Engelholm SA, Pedersen AT, DANISH 'PELVIC MASS' OVARIAN CANCER STUDY, et al. Risk of malignancy index (RMI) used as a diagnostic tool in a tertiary centre for patients with a pelvic mass. Acta Obstet Gynecol Scand. 2012;91:496–502.
176. Geomini P, Kruitwagen R, Bremer GL, Cnossen J, Mol BWJ. The accuracy of risk scores in predicting ovarian malignancy: a systematic review. Obstet Gynecol. 2009;113(2 Part 1):384–94.
177. Timmerman D, Testa AC, Bourne T, Ferrazzi E, Ameye L, Konstantinovic ML, International Ovarian Tumor Analysis Group, et al. Logistic regression model to distinguish between the benign and malignant adnexal mass before surgery: a multicenter study by the International Ovarian Tumor Analysis Group. J Clin Oncol. 2005;23(34):8794–801.
178. Van Holsbeke CD, Van Calster B, Bourne T, Ajossa S, Testa AC, Guerriero S, et al. External validation of diagnostic models to estimate the risk of malignancy in adnexal masses. Clin Cancer Res. 2011;18:815–25.
179. Hogdall C, Fung ET, Christensen IJ, Nedergaard L, Engelholm SA, Petri AL, et al. A novel proteomic biomarker panel as a diagnostic tool for patients with ovarian cancer. Gynecol Oncol. 2011;123:308–13.
180. Rice GE, Edgell TA, Autelitano DJ. Evaluation of midkine and anterior gradient 2 in a multimarker panel for the detection of ovarian cancer. J Exp Clin Cancer Res. 2010;29:62.
181. Lambeck AJ, Crijns AP, Leffers N, Sluiter WJ, ten Hoor KA, Braid M, et al. Serum cytokine profiling as a diagnostic and prognostic tool in ovarian cancer: a potential role for interleukin 7. Clin Cancer Res. 2007;13(8):2385–91.
182. Yip P, Chen TH, Seshaiah P, Stephen LL, Michael-Ballard KL, Mapes JP, et al. Comprehensive serum

profiling for the discovery of epithelial ovarian cancer biomarkers. PLoS One. 2011;6(12):e29533.
183. Petri AL, Simonsen AH, Høgdall E, Christensen IJ, Kjaer SK, Yip C, et al. Comparison of proteomic biomarker panels in urine and serum for ovarian cancer diagnosis. Proteomics Clin Appl. 2010;4(3):304–14.
184. Schaner ME, Ross DT, Ciaravino G, Sorlie T, Troyanskaya O, Diehn M, et al. Gene expression patterns in ovarian carcinomas. Mol Biol Cell. 2003;14(11):4376–86.
185. Moore RG, Brown AK, Miller MC, Skates S, Allard WJ, Verch T, et al. The use of multiple novel tumor biomarkers for the detection of ovarian carcinoma in patients with a pelvic mass. Gynecol Oncol. 2008;108(2):402–8.
186. Moore RG, McMeekin DS, Brown AK, DiSilvestro P, Miller MC, Allard WJ, et al. A novel multiple marker bioassay utilizing HE4 and CA125 for the prediction of ovarian cancer in patients with a pelvic mass. Gynecol Oncol. 2009;112(1):40–6.
187. Huhtinen K, Suvitie P, Hiissa J, Junnila J, Huvila J, Kujari H, et al. Serum HE4 concentration differentiates malignant ovarian tumours from ovarian endometriotic cysts. Br J Cancer. 2009;100(8):1315–9.
188. Nolen B, Velikokhatnaya L, Marrangoni A, De Geest K, Lomakin A, Bast Jr RC, Lokshin A. Serum biomarker panels for the discrimination of benign from malignant cases in patients with an adnexal mass. Gynecol Oncol. 2010;117(3):440–5.
189. Holcomb K, Vucetic Z, Miller MC, Knapp RC. Human epididymis protein 4 offers superior specificity in the differentiation of benign and malignant adnexal masses in premenopausal women. Am J Obstet Gynecol. 2011;205(4):358.e351–6.
190. Moore RG, Miller MC, Disilvestro P, Landrum LM, Gajewski W, Ball JJ, Skates SJ. Evaluation of the diagnostic accuracy of the risk of ovarian malignancy algorithm in women with a pelvic mass. Obstet Gynecol. 2011;118(2 Pt 1):280–8.
191. Moore RG, Jabre-Raughley M, Brown AK, Robison KM, Miller MC, Allard WJ, et al. Comparison of a novel multiple marker assay vs the risk of malignancy index for the prediction of epithelial ovarian cancer in patients with a pelvic mass. Am J Obstet Gynecol. 2010;203(3):228.e221–6.
192. Van Gorp T, Veldman J, Van Calster B, Cadron I, Leunen K, Amant F, et al. Subjective assessment by ultrasound is superior to the risk of malignancy index (RMI) or the risk of ovarian malignancy algorithm (ROMA) in discriminating benign from malignant adnexal masses. Eur J Cancer. 2012;48:1649–56.
193. Kadija S, Stefanovic A, Jeremic K, Radojevic MM, Nikolic L, Markovic I, Atanackovic J. The utility of human epididymal protein 4, cancer antigen 125, and risk for malignancy algorithm in ovarian cancer and endometriosis. Int J Gynecol Cancer. 2012;22:238–44.
194. Abdel-Azeez HA, Labib HA, Sharaf SM, Refai AN. HE4 and mesothelin: novel biomarkers of ovarian carcinoma in patients with pelvic masses. Asian Pac J Cancer Prev. 2010;11(1):111–6.
195. Chang X, Ye X, Dong L, Cheng H, Cheng Y, Zhu L, et al. Human epididymis protein 4 (HE4) as a serum tumor biomarker in patients with ovarian carcinoma. Int J Gynecol Cancer. 2011;21(5):852–8.
196. Kim YM, Whang DH, Park J, Kim SH, Lee SW, Park HA, et al. Evaluation of the accuracy of serum human epididymis protein 4 in combination with CA125 for detecting ovarian cancer: a prospective case-control study in a Korean population. Clin Chem Lab Med. 2011;49(3):527–34.
197. Ruggeri G, Bandiera E, Zanotti L, Belloli S, Ravaggi A, Romani C, et al. HE4 and epithelial ovarian cancer: Comparison and clinical evaluation of two immunoassays and a combination algorithm. Clin Chim Acta. 2011;412(15–16):1447–53.
198. Van Gorp T, Cadron I, Despierre E, Daemen A, Leunen K, Amant F, et al. HE4 and CA125 as a diagnostic test in ovarian cancer: prospective validation of the Risk of Ovarian Malignancy Algorithm. Br J Cancer. 2011;104(5):863–70.
199. Montagnana M, Danese E, Ruzzenente O, Bresciani V, Nuzzo T, Gelati M, et al. The ROMA (Risk of Ovarian Malignancy Algorithm) for estimating the risk of epithelial ovarian cancer in women presenting with pelvic mass: is it really useful? Clin Chem Lab Med. 2011;49(3):521–5.
200. Jacob F, Meier M, Caduff R, Goldstein D, Pochechueva T, Hacker N, et al. No benefit from combining HE4 and CA125 as ovarian tumor markers in a clinical setting. Gynecol Oncol. 2011;121(3):487–91.
201. U.S. Food and Drug Administration. FDA news release: FDA clears a test for Ovarian Cancer. http://www.fda.gov/NewsEvents/Newsroom/PressAnnouncements/ucm182057.htm. Accessed 14 May 2010.
202. Zhang Z, Chan DW. The road from discovery to clinical diagnostics: lessons learned from the first FDA-cleared in vitro diagnostic multivariate index assay of proteomic biomarkers. Cancer Epidemiol Biomarkers Prev. 2010;19(12):2995–9.
203. Miller R, Smith A, DeSimone CP, Van Hoorde K, Van Gorp T, Valentin L, Bourne T. Performance of the American College of Obstetricians and Gynecologists' ovarian tumor referral guidelines with a multivariate index assay. Obstet Gynecol. 2011;117(6):1298–306.
204. Ueland FR, Desimone CP, Seamon LG, Miller RA, Goodrich S, Podzielinski I, et al. Effectiveness of a multivariate index assay in the preoperative assessment of ovarian tumors. Obstet Gynecol. 2011;117(6):1289–97.
205. Moore LE, Pfeiffer RM, Zhang Z, Lu KH, Fung ET, Bast Jr RC. Proteomic biomarkers in combination with CA 125 for detection of epithelial ovarian cancer using prediagnostic serum samples from the Prostate, Lung, Colorectal, and Ovarian (PLCO) Cancer Screening Trial. Cancer. 2012;118(1):91–100.

Surface Epithelial Tumours of the Ovary

4

Purnima Makhija and Naveena Singh

Introduction

Surface epithelial tumours, or epithelial and stromal tumours as they are often referred to, form the majority of ovarian neoplasms. In fact the term 'ovarian cancer' is practically used almost synonymously with surface epithelial malignancies. The tumours include a number of distinct entities. Common to many of the tumour types in this category is the existence of benign and borderline in addition to malignant counterparts. These tumours are associated with nulliparity and obesity while pregnancies and oral contraception appear to play a protective role, hence suggesting a direct role of ovulation-related events in causing the disease. The non-specific nature of the presenting symptoms and inconsistent signs of early cancers result in greater than 70–75 % of cancers in this group presenting at a late stage when the tumours have already spread beyond the pelvis. Each year ovarian cancer afflicts 204,000 women worldwide and claims 125,000 lives.

P. Makhija, MD • N. Singh, MBBS, FRCPath (✉)
Department of Cellular Pathology,
Barts Health NHS Trust,
2nd Floor 80 Newark Street,
London E1 2ES, England, UK
e-mail: n.singh@bartshealth.nhs.uk

WHO Classification of Epithelial Ovarian Tumours

The World Health Organization (WHO) classification of epithelial ovarian tumours [1] divides the surface epithelial tumours into distinct disease entities which differ not just in their histologic appearances but also in molecular characteristics. Histotyping and classifying these tumours is important as they have different behaviours and different therapeutic options [2]:

- Serous
- Mucinous
- Endometrioid
- Clear cell
- Transitional
- Squamous
- Mixed epithelial
- Undifferentiated

Pathogenesis

Traditionally these tumours have been thought to arise from the surface epithelium which has undergone metaplasia into various cell types, namely, serous, endometrioid, clear, mucinous and transitional cells. These in turn undergo malignant transformation and give rise to the corresponding tumours. However, although scientists have demonstrated the ability of surface

S.A. Farghaly (ed.), *Advances in Diagnosis and Management of Ovarian Cancer*,
DOI 10.1007/978-1-4614-8271-0_4, © Springer Science+Business Media New York 2014

epithelium to transform into tumours in mouse models [3], in situ lesions have not been demonstrated in the surface epithelium. It was therefore suggested that cortical inclusion cysts, which may be acquired during reproductive life, undergo metaplasia and subsequent malignant transformation. These inclusions may originate either from invaginations of the surface epithelium or from the epithelium of the distal fallopian tube (endosalpingiosis). Alternatively, they may be formed as a result of implantation via retrograde menstruation (endometriosis) [4]. Again this hypothesis may explain the origin of some of the ovarian tumours, but not the majority, as only few reports have demonstrated dysplastic or in situ lesions in inclusion cysts [5]. Another theory is that surface epithelial tumours arise from secondary müllerian structures such as paratubal and paraovarian cysts. Once again precursors of surface epithelial tumours are rarely reported in these structures making this hypothesis less likely.

More recently it has been proposed that the vast majority of these tumours (in particular high-grade serous carcinomas) arise from intraepithelial carcinomas of the fallopian tube (Fig. 4.1) [6]. This has been supported by extensive sampling of the fimbrial ends of the fallopian tubes in high-grade serous tumours, which has revealed that greater than 70 % of sporadic ovarian high-grade serous tumours demonstrated mucosal tubal involvement [7]. A further recent finding has been the identification of secretory as opposed to ciliated tubal cells that express p53, in the fallopian tube. These lesions are termed as p53 signatures and are seen not only in association with tubal intraepithelial carcinomas but also in normal-appearing fallopian tubes in women who have no invasive cancer or intraepithelial carcinoma. p53 signatures are associated with lower parity and higher age at first childbirth, similar to risk factors associated with ovarian cancers. It is therefore believed that these and other recently described abnormalities may be cancer precursors [8].

While the concept of the fallopian tube epithelium being the origin of serous tumours is gaining popularity, it is suggested that most of the so-called ovarian primary non-serous epithelial tumours also have possible extraovarian origins. Endometrioid and clear cell tumours may actually originate from endometriotic tissue possibly from retrograde menstrual flow. Mucinous and Brenner tumours which are often linked to each other may originate from transitional-type epithelium found in paratubal and paraovarian locations [7, 9].

While the cell of origin of surface epithelial tumours remains a subject of debate, major advances have been made in the knowledge of

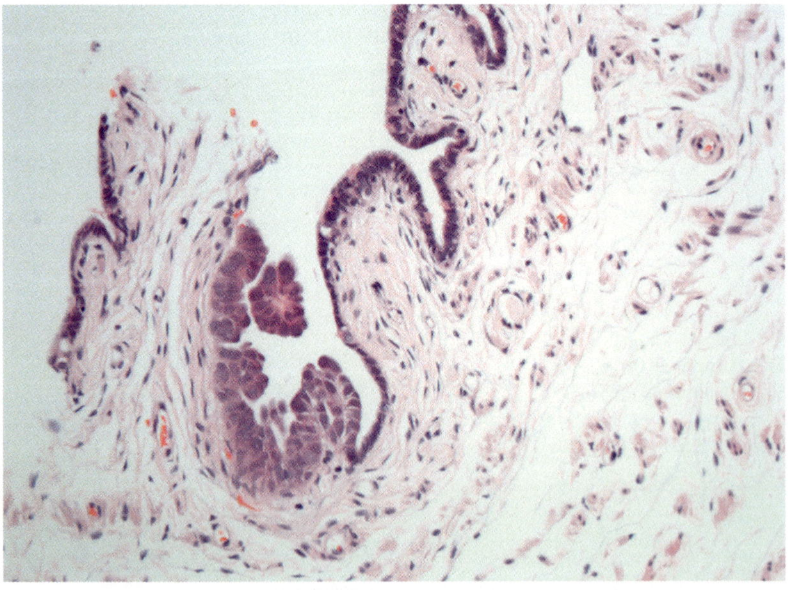

Fig. 4.1 Serous tubal intraepithelial carcinoma (STIC) at the fimbrial end of the Fallopian tube; the epithelial cells show enlarged and atypical nuclei with formation of tufts

the molecular basis of these tumours. These have highlighted that traditional morphology can predict specific molecular alterations likely to be present in a given tumour [10]. For example, *p53* and *BRCA* mutations are commonly seen in ovarian high-grade serous carcinomas. Mucinous carcinomas are characterised by a high prevalence of *KRAS* mutations. Mutations of *PIK3CA* are observed frequently in clear cell carcinomas. Mutations of *CTNNB1* are common in endometrioid carcinomas but rare in serous, mucinous and clear cell carcinomas.

It is thought that the candidate mechanism is oxidative genotoxic injury, perhaps a function of ovulation. Because ovulation occurs on the ovarian surface, both the ovarian surface and distal tube are targets [11, 12]. *BRCA* mutations and other genetic factors would increase the vulnerability to genotoxic injury and result in neoplastic transformation.

Given these advances in our understanding of the molecular alterations in the main types of ovarian epithelial malignancy, there has been a proposal for a dualistic pathway of ovarian epithelial carcinogenesis. This model divides the pathway of ovarian tumorigenesis into the type 1 pathway and the type 2 pathway [7]. Tumours in the type 1 pathway have in common frequent *BRAF/KRAS* mutations and rarely have a *p53* mutation. Other mutations characteristic of this group are *ERBB2*, *CTNNB1*, *PTEN*, *PIK3CA*, *ARID1A* and *PPP2R1A*. They have lower cellular proliferation. These tumours are considered to arise via a well-defined adenoma-carcinoma sequence in a stepwise fashion and are genetically stable. These tumours have in common the fact that they all appear to arise from a benign precursor lesion. The cancers included within this group are low-grade serous, mucinous, endometrioid and clear cell carcinomas. All these tumours have a better 5-year survival but are not as chemosensitive as tumours in the type 2 group. Tumours in the type 2 pathway exhibit frequent *p53* mutations and are genetically unstable. They show higher cellular proliferation, i.e. they are high-grade tumours which arise from less clearly defined precursor lesions. They have a poorer 5-year survival but are in general more chemosensitive compared to tumours in the type 1 group. They include high-grade serous carcinomas, carcinosarcomas and undifferentiated carcinomas.

Serous Tumours of the Ovary

General Features

These tumours are the commonest subtype of epithelial tumours. They are composed of cells which are ciliated or secretory and resemble fallopian tube epithelium (Fig. 4.2). These tumours are morphologically similar to tumours arising in the fallopian tube and müllerian epithelial rests in the pelvis (primary peritoneal carcinomas).

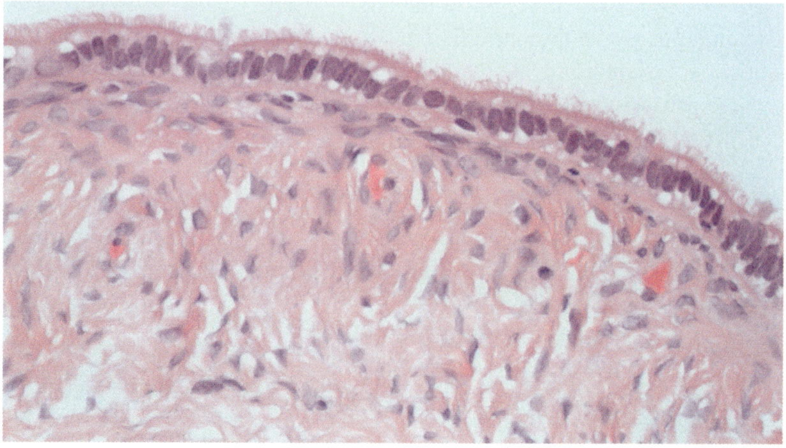

Fig. 4.2 Normal serous-type epithelium is composed of columnar cells with a ciliated luminal surface

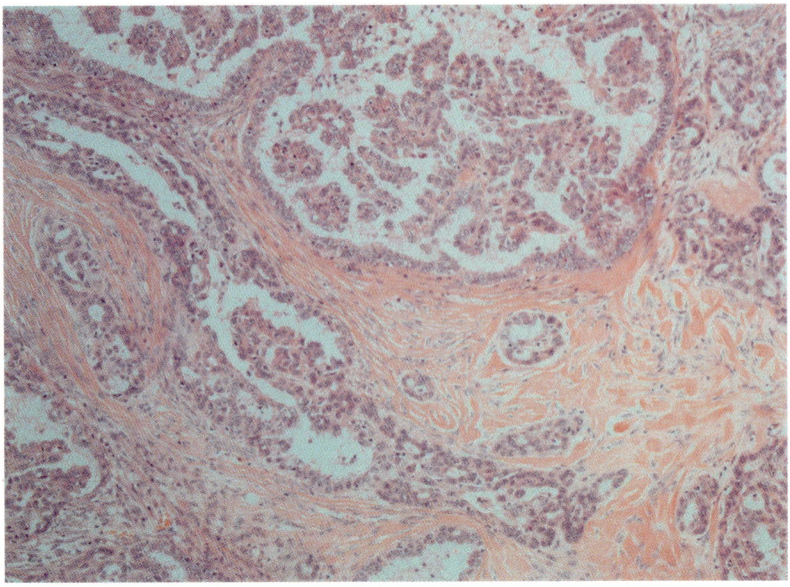

Fig. 4.3 Low-grade serous carcinoma is composed of tumour cell in a delicate papillary architecture

Serous Carcinomas

These tumours account for 80–85 % of all ovarian carcinomas; 95 % of stage III to IV tumours are serous carcinomas. Fewer than 5 % of serous carcinomas present at stage I [13].

Macroscopically, these tumours range in size from being undetectable to greater than 20 cm. Two-thirds of the tumours are bilateral. Most are solid and friable with areas of necrosis and haemorrhage. Variable proportions of cystic change are seen. On microscopy the tumours have a glandular, papillary and solid architecture. The glands are slit-like and irregular, and the papillae show complex branching. Solid areas are extensive in high-grade tumours. There are varying amounts of psammoma bodies, ranging from few to numerous (psammocarcinoma).

Currently a two-tier grading system is most widely used [14, 15]. This separates the tumour into two distinct subtypes with different genetic features, pathology and behaviour. Although low-grade and high-grade serous carcinomas follow independent pathways and are currently believed to be totally different biological entities, infrequently high-grade serous carcinomas evolve from low-grade tumours. Up to 3 % of high-grade serous carcinomas in one series were associated with low-grade components [7]. Molecular studies of low-grade and high-grade components showed identical *KRAS* mutations in a few cases, suggesting a clonal relationship between low-grade and high-grade tumours in select cases. The above findings show that a small minority of high-grade serous carcinomas may evolve from low-grade tumours.

Low-Grade Serous Carcinoma

Low-grade serous carcinomas are most often seen in conjunction with a pre-existing borderline tumour, either serous adenofibroma, typical serous borderline tumour or micropapillary borderline tumour. These tumours consistently show mutations of *BRAF*, *KRAS* or *ERBB2*. Very few tumours (8 % of all tumours) show *p53* mutations.

Microscopy

These tumours show a micropapillary architecture and lack necrosis (Fig. 4.3). They often contain many psammoma bodies (Figs. 4.4 and 4.5). Stromal invasion is seen in the form of glands or papillae surrounded by a non-epithelial lined space. Large complex papillae are seldom seen.

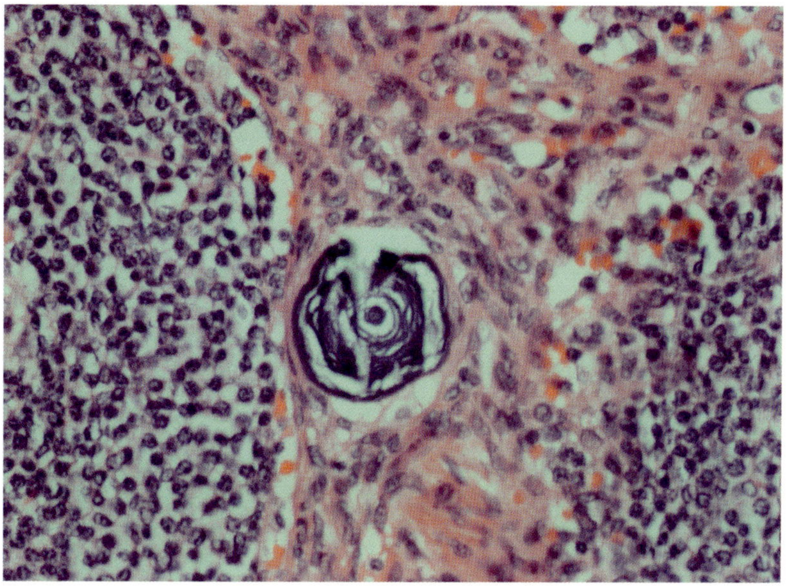

Fig. 4.4 Psammoma body; these are laminated calcified structures found in a variety of tumours which have papillary architecture, including serous ovarian carcinomas

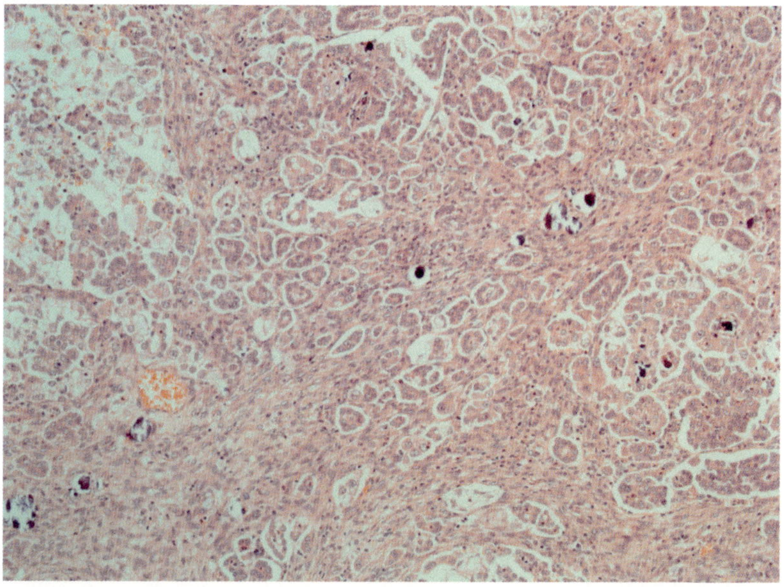

Fig. 4.5 Low-grade serous carcinoma with numerous psammoma bodies

The cells are bland with round to oval nuclei showing evenly distributed chromatin, sometimes containing a prominent nucleolus (Fig. 4.6). The cells should not show more than threefold variation in nuclear size. Multinucleated giant cells and bizarre cells are not a feature. Mitotic rate is low (less than 12/10 hpf) [15]. Rarely these tumours show an inverted macropapillary pattern which may be mistaken for a borderline serous adenofibroma but can be recognised to be an invasive tumour by the space surrounding medium-sized papillae. These tumours are often associated with pre-existing benign or borderline tumours.

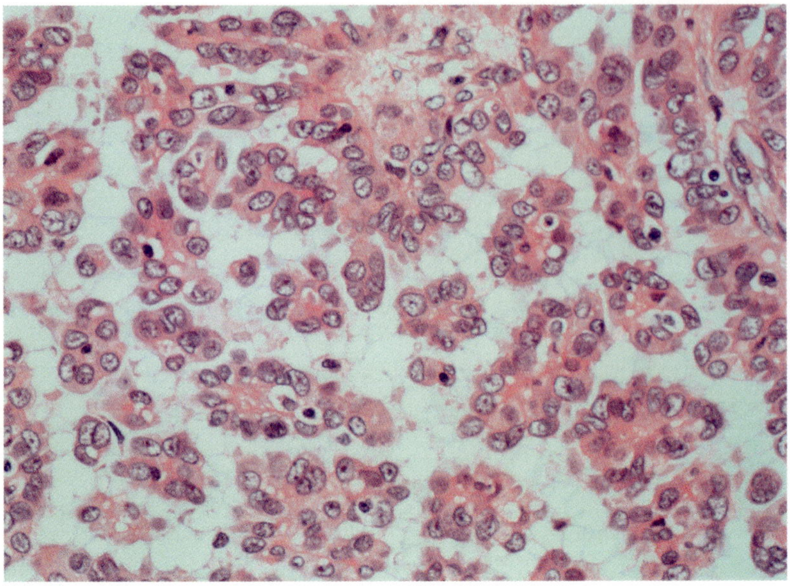

Fig. 4.6 Low-grade serous carcinoma: nuclei appear monotonous; though these can show some variation in size mitotic activity is low and atypia is not a feature

Immunohistochemistry of Low-Grade Carcinoma

These tumours are often WT1 positive and oestrogen (ER)/progesterone (PR) positive. The Ki-67 proliferation index is significantly lower in low-grade tumours compared to high-grade tumours (average, 23 %). p53 immunostaining (which is not the most reliable indicator of *p53* mutations) is strongly positive in only 18 % cases. p16 is sometimes useful in differentiating between low-grade and high-grade serous carcinomas, and strong positivity (>75 % of tumour cells) is seen only in 27 % cases [16].

High-Grade Serous Carcinoma

The high-grade tumours are the more common type and constitute 90 % of all serous carcinomas [14]. These tumours are generally not seen adjacent to a borderline tumour. Roughly half these tumours are associated with intraepithelial carcinoma in the fallopian tube, almost always in the fimbrial end [17]. The rest of the high-grade serous tumours are believed to arise either from the ovarian surface or the peritoneum. These tumours are seldom associated with mutations of *KRAS*, *BRAF* or *ERBB2*. In contrast, *p53* mutations occur in 50 % of these tumours. In addition, these tumours are associated with a high level of chromosomal instability. Another association is with germline *BRCA1* or *BRCA2* mutations. Roughly 15 % of ovarian serous carcinomas have a germline *BRCA* mutation, and almost all of these are high grade.

Microscopy

These neoplasms typically show complex papillae (Fig. 4.7). Psammoma bodies may be numerous, few or absent (Fig. 4.8). These tumours are often associated with variable amounts of necrosis. Other patterns encountered are glandular and solid and tumours with intracytoplasmic lumina and mucinous inclusions. They share high-grade nuclear features, large nuclei and often prominent nucleoli. Bizarre cells and multinucleated giant cells are often seen. Mitotic activity is high, and atypical mitotic figures are often seen (Fig. 4.9).

Immunohistochemistry of high-grade carcinoma: These tumours are often WT1 positive and variably ER/PR positive. The Ki-67 proliferation index is significantly higher in high-grade tumours (average 55 %). p53 immunostaining is strongly positive in 64 % cases. p16 is strongly positive (>75 % tumour cells) in 83 % cases [16].

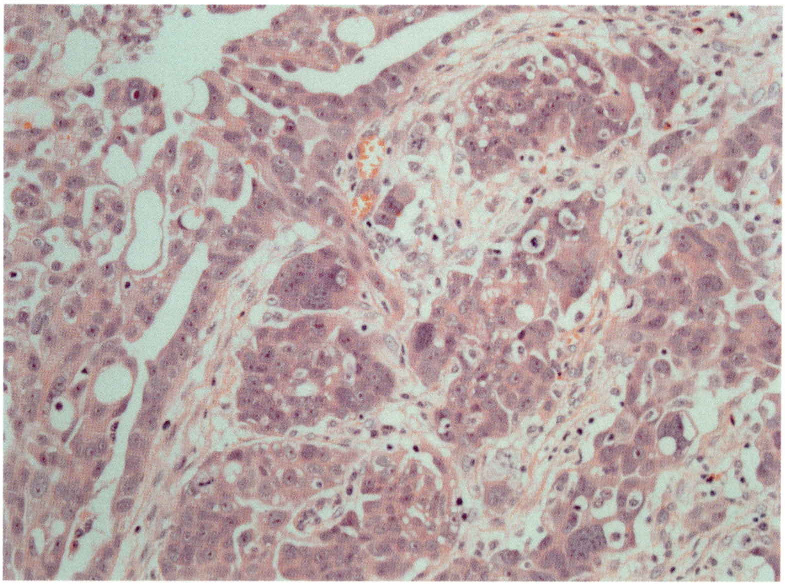

Fig. 4.7 High-grade serous carcinoma: In addition to papillae, the cells are arranged in solid masses

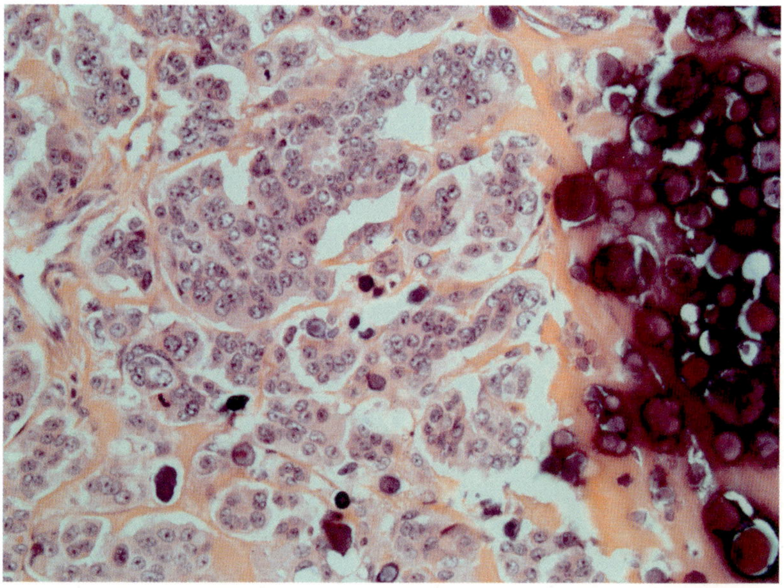

Fig. 4.8 High-grade serous carcinoma; large numbers of psammoma bodies may be seen

Serous Borderline Tumour

These tumours account for 10–15 % of serous tumours. They are tumours of low malignant potential with atypical proliferation of serous-type cells (accounting for more than 10 % of the total tumour) and no evidence of destructive stromal invasion. These tumours occur in patients 10–15 years younger than serous carcinomas (average age 45 years); however, the age range is broad (12–89 years). Borderline tumours of the ovary are associated with extraovarian disease in the form of peritoneal implants in 20–46 % of cases. The remaining cases are confined to the ovary. The prognosis of tumours confined to the ovary or those with associated noninvasive

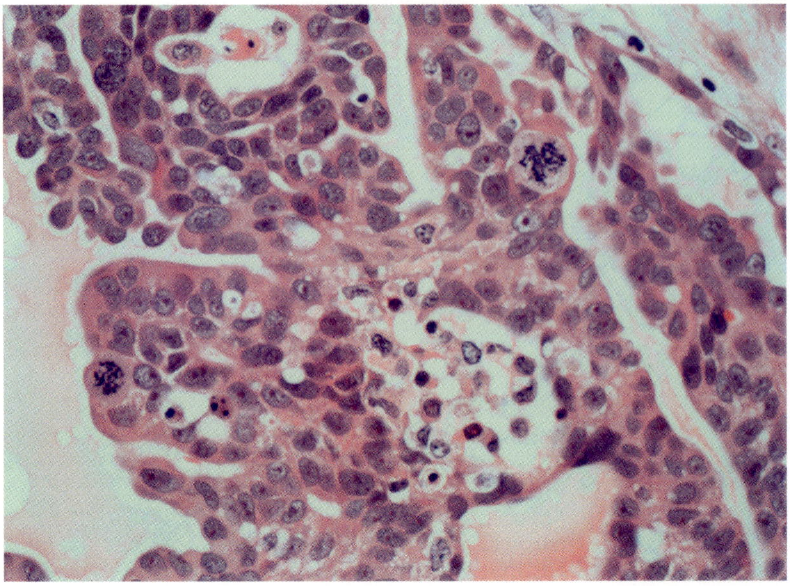

Fig. 4.9 High-grade serous carcinoma: cells have coarse chromatin and prominent large nucleoli and show frequent and atypical mitotic activity

peritoneal implants is excellent (10-year survival between 92 and 100 %) [18]. The survival drops significantly if the implants are invasive [19].

Macroscopically serous borderline tumours (SBTs) are cystic with variable numbers of intracystic or surface excrescences. These excrescences are covered by fine papillae giving them a velvety appearance. They are more extensive than the smooth more polypoid excrescences of benign tumours. The tumours are bilateral in 25–40 % of cases. Microscopically the typical borderline tumours (which make up 90 % of all SBTs) are characterised by broad papillae showing hierarchical branching, covered by stratified epithelial cells showing mild to moderate atypia (Figs. 4.10 and 4.11). Mitotic figures are infrequent. The stroma is fibrous but may be oedematous. There may be surface involvement in up to 50 % of all cases. These surface tumours (auto implants) are identical to noninvasive extraovarian desmoplastic implants. Although autoimplants are seen more frequently in high-stage tumours (those with extraovarian disease), they do not alter the prognosis in stage I tumours.

Stromal microinvasion (invasion <3 mm or <10 mm^2 in greatest dimension) may be seen in 10–15 % of SBT as individual cells, small clusters of eosinophilic cells, cribriform nests or small papillary structures within the cyst wall or the stroma of papillae with minimal stromal response. This is in contrast to the destructive stromal invasion in serous carcinomas in which the invasion by neoplastic epithelium is irregular, haphazard and associated with effacement of ovarian stroma and/or a stromal fibroblastic reaction [20]. Microinvasion is more commonly seen in pregnancy (eight- to nine-fold more frequently). Until quite recently it was believed that microinvasion in a borderline serous tumour does not confer a worse prognosis; however, large studies have now shown that with the exception of microinvasion in SBT occurring in pregnancy, tumours with microinvasion have poorer clinical outcomes worse than those without [19, 21].

Approximately 10 % of serous borderline tumours show micropapillary morphology. These tumours are characterised by filiform, nonbranching micropapillae without fibrovascular cores which emanate from a fibrous stalk in a nonhierarchical 'Medusa head-like' pattern (Fig. 4.12). This proliferation can sometimes have a cribriform pattern. The tumour cells are monomorphic, cuboidal to columnar and sometimes show a hobnail appearance. They show mild to moderate atypia and often contain small nucleoli. The micropapillary area should be at least 5 mm in

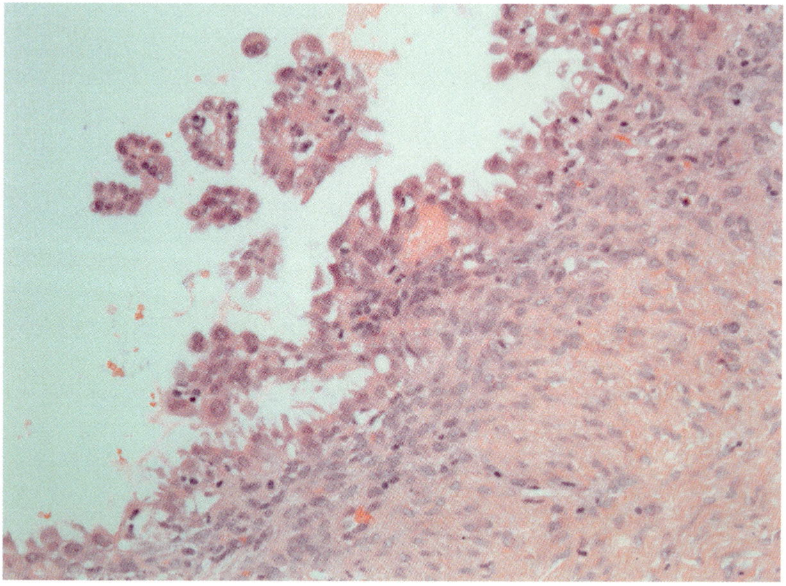

Fig. 4.10 Serous borderline tumour: the diagnosis depends on the presence of atypical proliferation in the form of tufts of cells and detachment of cell clusters into the luminal space, accompanied by cytological atypia

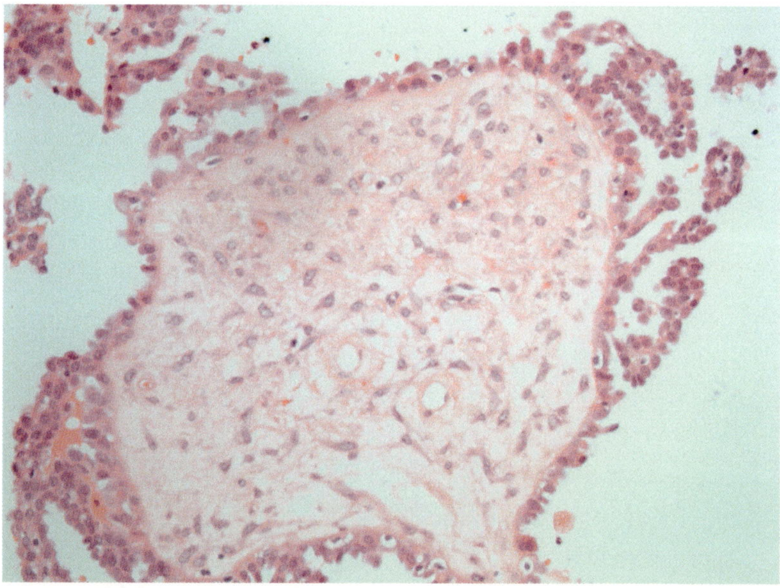

Fig. 4.11 Serous borderline tumour: tuft formation and cell detachment from the surface of a broad fibrous papilla

size before the tumour is labelled as a micropapillary variant. Micropapillary variants of SBT are different from typical SBT in that they are more often bilateral, have a higher incidence of extra-ovarian implants which may be invasive, have a higher frequency of surface involvement and a higher stage at presentation. These tumours have an overall poorer survival largely due to association with invasive implants. Although it has been suggested that micropapillary tumours be classed as cancers, currently the preferred term for these tumours is SBT with micropapillary features [22].

Extraovarian implants are seen in 20–46 % of all SBTs [23]. They are more frequent in micropapillary variants and in borderline tumours with

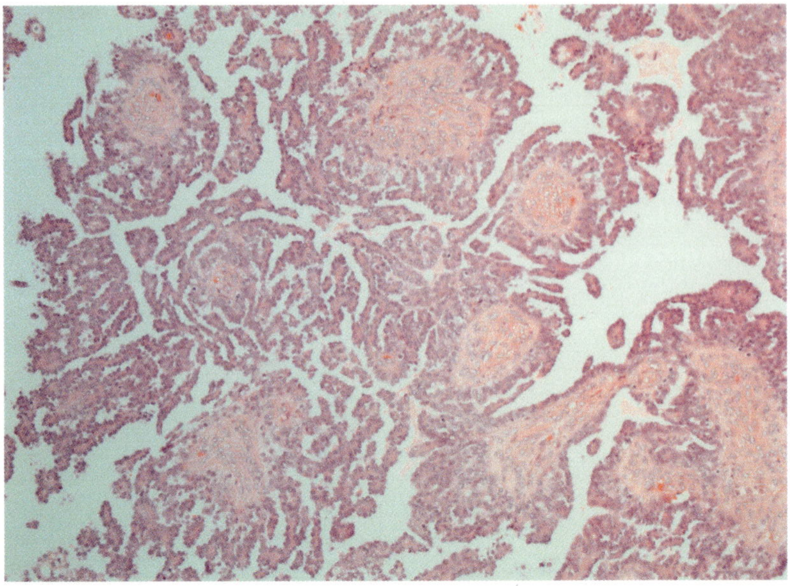

Fig. 4.12 Micropapillary pattern in a serous borderline tumour: the entire circumference of the fibrous papillae is covered by long and slender tufts of cells; this is also described as 'nonhierarchical' branching as the tiny micropapillae emanate directly from a broad fibrous papilla rather than the formation of progressively smaller calibre branches

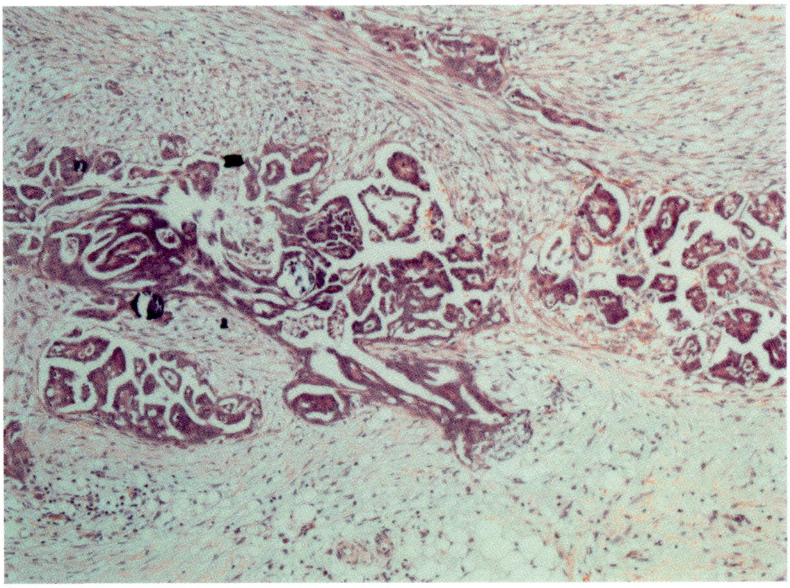

Fig. 4.13 Invasive implant from a case of serous borderline tumour: there is haphazard infiltration of adipose tissue by tumour-forming glands and papillae

surface involvement. In fact, 94 % of patients with implants have borderline tumours with an exophytic surface component. The type of implant, invasive or noninvasive, is the most important prognostic factor in SBT. Over 80 % of implants are noninvasive; 10–15 % are invasive and 5 % are indeterminate.

Invasive implants are characterised by the presence of irregular, haphazard infiltration into normal tissue by glands or small solid epithelial nests (Fig. 4.13). Invasive implants sometimes engulf or replace omental adipose tissue. In addition to invasion of underlying normal tissue, a micropapillary architecture and solid epithelial nests surrounded by clefts are also considered by some as criteria for invasive implants [24].

Noninvasive implants are further classified as desmoplastic or epithelial, based upon the

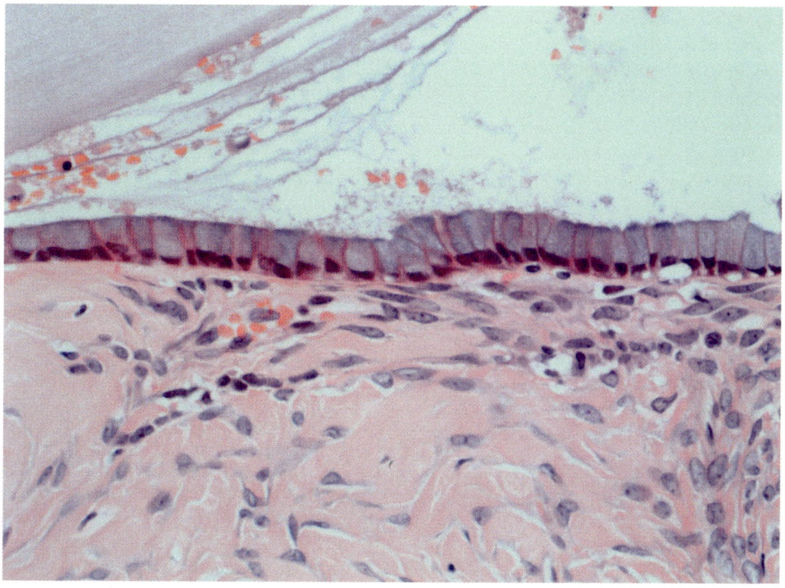

Fig. 4.14 Mucinous epithelium of intestinal type consists of mucin-secreting columnar epithelial cells with basally located bland nuclei

presence or absence of a marked stromal reaction. The noninvasive epithelial implants comprise glands and papillae which sometimes show hierarchical branching and epithelial tufting. They resemble the papillary proliferation of the primary borderline ovarian tumour with minimal or absent stromal response. Desmoplastic noninvasive implants are composed of peritoneal plaques and nodules composed of glands and papillae embedded in a fibroblastic stroma. The individual papillae and glandular structures are often associated with psammoma bodies. When the distinction between invasive and noninvasive implants is problematic, the implants are classified as indeterminate [19].

Although it has been established that it is the invasive implants that confer an adverse prognosis to serous borderline tumours, noninvasive implants also do impart a slightly greater risk of adverse outcome than when absent [19]. Noninvasive implants should be differentiated from endosalpingiosis, which is characterised by the presence of well-formed glands lined by tubal-type epithelium. Various theories regarding the origins of implants have been proposed. Transcoelomic spread from SBT is the most popular because of the frequent association with ovarian surface involvement and clonality studies showing similarities between ovarian tumours and implants [25]. Alternative theories that they develop from endosalpingiosis or synchronously directly from the peritoneum have also been suggested.

Lymph node involvement is seen in 20–30 % of patients with SBT who undergo a lymphadenectomy for staging. The lymph node involvement is typically in the sinuses and not in the lymph node parenchyma, a feature which helps to differentiate these from endosalpingiosis which is a close differential diagnosis. The presence of lymph node involvement does not alter the prognosis of these tumours [26].

Mucinous Tumours of the Ovary

This group of tumours (including their benign, borderline and malignant counterparts) represents the second most common type of epithelial tumours. These are characterised by mucin-containing epithelium that resembles either gastrointestinal epithelium (intestinal type) or endocervix (endocervical type) (Fig. 4.14). About 80 % of the tumours are benign, 10 % are borderline and 10 % are malignant. Occasionally, they are mixed with other types of surface epithelial neoplasms, including benign Brenner tumour.

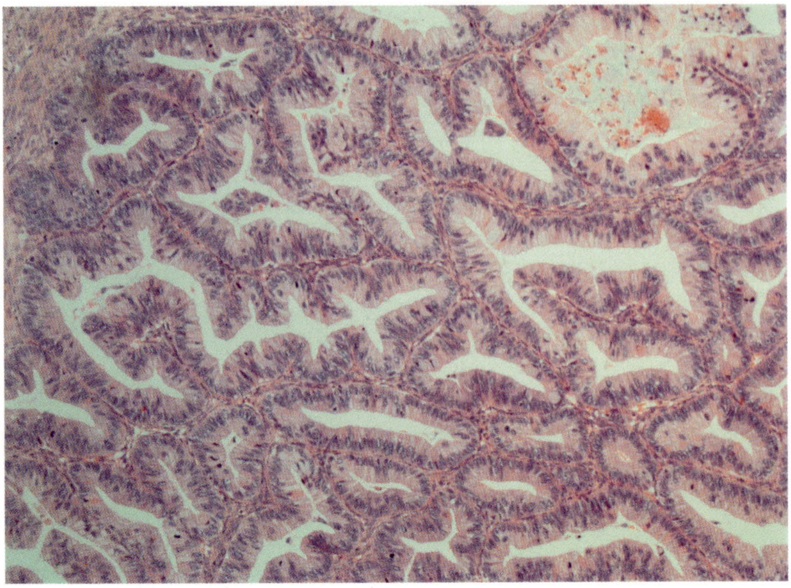

Fig. 4.15 Mucinous carcinoma of the ovary consists of glands lined by mucinous epithelium crowded together with no intervening stroma

Three to five percent develop in association with dermoid cysts [27] . The most common molecular genetic alteration in mucinous borderline tumours and mucinous carcinomas is a point mutation of KRAS. In fact an increasing frequency of KRAS mutations at codons 12 and 13 is described in mucinous cystadenomas, mucinous borderline tumours and mucinous carcinomas, respectively, suggesting a stepwise transition from benign precursors [17].

Mucinous Carcinoma

Primary ovarian mucinous carcinomas are relatively rare. The incidence is much lower than was previously believed to be the case. Mucinous carcinomas account for less than 3 % of all ovarian carcinomas [13, 28]. The main reason for the apparent reduction in incidence is the recognition of the fact that many of the tumours believed to be primary ovarian mucinous carcinoma in the past were in fact secondary adenocarcinomas. Also the distinction between a borderline tumour with intraepithelial carcinoma and microinvasion and a frankly invasive adenocarcinoma has become more clearly defined allowing many more tumours to be classified as borderline tumours [13]. Most tumours are stage I at presentation.

Macroscopically these tumours are variably cystic with solid areas. Microscopically the epithelium may be of gastrointestinal type or endocervical type. Most primary ovarian mucinous carcinomas are of gastrointestinal type [29]. These tumours are characterised by glandular and cystic spaces lined by columnar or polygonal epithelial cells with cytoplasmic mucin, sometimes containing goblet cells (Fig. 4.15). The endocervical-type tumours show papillae and glands lined by endocervical-type mucinous epithelium. Minor components of serous epithelium may be present, but, when these are prominent, the tumours are labelled seromucinous carcinomas. The endocervical-type mucinous tumours are often bilateral and may be associated with endometriosis. Mucinous tumours are graded using a three-tier grading system. Some use the Shimizu and Silverberg grading system [30]; others use a grading system similar to International Federation of Gynecology and Obstetrics (FIGO) grading of endometrioid carcinoma [31]. Most tumours (90–95 %) are morphologically heterogeneous with benign and borderline components present, and only rarely are they uniformly malignant. Mucinous tumours are considered invasive if one

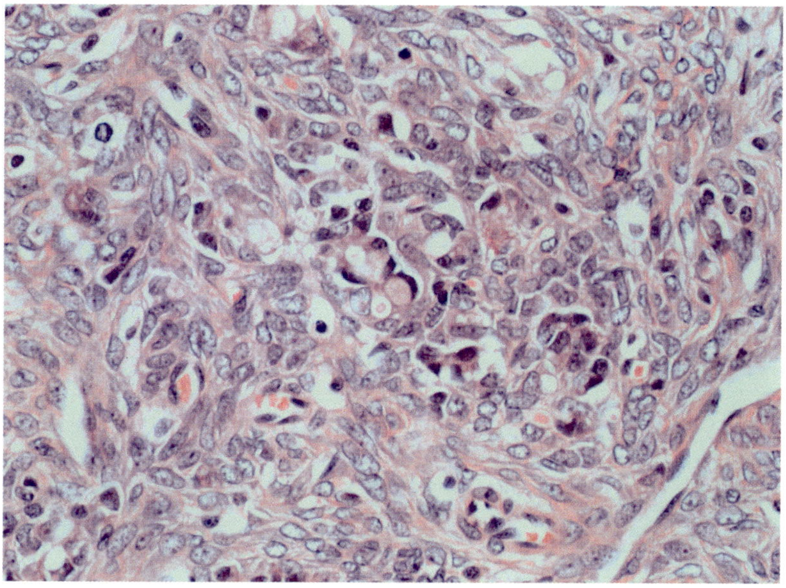

Fig. 4.16 Krukenberg tumour: Signet ring cell carcinoma shows very monotonous epithelial cells with eccentric nuclei displaced to the periphery by a large mucin vacuole (an example is seen at the centre of this field). Tumour cells are surrounded by a prominent reactive stromal component which may mask the true nature of this neoplasm

of two patterns of stromal invasion is present, infiltrative or expansile. An infiltrative pattern is defined as disorderly penetration of the stroma by neoplastic cells with or without an associated desmoplastic response. Infiltrative invasion >3 mm in two linear dimensions or with a total area >10 mm^2 is considered frankly invasive. Tumours with less infiltration are classified as borderline with microinvasion. An expansile pattern is defined as a complex arrangement of glands, cysts or papillae lined by malignant epithelium with minimal or no recognisable intervening stroma.

A major consideration in the diagnosis of mucinous carcinomas and borderline tumours is the exclusion of metastasis from the gastrointestinal tract, including biliary tract and pancreas. Findings favouring a primary tumour over a metastatic carcinoma are unilaterality, size >10 cm, a smooth tumour surface with absence of surface or hilar involvement, benign-appearing or borderline-appearing areas (either with atypia only or with intraepithelial carcinoma), absence of extensive vascular invasion, absence of necrosis in the absence of torsion and finally an 'expansile' rather than a destructive infiltrative invasive pattern. Extensive intra-abdominal disease as well as a multinodular appearance of the tumour with intervening normal parenchyma favours a metastatic carcinoma, as does resemblance of the tumour to a known primary [32]. The possibility of metastasis should always be strongly considered in cases with a known extraovarian primary. The index of suspicion for an extraovarian primary should be high in a widely disseminated mucinous malignancy. It must be noted that algorithms based on size and laterality alone will identify about 85 % of cases correctly, but the remainder could be wrongly categorised so other features should be taken into account. Certain patterns, such as signet ring morphology and abundant extracellular pools of mucin, are almost exclusively seen in metastases (Figs. 4.16 and 4.17).

Immunohistochemistry can help distinguish between primary and metastatic carcinomas from the gastrointestinal tract, although an overlap exists between the various markers. As stated, most primary ovarian mucinous carcinomas are of the intestinal or enteric type, and therefore they are negative for oestrogen and progesterone receptors and commonly positive for cytokeratin (CK) 20, carcinoembryonic antigen (CEA), cancer antigen (CA) 19.9 and CDX2. CA 19.9 is often diffusely positive while CK20, CEA and CDX2 are most commonly focally positive, but exceptions may sometimes exist where these markers are either negative or even diffusely

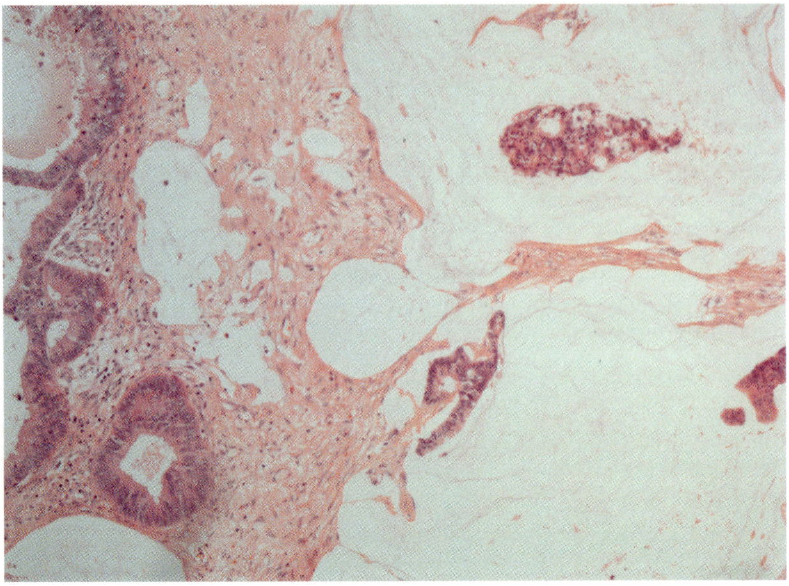

Fig. 4.17 Metastatic mucinous carcinoma within the ovary; a pattern characterised by abundant extracellular pools of mucin suggests extraovarian origin

positive. Positivity with these markers may be reflected in increased serum levels. For example, serum CA 19.9 may be massively elevated in primary ovarian mucinous neoplasms of intestinal type. These tumours are usually, although not always, diffusely CK7 positive. Although most colorectal carcinomas are CK7 negative, rectal carcinomas may often be CK7 positive [29]. Racemase and beta-catenin (β-catenin) may also be useful markers as they are more often positive in metastatic colorectal carcinomas compared to primary ovarian carcinomas [33]. SMAD4 can sometimes be useful in differentiating ovarian mucinous tumours from metastatic pancreatobiliary tumours as it is almost invariably positive in primary ovarian mucinous neoplasms while approximately 50 % of pancreatic and some biliary tract adenocarcinomas are negative. p16 is positive in endocervical tumours and negative in primary mucinous carcinomas. Oestrogen receptor (ER) is positive in metastatic breast carcinomas and endometrioid tumours.

Mucinous Borderline Tumour

Macroscopically mucinous borderline tumours (MBTs) are large multiloculated cysts (mean diameter, 17 cm) with fleshy polypoid areas, excrescences or sometimes solid areas. Around 90 % of MBTs are unilateral [23, 27]. Microscopically, as with invasive mucinous carcinomas, MBT can be either of intestinal or endocervical type.

The endocervical-like-type tumours are closely related to serous borderline tumours with which they are often mixed (also known as seromucinous borderline tumours or müllerian borderline mucinous tumours). These account for only 5–14 % of müllerian borderline mucinous tumours and have little in common with intestinal-type mucinous tumours. These tumours are often associated with background endometriosis and may even arise from an endometriotic cyst. They are characterised as broad papillae covered by endocervical-type epithelium admixed with rounded or polygonal cells with abundant eosinophilic cytoplasm (so-called indifferent cells) which are commonly seen at the tips of the papillae. Also seen are numerous acute inflammatory cells within the cytoplasm and in the extracellular mucin. The neoplastic cells show minimal nuclear atypia, but rare cases of intraepithelial carcinoma and microinvasion are reported which have overall benign behaviour. Around 6 % of these tumours are associated with noninvasive or

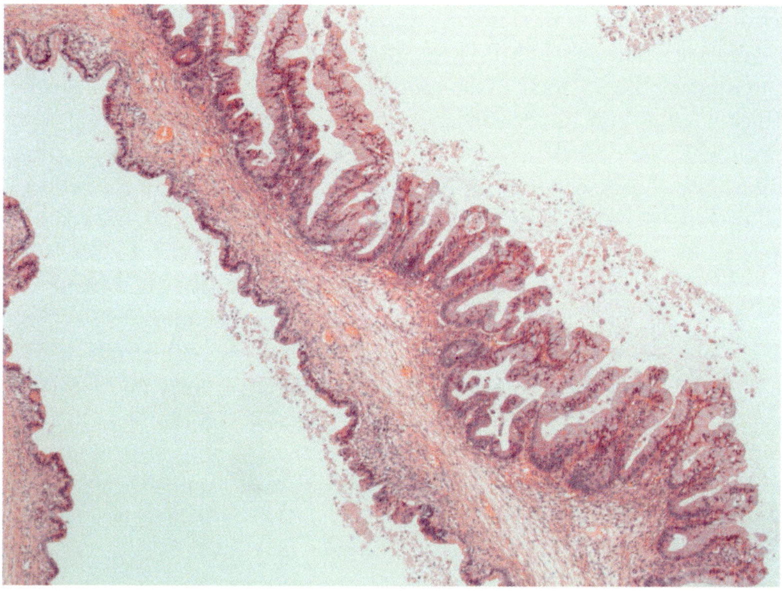

Fig. 4.18 Mucinous borderline tumour; variation in the appearance of the epithelium lining the cystic and glandular spaces: the lower space is lined by monolayered epithelium while the upper part shows multilayering and atypia

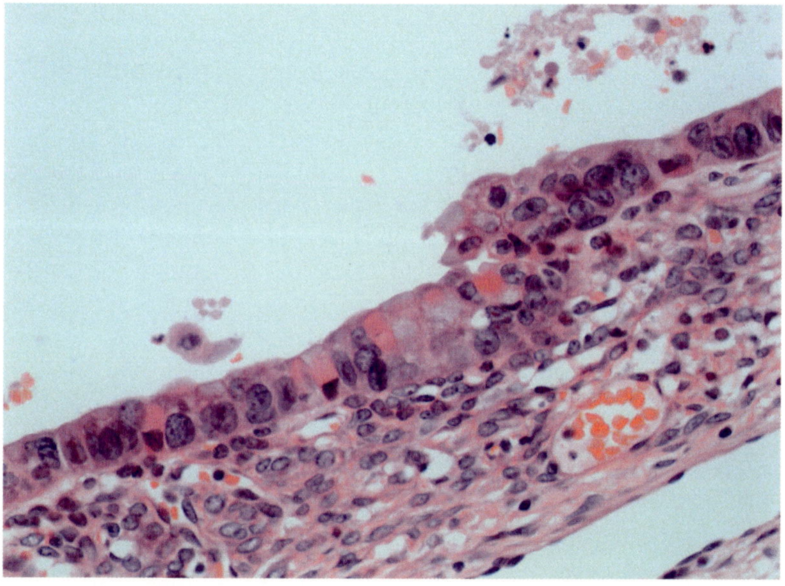

Fig. 4.19 Pronounced cytological atypia in a mucinous borderline tumour: there is nuclear pleomorphism, nucleoli are prominent and have lost their basal orientation (compare with Fig. 4.14.)

invasive implants in the peritoneum and rare lymph node metastasis [34, 35]. These tumours are bilateral in 15–40 % of cases.

The vast majority (85 %) of MBT are of intestinal type [35]. These tumours contain benign areas lined by a single layer of mucinous epithelium with basally placed nuclei and areas where the epithelial cells show stratification and crowding and a papillary architecture (Fig. 4.18). Cytological atypia is seen in the form of nuclear hyperchromasia and pleomorphism (Fig. 4.19). Mitotic figures are seen especially at the base of the papillae. The lumen contains mucin, and the cyst wall shows mucin extravasation with secondary inflammation. The cells are similar to gastric or intestinal epithelium, often associated with goblet cells and sometimes even paneth cells. When the lining epithelium shows severe cytological atypia with marked stratification, the tumours are classified as MBT with intraepithelial carcinoma. Small foci of invasion less than 10 mm^2 or 3 mm in two linear dimensions are classified as MBT with microinvasion. Microinvasion is seen 9 % of MBT, and tumours with this feature show no adverse clinical behaviour.

Rarely, mucinous tumours, benign, borderline or malignant and generally of intestinal type, show one or more discrete well-circumscribed mural nodules that protrude into the lumen of the cystic neoplasms. These nodules have a distinctly different gross and microscopic appearance from the mucinous tumour. The nodules may be reactive or neoplastic or a mixtures of both types. The reactive nodules are multiple and red-brown and range from 0.2 to 4 cm in diameter. They consist of a heterogeneous admixture of spindle cells, osteoclast-like multinucleated giant cells and inflammatory cells, often with cholesterol clefts and haemorrhage [27]. Reactive nodules do not confer a worse prognosis on the tumour. The neoplastic nodules are composed of anaplastic carcinoma [36], spindle cell sarcoma or combined carcinoma and sarcoma. These have been reported in to have a 50 % mortality rate, according to one compilation of reported cases [37]. Others have reported that their presence in an unruptured stage I neoplasm does not necessarily carry an adverse prognosis [38].

Pseudomyxoma Peritonei

Pseudomyxoma peritonei (PMP) is primarily a clinical or surgical designation for localised or widespread intraperitoneal deposits of extracellular mucin associated with fibrosis caused by rupture or leakage of a mucinous neoplasm. Recent evidence suggests that PMP most often results from dissemination of an appendiceal mucinous neoplasm with microscopic features of an adenoma, cystadenoma or villous adenoma. The ovarian involvement which is often seen in PMP is therefore now believed to be secondary, unless there is a dermoid cyst present giving rise to a low-grade mucinous neoplasm. The suggested guidelines for categorisation are: if there is a mucinous appendiceal tumour, this should be considered primary with ovarian metastases, even if the ovarian tumour has an accompanying dermoid cyst; if the ovarian tumour is unilateral and associated with a dermoid cyst with no evidence of appendiceal tumour, the ovarian tumour should be considered primary; and if the appendix has been removed previously with no evidence of PMP at surgery and no other primary site is identified, then the ovarian tumour should be considered primary [39].

Although PMP follows a variable clinical course and may lead to significant morbidity and mortality, it has a considerably more favourable prognosis than does peritoneal carcinomatosis from a metastatic mucinous carcinoma. Thus the distinction is an important one and based on the microscopic assessment of the neoplastic epithelial cells in the peritoneal mucinous deposits and in the primary tumour.

Endometrioid Tumours of the Ovary

These surface epithelial tumours resemble their endometrial counterparts. Endometrioid tumours account for 8–21 % of all surface epithelial tumours. Most endometrioid tumours are carcinomas while benign and borderline endometrioid tumours are rare (less than 1 %) [40, 41]. This is in contrast to serous and mucinous tumours where the vast majority are benign. These tumours occur in the fifth and sixth decades of life. Associated endometriosis can be demonstrated in 25–36 % of tumours, either in the same ovary or elsewhere in the pelvis [42]. Residual ipsilateral endometriosis is present in 13 % of endometrioid carcinomas. When the tumours occur in association with ovarian endometriosis, they tend to occur in women 5–10 years younger than those without ovarian endometriosis [43]. Although borderline endometrioid tumours have an excellent prognosis and almost never behave in a malignant fashion, these are often associated with endometrioid carcinomas, suggesting a possible transition from borderline to malignant tumours.

Molecular genetic studies of endometrioid carcinomas reveal mutations of *KRAS* and *BRAF*

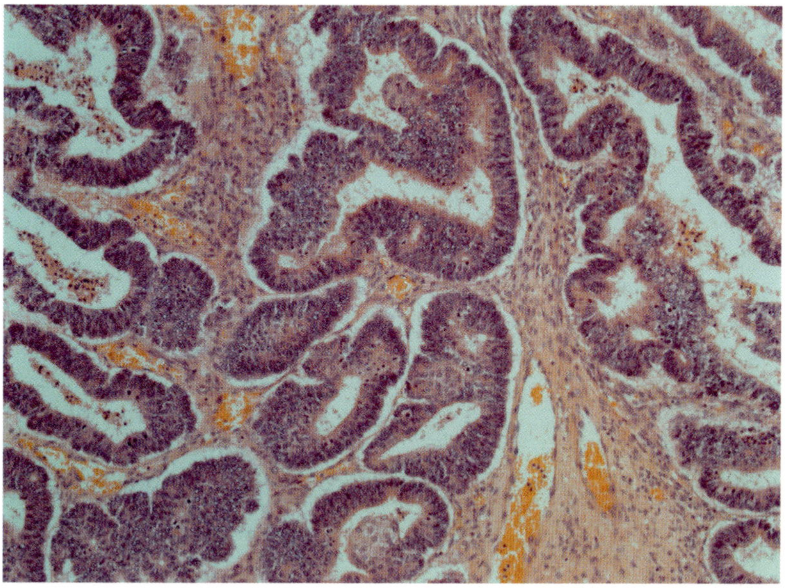

Fig. 4.20 Endometrioid carcinoma of the ovary is identical to that occurring in the endometrium: a typical appearance is seen here with crowded glands line by tall columnar epithelium with pseudostratified nuclei

in approximately 10 % of carcinomas [17]. In addition, *PTEN* is mutated in 21 % of endometrioid ovarian tumours and in 46 % of those with 10q23 loss of heterozygosity (LOH), making PTEN the most common gene mutation reported so far in these tumours. Similar molecular genetic alterations including loss of heterozygosity at 10q23 and mutations in *PTEN* have been reported in endometriosis suggesting that endometriosis may be a precursor to endometrioid carcinoma [44]. Mutations of β-*catenin* have been detected in more than 60 % of ovarian well-differentiated endometrioid carcinomas and in endometrioid borderline tumours but in less than 3 % of grade III tumours [45]. These molecular changes suggest stepwise tumour progression in the development of endometrioid carcinoma from a precursor lesion. *ARID1A* mutations may be seen in up to 30 % of endometrioid carcinomas [46]. Endometrioid tumours may also be linked to the Lynch syndrome characterised by germline mutations of mismatch repair genes [47].

Endometrioid Carcinoma

This tumour closely resembles the common variants of endometrioid endometrial carcinoma. The most common stage at presentation for these tumours is stage I or II. High-stage endometrioid ovarian carcinomas are rare.

Macroscopically the tumours measure 10–20 cm in diameter and are solid or cystic with solid areas. The solid areas show necrotic foci giving the tumour a variegated appearance. The cysts contain haemorrhagic fluid. They are bilateral in about 10 % cases [28]. Microscopically the tumours are similar to their endometrial counterparts (Fig. 4.20). They are graded using a three-tier grading system. Most commonly the three-tier FIGO grading system developed for endometrial carcinomas is used, whereby grade 1 tumours are those with less than 5 % solid areas, grade 2 have 5–50 % solid areas, and grade 3 tumours have more than 50 % solid areas. Some use the Shimizu and Silverberg grading system, which is similar to the grading system used for breast cancers. In this grading system, the features used to assess grade are architecture (score 1 for glandular pattern, score 2 for papillary pattern and score 3 for solid pattern), nuclear pleomorphism (score 1 for mild, score 2 for moderate and score 3 for severe) and mitotic activity (score 1: 0–9/10 hpf, score 2: 10–24/10 hpf, score 3: >24 mitotic figures/10 hpf). The grade is based on the total score: grade 1 (3–5 points), grade 2

(6–7 points) and grade 3 (8–9 points) [48]. Although this grading system is no longer used for serous carcinomas where a two-tier system is more widely used, it correlates well with survival for all ovarian carcinomas with the exception of clear cell carcinomas [30].

The low-grade tumours of either grading system are composed of back-to-back glands with stratification of epithelial cells similar to low-grade endometrial carcinomas. Squamous differentiation is commonly seen in the form of morules or sheets. In high-grade endometrioid carcinomas, the glands merge and the tumour cells are dispersed in solid sheets. The tumour cells become more pleomorphic with prominent nucleoli, and areas of necrosis are seen. High-grade endometrioid ovarian carcinomas are extremely rare, and many tumours labelled as such may actually represent high-grade serous carcinomas. WT1 staining may be of value in distinguishing high-grade endometrioid from high-grade serous tumours. Most (80–90 %) serous carcinomas exhibit diffuse nuclear positivity with WT1 while most endometrioid adenocarcinomas are negative or at the most focally positive [49, 50].

Uncommon features seen in these tumours are a secretory pattern where glands show presence of subnuclear vacuolation resembling early secretory endometrium, sex cord-stromal pattern where granulosa cell-like or sertoliform areas may be seen, or luteinised stromal cells that resemble Leydig cells or luteinised granulosa cells are seen. Oxyphilic tumour cells, spindle-shaped cells and ciliated cells may also rarely be seen in endometrioid carcinomas. A yolk sac component which stains positively for alpha-fetoprotein may be seen in association with otherwise typical endometrioid carcinomas [51]. Other unusual patterns seen in endometrial carcinomas may be seen here such as small non-villous papillae or a corded and hyalinised pattern (CHEC pattern).

Endometrioid carcinomas must be differentiated from a variety of other carcinomas. The most helpful feature is finding foci of well-differentiated endometrioid carcinoma. Endometrioid carcinomas are ER and PR positive (>75 %) which helps in differentiating them from mucinous and clear cell carcinomas, which are generally negative for ER and PR. As mentioned above, they are generally negative for WT1 (positive in <5 % of cases). This helps to differentiate them from serous carcinomas. Approximately 30 % of tumours express nuclear β-catenin. p53 is positive in high-grade examples.

Another challenge faced by pathologists is differentiating primary ovarian endometrioid carcinoma from metastatic carcinoma. This arises for two distinct reasons. Some metastatic carcinomas, typically of colorectal origin, are notorious for showing endometrioid morphology (Fig. 4.21). The ovarian tumour may arise before, simultaneously, or years after presentation of the colorectal malignancy. A good clinical history and regard to even focal mucin secretion, as well as the other characteristics of metastatic tumours mentioned in the section on mucinous neoplasms, can help avoid misdiagnosis.

The second reason is that while 15–23 % of all metastatic ovarian tumours arise from endometrial primaries, around 10 % of ovarian endometrioid carcinomas are associated with independent *synchronous* endometrial carcinomas. Distinguishing metastasis from simultaneous low-stage disease is often difficult but crucial owing to the striking differences in prognosis and management. Of the synchronous tumours, 86 % have endometrioid morphology in both the endometrium and the ovary [52]. When the endometrial carcinoma invades the myometrium deeply or is associated with lymphovascular space invasion or lymph node metastasis, the most likely diagnosis is metastasis of a primary endometrial carcinoma to the ovary. Other factors that may also point towards ovarian metastasis are bilateral and multinodular ovarian tumours and ovarian surface involvement, absence of endometriosis and presence of atypical hyperplasia in the endometrium.

Borderline Endometrioid Tumours

These are rare endometrioid tumours with architectural and cytological atypia which lack destructive stromal invasion. Macroscopically these

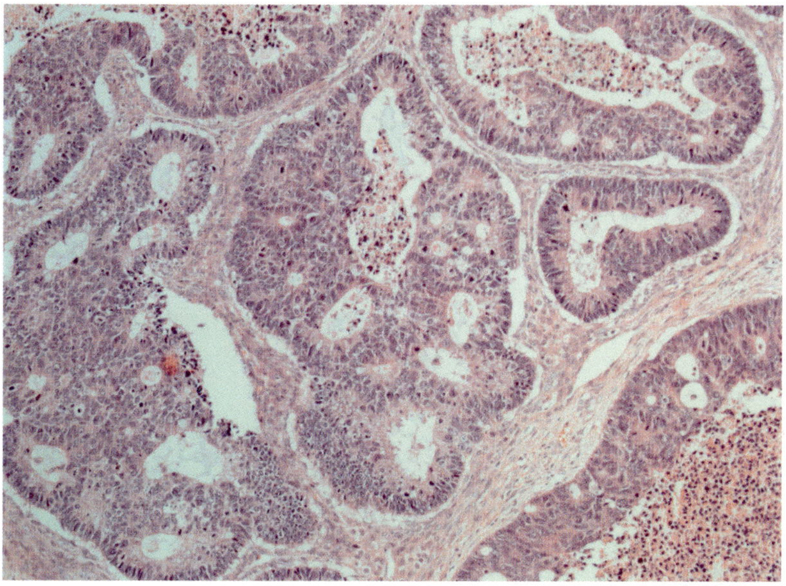

Fig. 4.21 Metastatic colorectal carcinoma can resemble endometrioid carcinoma, a recognised pitfall in ovarian pathology

tumours are predominantly solid with cystic areas. They are almost always unilateral. On microscopy, these tumours are characterised by a proliferation of glands lined by endometrioid-type epithelium. Glands may be densely packed with little stroma, but there may be areas with abundant, cellular or fibrous stroma. Borderline tumours closely resemble benign adenofibromas but unlike adenofibromas show more complex glandular contours and less separation of glands. Cytological atypia which is seen in these tumours is typically absent in adenofibromas. Those with severe cytological atypia are classed as borderline tumours with intraepithelial carcinoma. By definition there is no destructive stromal invasion; however, small foci of infiltration or foci of confluent glands are considered to be microinvasive if they do not exceed 10 mm^2 or 5 mm in greatest dimension. As with all borderline tumours, those with microinvasion and intraepithelial carcinomas do not behave badly, and these tumours, with rare exceptions, have an excellent prognosis. The frequent presence of squamous metaplasia allows distinction from borderline serous tumours.

Among all reported cases of borderline endometrioid tumours, only very few are described as having advanced-stage disease at diagnosis, with reported peritoneal implants of bland endometrioid epithelium outside of the ovary in the absence of haemorrhage or endometrial-type stroma. Endometrial stroma, however, is often difficult to identify even in what is otherwise clearly endometriosis, and therefore it is possible that some if not all reported cases of implants actually represent endometriosis, rather than a metastasis from the ovarian tumour.

Clear Cell Tumours of the Ovary

These tumours are almost always malignant; benign and borderline counterparts are very rare. Ovarian clear cell carcinomas (CCCs) are believed to occur with approximate equal frequency to endometrioid adenocarcinomas. Most of these tumours are diagnosed at an early stage (stage I or II) [28]. These tumours are believed to arise from ovarian endometriosis and a careful search for endometriosis is often rewarding either on the same side or in the contralateral ovary. For as yet unknown reasons these tumours are more prevalent in Japan. When corrected for stage, these are among the most lethal types of ovarian cancer with a 5-year survival rate (all stages) of less than 35 % in a large multicentre Japanese series [53]. They are often resistant to

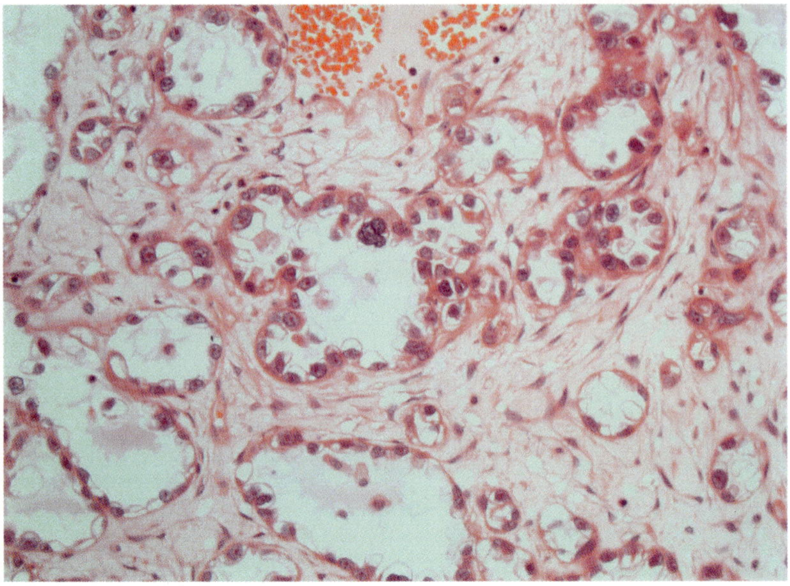

Fig. 4.22 Clear cell carcinoma: glandular spaces are lined by cells with a 'hobnail' luminal outline; these have distinct cytoplasmic outlines and clear cytoplasm with atypical nuclei

platinum-based chemotherapy. In their clinical picture they show a greater propensity than other carcinoma subtypes for thromboembolic complications and nodal involvement, the latter especially in recurrences. Although they share some similarities with mucinous and endometrioid tumours such as development from a benign precursor, there are significant differences such as a higher degree of genetic instability in these tumours [17]. Sequence mutations of *PIK3CA* are detected in one-third of all CCCs [9]. In addition, 46 % of patients with ovarian CCC have mutations in *ARID1A*. Loss of *ARID1A* expression is associated with loss of nuclear BAF250a expression in tumour cells. *ARID1A* mutations are not seen in high-grade serous carcinomas but may be seen in up to 30 % of endometrioid carcinomas [46].

Mutations in *TP53*, *KRAS*, *PTEN, CTNNB1* and *BRAF* are detected in fewer cases. This is in contrast to endometrioid carcinomas which are also thought to develop from endometriosis but have a high frequency of *PTEN* and *CTNNB1* mutations. A proportion of CCCs are linked to Lynch syndrome and are therefore characterised by germline mutations of mismatch repair genes [47].

Clear Cell Carcinoma

Macroscopically these tumours are large, typically cystic with solid areas. The cystic areas may contain haemorrhagic, serous or mucinous fluid. Areas of haemorrhage and necrosis may be present in the solid areas giving the tumours a variegated appearance. Associated endometriosis may be seen as haemorrhagic areas adjacent to the tumour. Microscopically, these tumours are composed of cells arranged in papillary, solid and tubulocystic patterns. The lining epithelial cells have a moderate amount of clear cytoplasm with distinct cell membranes and eccentric nuclei (Fig. 4.22). Hobnail cells are commonly seen; this appearance results from the bulbous, dark appearance of nuclei in cells which protrude into a cystic space. An oxyphilic variant, characterised by cells with abundant eosinophilic cytoplasm, may form a minor component or the exclusive element in up to 5 % of cases. Mitoses are generally infrequent in these tumours, ranging from 0 to 13/10 hpf with a mean of 3.78 [54]. The stroma surrounding the tumour cells may be hyalinised, oedematous or myxoid. Necrosis, lymphoplasmacytic infiltration and sometimes psammoma bodies may also be seen.

One challenge faced by pathologists when diagnosing ovarian clear cell carcinoma is differentiating these tumours from serous and, to a lesser extent, endometrioid carcinomas, which may also show similar architectural features and clear cytoplasm. The distinctive morphology and immunophenotype allow these tumours to be diagnosed reproducibly. Morphologic features that help differentiating these tumours from serous carcinomas include lower mitotic index and lower degree of nuclear pleomorphism compared to high-grade serous carcinomas. Absence of a cribriform architecture, columnar cell shape and squamoid areas helps differentiate these tumours from endometrioid tumours. On immunohistochemistry, these tumours are positive for hepatocyte nuclear factor-1beta (HNF1β), cytokeratin 7, leuM1 and epithelial membrane antigen (EMA). Up to 80–85 % of these tumours stain for HNF1β, as opposed to less than 5 % of serous carcinomas. Few CCCs show positive staining for WT1, p53 and oestrogen receptor compared with serous carcinomas. The proliferative index on Ki-67 staining is also significantly lower in CCC (mean, 12.7) when compared with high-grade serous carcinomas (mean, 27.5 %) [55].

There are other morphological mimics of CCC. These tumours can resemble SBTs, especially at frozen section; a high index of suspicion and due consideration to all morphological parameters including bilaterality can help in this distinction. Yolk sac tumours of the ovary can have clear cell areas but are generally seen in a younger age group and are positive for alpha-fetoprotein and negative for leuM1. Dysgerminomas may also have cytoplasmic clearing but are positive for PLAP and negative for keratins and epithelial membrane antigen. Ovarian CCCs can be differentiated from metastatic renal cell carcinomas by the presence of hobnail cells or endometriosis. Also, unlike ovarian CCCs, renal cell carcinomas are typically CK7 negative and diffusely positive with CD10 and renal cell carcinoma antibody [56]. Sex cord-stromal tumours such as juvenile granulosa cell tumours and Sertoli-Leydig cell tumours may also show clear cell change. These are often inhibin positive which helps differentiate these from CCC.

Borderline Clear Cell Tumour

There are very few reported cases of borderline clear cell tumours. These are similar morphologically to the benign clear cell adenofibroma but show moderate to marked degrees of epithelial proliferation and atypia [57]. Of all cases reported, most patients had a good prognosis, with the exception of a few including one patient with a borderline adenofibroma who developed a questionable lung metastasis and another patient who had a microinvasive tumour who subsequently went on to have a pelvic recurrence [58].

Transitional Cell Carcinomas of the Ovary

This broad category includes benign, borderline and malignant Brenner tumours and transitional cell carcinomas. Although these tumours are considered surface epithelial in origin, some of these have been found in association with dermoid cysts and may be of germ cell origin.

Transitional Cell Carcinoma

Transitional cell carcinomas of the ovary are rare and comprise about 1–2 % of all surface epithelial tumours of the ovary tumour [59]. These tumours are large solid and cystic masses. Microscopically they are similar to transitional cell carcinomas of the bladder and lack an associated benign or borderline Brenner tumour [60]. Interestingly, these tumours differ from their counterparts in the bladder in that they are negative for urothelial markers, such as uroplakin III and thrombomodulin, and do not coexpress CK 7 and CK 20 as do urothelial transitional cell carcinomas [61]. In fact most ovarian transitional cell carcinomas are WT1 positive, and this observation has led to a belief that many of these tumours are in fact variants of high-grade serous carcinomas and are not true transitional cell carcinomas [56]. The tumours are also often positive for p53 and p16. Antibodies to placental S100 and GATA3 expression which have all been demonstrated in bladder tumours have also been studied in ovarian transitional cell tumours, and, while these markers are expressed in most cases of benign Brenner tumour, they are either weakly positive or negative in transitional cell carcinomas [62]. This immunohistochemical profile allows differentiation from metastatic urothelial carcinomas which express CK7, CK20 and urothelial markers and are negative for WT1. Molecular analysis of a small group of tumours shows that they often harbour *p53* mutations [63]. It has been reported that these carcinomas usually behave more favourably than poorly differentiated carcinomas of the other types, apparently due to their better response to chemotherapy.

Malignant Brenner Tumour

Grossly these tumours are solid and cystic masses. Microscopically, malignant Brenner tumours are characterised by invasive transitional carcinomas along with a benign or borderline Brenner tumour component. Mucinous elements and/or squamous cell carcinoma may be associated with the transitional component. Studies have shown that in Brenner tumours, protein expression for epidermal growth factor receptor (EGFR) parallels the degree of malignancy: expression is weak in benign, intermediate in borderline and strong in malignant Brenner tumours but negative in transitional cell carcinomas. Immunoreactivity for cyclin D1 is strong in malignant Brenner tumours and weak in benign and borderline Brenner tumours and transitional cell carcinomas [63]. This is in contrast to urothelial markers such as uroplakin III and thrombomodulin which are more commonly seen in benign Brenner tumours and are weak to absent in borderline and malignant Brenner tumours and transitional cell carcinomas. Most malignant Brenner tumours are stage I and have an excellent prognosis with an 88 % 5-year survival; about one fifth, however, present with extraovarian spread and behave similarly to other ovarian cancers [64].

Borderline Brenner Tumour

These tumours are almost always unilateral. Typically these are solid and cystic masses. The solid areas are similar to those seen in benign Brenner tumours and are firm and yellow-white with gritty areas due to calcification. Microscopically the tumours are composed of confluent nests and papillae of transitional cells that resemble urothelial papillary transitional cell carcinomas, but there is no evidence of destructive stromal invasion. These tumours are generally negative for urothelial markers such as uroplakin III and thrombomodulin compared with benign Brenner tumours.

Squamous Cell Carcinomas of the Ovary

Primary squamous cell carcinomas (SCCs) of the ovary are uncommon, most arising in dermoid cysts and therefore classified as germ cell tumours. A minority are associated with endometriosis, arise in a Brenner tumour or appear in pure form. The last three types of SCC belong to the surface epithelial–stromal category of tumours [65]. SCC seen in association with endometriosis arises from neoplastic transformation of pre-existing endometrial epithelium. Cases of pure primary SCC of the ovary are believed to arise as a result of seeding from an occult premalignant or fully malignant squamous lesions located outside the ovary [66]. This observation has been put forward based on the finding of associated cervical carcinoma in situ in some cases of primary SCC.

Primary SCC tend to be smaller than other aggressive ovarian neoplasms with an average size of approximately 10–12 cm. These lesions may be solid and cystic with cysts showing sebaceous contents and areas of necrosis. Those arising from endometriosis may show endometriotic cysts on gross examination. Histologic examination shows invasive SCC often with obvious keratin pearl formation [65]. The differential diagnoses are metastatic SCC from cervix and other sites and squamous differentiation in endometrioid carcinoma.

In terms of clinical behaviour, both stage and grade correlate with outcome, and SCC associated with endometriosis have a poorer outcome than those arising in dermoids [65].

Mixed Carcinomas of the Ovary

A mixed carcinoma should be diagnosed when the tumour is composed of two or more of the epithelial subtypes described and where the minor component makes up at least 10 % of the neoplasm [1]. However, it is recommended that all morphological subtypes within an ovarian carcinoma should be documented and the percentages listed, even if the minor component accounts for less than 10 % [28]. These may be benign (e.g. mixed Brenner and mucinous tumour), borderline (such as borderline seromucinous tumour) or malignant. Unlike endometrial carcinomas, true mixed carcinomas of the ovary are relatively uncommon. A combination of endometrioid and CCC may rarely occur as both tumours arise in endometriosis. The combinations of serous and undifferentiated or endometrioid and undifferentiated carcinoma are discussed below. It is believed that combinations of serous and clear cell carcinoma and serous and endometrioid carcinoma probably represent serous carcinomas. Some feel that the seromucinous subtype of tumours is better categorised as a type of mixed epithelial tumour, rather than grouped with mucinous neoplasms. The clinical behaviour of mixed epithelial tumours is dependent on the components present.

Undifferentiated Carcinomas of the Ovary

Undifferentiated carcinomas are high-grade tumours which present at a high stage, 91 % of tumours presenting at stage III or IV. They have an extremely aggressive clinical course. They show either no differentiating features whatsoever or small foci of differentiation. When defined as carcinomas in which 50 % of the tumour is undifferentiated, the incidence is 4.1 % of all ovarian malignancies [67]. Adequate sampling of these tumours is essential as this may reveal areas diagnostic of high-grade serous carcinoma, such as papillary formations, slit-like spaces or psammoma bodies or areas of better-differentiated endometrioid carcinoma with squamous differentiation. When there is a component of better-differentiated carcinoma, the tumours are labelled as combined undifferentiated and differentiated carcinomas. The presence of even a small undifferentiated component in tumours with associated differentiated components should be documented, as it appears to be associated with a poor clinical outcome [68].

Macroscopically these are predominantly solid with large areas of necrosis. Microscopically they are composed of solid sheets of highly pleomorphic tumour cells with numerous mitoses and areas of necrosis. Sometimes the tumour cells can have spindle cell morphology. These tumours have no specific immunophenotype but stain for cytokeratins, especially CK18, and EMA. The differential diagnosis includes granulosa cell tumours which can sometimes have bizarre nuclei. Positive staining for inhibin and negative staining for EMA help make the diagnosis of granulosa cell tumours. Transitional cell carcinomas are another differential diagnosis. These are recognised by the presence of thick papillae with smooth luminal borders in contrast to the pseudopapillae secondary to tumour necrosis that is often seen in undifferentiated carcinomas [64]. Small cell carcinoma either of the hypercalcemic type or the pulmonary type can also be confused with undifferentiated carcinomas. The former is seen in younger women, and the pulmonary-type small round cell tumours generally show positive staining for neuroendocrine markers [69].

Miscellaneous Epithelial Malignancies of the Ovary

Carcinosarcoma

Carcinosarcomas (malignant mixed Müllerian tumours [MMMTs]) are included in the group of epithelial tumours. These are believed to

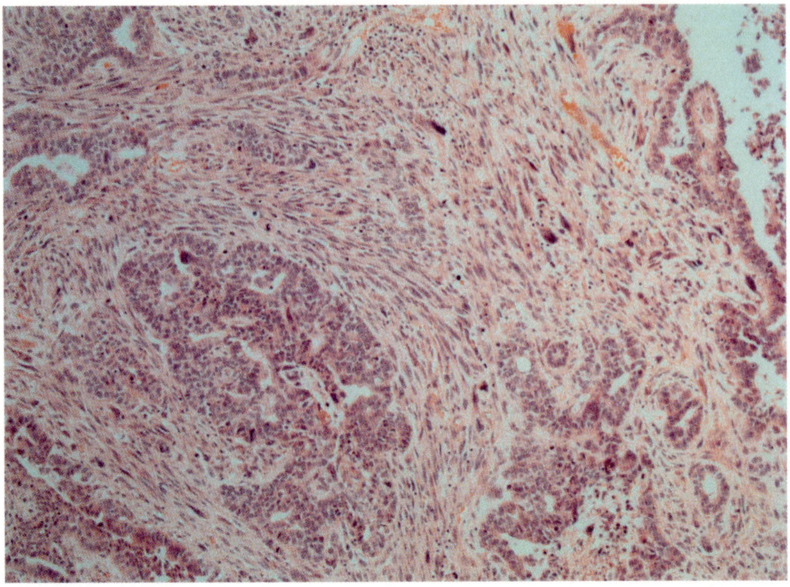

Fig. 4.23 High-grade carcinosarcoma (malignant mixed Müllerian tumour) is characterised by a biphasic pattern of adenocarcinoma and sarcoma; in this example malignant glandular elements are separated by an atypical spindle cell component

develop from ovarian surface epithelium or foci of endometriosis and to represent metaplastic sarcomatous differentiation in high-grade carcinomas. These are morphologically similar to uterine carcinosarcomas with monoclonal malignant epithelial and stromal components (Fig. 4.23) [70]. These tumours generally present at a high stage [13] and are associated with a poor outcome.

Small Cell Carcinoma, Hypercalcemic Type

This is an undifferentiated subtype of ovarian carcinoma with a wide age range at presentation but occurring commonly in young women [69, 71]. Two-thirds of cases are associated with increased serum calcium levels. Most patients present with symptoms and signs related to the pelvic mass. The tumours are predominantly solid, with areas of necrosis and haemorrhage. On histology these are composed of a uniform population of undifferentiated cells with scanty cytoplasm and hyperchromatic nuclei with prominent nucleoli (Fig. 4.24). There is very high mitotic activity. The tumour cells are arranged in solid sheets or in a trabecular pattern. Formation of follicle-like spaces is common, giving rise to an appearance resembling granulosa cell tumour, particularly at frozen section. The histogenesis of these tumours is not established, as ultrastructurally and genetically they do not appear to be related to epithelial or germ cell tumours [72].

Small Cell Carcinoma, Pulmonary Type

Small cell carcinomas of pulmonary type characterised by neuroendocrine differentiation can occur in the ovary as at many other sites. These usually occur in the postmenopausal age group and present as solid pelvic masses with an aggressive clinical course. Morphological and immunohistochemical features are as for the typical pulmonary tumours with solid sheets of cells with scanty cytoplasm and nuclei with a 'salt and pepper' chromatin pattern. Behaviour is uniformly aggressive.

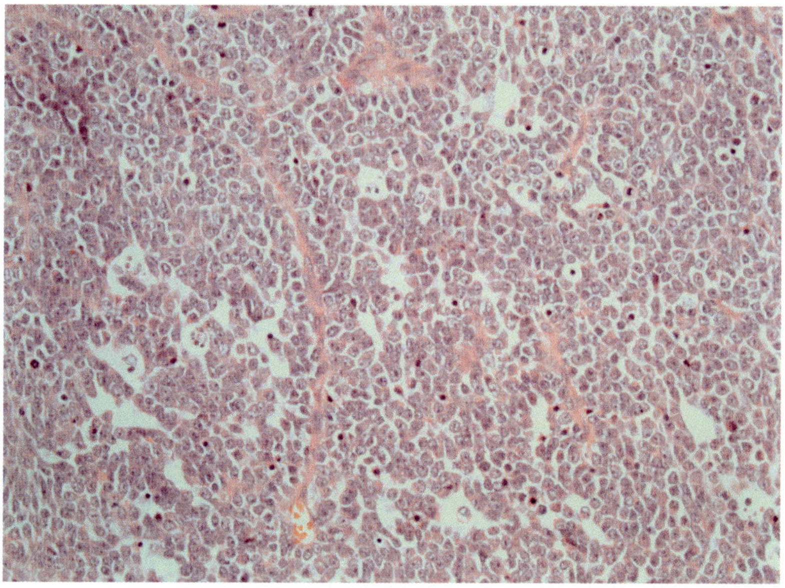

Fig. 4.24 Ovarian small cell carcinoma characterised by sheets of monotonous epithelial cells with scanty cytoplasm and atypical nuclei with high mitotic activity

Conclusion

Primary epithelial malignancies of the ovary are of five major subtypes, as distinguished by their morphology, pathogenesis, molecular and immunohistohemical characteristics, clinical behaviour and response to treatment. In approximate order of frequency these are: high grade serous, clear cell, endometrioid, low grade serous and mucinous carcinomas. Rarer subtypes exist which have distinctive features. As newer treatment regimens appear it is vital to distinguish these tumours from one another, and also from metastases to the ovary.

References

1. Lee KR, et al. Tumors of the ovary and peritoneum. In: Tavassoli FA, Devilee P, editors. Pathology and genetics of tumours of the breast and female genital organs. Lyon: IARC Press; 2003.
2. Prat J. Ovarian carcinomas: five distinct diseases with different origins, genetic alterations, and clinicopathological features. Virchows Arch. 2012;460(3): 237–49.
3. Cheng W, Liu J, Yoshida H, Rosen D, Naora H. Lineage infidelity of epithelial ovarian cancers is controlled by HOX genes that specify regional identity in the reproductive tract. Nat Med. 2005;11(5):531–7.
4. Crum CP, Drapkin R, Kindelberger D, Medeiros F, Miron A, Lee Y. Lessons from BRCA: the tubal fimbria emerges as an origin for pelvic serous cancer. Clin Med Res. 2007;5(1):35–44.
5. Hutson R, Ramsdale J. WellsM. p53 protein expression in putative precursor lesions of epithelial ovarian cancer. Histopathology. 1995;27(4):367–71.
6. Crum CP, Drapkin R, Miron A, Ince TA, Muto M, Kindelberger DW, Lee Y. The distal fallopian tube: a new model for pelvic serous carcinogenesis. Curr Opin Obstet Gynecol. 2007;19(1):3–9.
7. Kurman RJ, Shih IM. The origin and pathogenesis of epithelial ovarian cancer: a proposed unifying theory. Am J Surg Pathol. 2010;34(3):433–43.
8. Chen EY, Mehra K, Mehrad M, Ning G, Miron A, Mutter GL, et al. Secretory cell outgrowth, PAX2 and serous carcinogenesis in the Fallopian tube. J Pathol. 2010;222(1):110–6.
9. Kurman RJ, Shih IM. Molecular pathogenesis and extraovarian origin of epithelial ovarian cancer–shifting the paradigm. Hum Pathol. 2011;42(7):918–31.
10. Cho KR. Ovarian cancer update: lessons from morphology, molecules, and mice. Arch Pathol Lab Med. 2009;133(11):1775–81.
11. Murdoch WJ. Carcinogenic potential of ovulatory genotoxicity. Biol Reprod. 2005;73(4):586–90.
12. Murdoch WJ, Murphy CJ, Van Kirk EA, Shen Y. Mechanisms and pathobiology of ovulation. Soc Reprod Fertil Suppl. 2010;67:189–201.
13. Seidman JD, Horkayne-Szakaly I, Haiba M, Boice CR, Kurman RJ, Ronnett BM. The histologic type and

stage distribution of ovarian carcinomas of surface epithelial origin. Int J Gynecol Pathol. 2004; 23(1):41–4.
14. Vang R, Shih Ie M, Kurman RJ. Ovarian low-grade and high-grade serous carcinoma: pathogenesis, clinicopathologic and molecular biologic features, and diagnostic problems. Adv Anat Pathol. 2009;16(5): 267–82.
15. Malpica A, Deavers MT, Tornos C, Kurman RJ, Soslow R, Seidman JD. Grading ovarian serous carcinoma using a two-tier system. Am J Surg Pathol. 2004;28(4):496–504.
16. O'Neill CJ, Deavers MT, Malpica A, Foster H, McCluggage WG. An immunohistochemical comparison between low-grade and high-grade ovarian serous carcinomas: significantly higher expression of p53, MIB1, BCL2, HER-2/neu, and C-KIT in high-grade neoplasms. Am J Surg Pathol. 2005;29(8):1034–41.
17. Kurman RJ, Shih IM. Pathogenesis of ovarian cancer: lessons from morphology and molecular biology and their clinical implications. Int J Gynecol Pathol. 2008;27(2):151–60.
18. Uzan C, Kane A, Rey A, Gouy S, Duvillard P, Morice P. Outcomes after conservative treatment of advanced-stage serous borderline tumors of the ovary. Ann Oncol. 2010;21(1):55–60.
19. Longacre TA, McKenney JK, Tazelaar HD, Kempson RL, Hendrickson MR. Ovarian serous tumors of low malignant potential (borderline tumors): outcome-based study of 276 patients with long-term (> or =5-year) follow-up. Am J Surg Pathol. 2005;29(6): 707–23.
20. McKenney JK, Balzer BL, Longacre TA. Patterns of stromal invasion in ovarian serous tumors of low malignant potential (borderline tumors): a reevaluation of the concept of stromal microinvasion. Am J Surg Pathol. 2006;30(10):1209–21.
21. Buttin BM, Herzog TJ, Powell MA, Rader JS, Mutch DG. Epithelial ovarian tumors of low malignant potential: the role of microinvasion. Obstet Gynecol. 2002;99(1):11–7.
22. Bell DA, Longacre TA, Prat J, Kohn EC, Soslow RA, Ellenson LH, et al. Serous borderline (low malignant potential, atypical proliferative) ovarian tumors: workshop perspectives. Hum Pathol. 2004;35(8): 934–48.
23. Hart WR. Borderline epithelial tumors of the ovary. Mod Pathol. 2005;18 Suppl 2:S33–50.
24. Bell KA, Smith Sehdev AE, Kurman RJ. Refined diagnostic criteria for implants associated with ovarian atypical proliferative serous tumors (borderline) and micropapillary serous carcinomas. Am J Surg Pathol. 2001;25(4):419–32.
25. Sieben NL, Roemen GM, Oosting J, Fleuren GJ, van Engeland M, Prat J. Clonal analysis favours a monoclonal origin for serous borderline tumours with peritoneal implants. J Pathol. 2006;210(4):405–11.
26. Lesieur B, Kane A, Duvillard P, Gouy S, Pautier P, Lhommé C, Morice P, Uzan C. Prognostic value of lymph node involvement in ovarian serous borderline tumors. Am J Obstet Gynecol. 2011;204(5):438.e1–7.
27. Hart WR. Mucinous tumors of the ovary: a review. Int J Gynecol Pathol. 2005;24(1):4–25.
28. McCluggage WG. Morphological subtypes of ovarian carcinoma: a review with emphasis on new developments and pathogenesis. Pathology. 2011;43(5): 420–32.
29. McCluggage WG. Immunohistochemistry in the distinction between primary and metastatic ovarian mucinous neoplasms. J Clin Pathol. 2012;65: 596–600.
30. Shimizu Y, Kamoi S, Amada S, Akiyama F, Silverberg SG. Toward the development of a universal grading system for ovarian epithelial carcinoma: testing of a proposed system in a series of 461 patients with uniform treatment and follow-up. Cancer. 1998;82(5): 893–901.
31. Lee KR, Scully RE. Mucinous tumors of the ovary: a clinicopathologic study of 196 borderline tumors (of intestinal type) and carcinomas, including an evaluation of 11 cases with 'pseudomyxoma peritonei'. Am J Surg Pathol. 2000;24(11):1447–64.
32. Lee KE, Young RH. The distinction between primary and metastatic mucinous carcinomas of the ovary: gross and histologic findings in 50 cases. Am J Surg Pathol. 2003;27(3):281–92.
33. Chou YY, Jeng YM, Kao HL, Chen T, Mao TL, Lin MC. Differentiation of ovarian mucinous carcinoma and metastatic colorectal adenocarcinoma by immunostaining with beta-catenin. Histopathology. 2003; 43(2):151–6.
34. Rutgers JL, Scully RE. Ovarian mullerian mucinous papillary cystadenomas of borderline malignancy. A clinicopathologic analysis. Cancer. 1988;61(2): 340–8.
35. Siriaunkgul S, Robbins KM, McGowan L, Silverberg SG. Ovarian mucinous tumors of low malignant potential: a clinicopathologic study of 54 tumors of intestinal and mullerian type. Int J Gynecol Pathol. 1995;14(3):198–208.
36. Provenza C, Young RH, Prat J. Anaplastic carcinoma in mucinous ovarian tumors: a clinicopathologic study of 34 cases emphasizing the crucial impact of stage on prognosis, their histologic spectrum, and overlap with sarcomalike mural nodules. Am J Surg Pathol. 2008;32(3):383–9.
37. Baergen RN, Rutgers RL. Mural nodules in common epithelial tumors of the ovary. Int J Gynecol Pathol. 1994;13(1):62–72.
38. Rodriguez IM, Prat J. Mucinous tumors of the ovary: a clinicopathologic analysis of 75 borderline tumors (of intestinal type) and carcinomas. Am J Surg Pathol. 2002;26(2):139–52.
39. Ronnett BM, Shmookler BM, Sugarbaker PH, Kurman RJ. Pseudomyxoma peritonei: new concepts in diagnosis, origin, nomenclature, and relationship to mucinous borderline (low malignant potential) tumors of the ovary. Anat Pathol. 1997;2:197–226.

40. Kline RC, Wharton JT, Atkinson EN, Burke TW, Gershenson DM, Edwards CL. Endometrioid carcinoma of the ovary: retrospective review of 145 cases. Gynecol Oncol. 1990;39(3):337–46.
41. Bell KA, Kurman RJ. A clinicopathologic analysis of atypical proliferative (borderline) tumors and well-differentiated endometrioid adenocarcinomas of the ovary. Am J Surg Pathol. 2000;24(11):1465–79.
42. DePriest PD, Banks ER, Powell DE, van Nagell Jr JR, Gallion HH, Puls LE, et al. Endometrioid carcinoma of the ovary and endometriosis: the association in postmenopausal women. Gynecol Oncol. 1992;47(1): 71–5.
43. McMeekin DS, Burger RA, Manetta A, DiSaia P, Berman ML. Endometrioid adenocarcinoma of the ovary and its relationship to endometriosis. Gynecol Oncol. 1995;59(1):81–6.
44. Jiang X, Hitchcock A, Bryan EJ, Watson RH, Englefield P, Thomas EJ, Campbell IG. Microsatellite analysis of endometriosis reveals loss of heterozygosity at candidate ovarian tumor suppressor gene loci. Cancer Res. 1996;56(15):3534–9.
45. Oliva E, Sarrió D, Brachtel EF, Sánchez-Estévez C, Soslow RA, Moreno-Bueno G, Palacios J. High frequency of beta-catenin mutations in borderline endometrioid tumours of the ovary. J Pathol. 2006; 208(5):708–13.
46. Wiegand KC, Shah SP, Al-Agha OM, Zhao Y, Tse K. Zeng, et al. TARID1A mutations in endometriosis-associated ovarian carcinomas. N Engl J Med. 2010;363(16):1532–43.
47. Ketabi Z, Bartuma K, Bernstein I, Malander S, Grönberg H, Björck E, et al. Ovarian cancer linked to Lynch syndrome typically presents as early-onset, non-serous epithelial tumors. Gynecol Oncol. 2011; 121(3):462–5.
48. Shimizu Y, Kamoi S, Amada S, Hasumi K, Akiyama F, Silverberg SG. Toward the development of a universal grading system for ovarian epithelial carcinoma. I. Prognostic significance of histopathologic features–problems involved in the architectural grading system. Gynecol Oncol. 1998;70(1):2–12.
49. Al-Hussaini M, Stockman A, Foster H, McCluggage WG. WT-1 assists in distinguishing ovarian from uterine serous carcinoma and in distinguishing between serous and endometrioid ovarian carcinoma. Histopathology. 2004;44(2):109–15.
50. McCluggage WG. WT1 is of value in ascertaining the site of origin of serous carcinomas within the female genital tract. Int J Gynecol Pathol. 2004;23(2): 97–9.
51. Nogales FF, Bergeron C, Carvia RE, Alvaro T, Fulwood HR. Ovarian endometrioid tumors with yolk sac tumor component, an unusual form of ovarian neoplasm. Analysis of six cases. Am J Surg Pathol. 1996;20(9):1056–66.
52. Zaino R, Whitney C, Brady MF, DeGeest K, Burger RA, Buller RE. Simultaneously detected endometrial and ovarian carcinomas–a prospective clinicopathologic study of 74 cases: a gynecologic oncology group study. Gynecol Oncol. 2001;83(2):355–62.
53. Takano M, Kikuchi Y, Yaegashi N, Kuzuya K, Ueki M, Tsuda H, et al. Clear cell carcinoma of the ovary: a retrospective multicentre experience of 254 patients with complete surgical staging. Br J Cancer. 2006; 94(10):1369–74.
54. DeLair D, Oliva E, Köbel M, Macias A, Gilks CB, Soslow RA. Morphologic spectrum of immunohistochemically characterized clear cell carcinoma of the ovary: a study of 155 cases. Am J Surg Pathol. 2011;35(1):36–44.
55. Kobel M, Kalloger SE, Carrick J, Huntsman D, Asad H, Oliva E, et al. A limited panel of immunomarkers can reliably distinguish between clear cell and high-grade serous carcinoma of the ovary. Am J Surg Pathol. 2009;33(1):14–21.
56. McCluggage WG. My approach to and thoughts on the typing of ovarian carcinomas. J Clin Pathol. 2008;61(2):152–63.
57. Roth LM, Langley FA, Fox H, Wheeler JE, Czernobilsky B. Ovarian clear cell adenofibromatous tumors. Benign, of low malignant potential, and associated with invasive clear cell carcinoma. Cancer. 1984;53(5):1156–63.
58. Bell DA, Scully RE. Benign and borderline clear cell adenofibromas of the ovary. Cancer. 1985;56(12): 2922–31.
59. Eichhorn JH, Young RH. Transitional cell carcinoma of the ovary: a morphologic study of 100 cases with emphasis on differential diagnosis. Am J Surg Pathol. 2004;28(4):453–63.
60. Logani S, Oliva E, Amin MB, Folpe AL, Cohen C, Young RH. Immunoprofile of ovarian tumors with putative transitional cell (urothelial) differentiation using novel urothelial markers: histogenetic and diagnostic implications. Am J Surg Pathol. 2003;27(11): 1434–41.
61. Soslow RA, Rouse RV, Hendrickson MR, Silva EG, Longacre TA. Transitional cell neoplasms of the ovary and urinary bladder: a comparative immunohistochemical analysis. Int J Gynecol Pathol. 1996;15(3): 257–65.
62. Esheba GE, Longacre TA, Atkins KA, Higgins JP. Expression of the urothelial differentiation markers GATA3 and placental S100 (S100P) in female genital tract transitional cell proliferations. Am J Surg Pathol. 2009;33(3):347–53.
63. Cuatrecasas M, Catasus L, Palacios J, Prat J. Transitional cell tumors of the ovary: a comparative clinicopathologic, immunohistochemical, and molecular genetic analysis of Brenner tumors and transitional cell carcinomas. Am J Surg Pathol. 2009;33(4):556–67.
64. Prat J. Ovarian carcinomas, including secondary tumors: diagnostically challenging areas. Mod Pathol. 2005;18 Suppl 2:S99–111.
65. Pins MR, Young RH, Daly WJ, Scully RE. Primary squamous cell carcinoma of the ovary. Report of 37 cases. Am J Surg Pathol. 1996;20(7):823–33.

66. Mahe E, Sur M. Squamous lesions of the ovary. Arch Pathol Lab Med. 2011;135(12):1611–4.
67. Silva EG, Tornos C, Bailey MA, Morris M. Undifferentiated carcinoma of the ovary. Arch Pathol Lab Med. 1991;115(4):377–81.
68. Tafe LJ, Garg K, Chew I, Tornos C, Soslow RA. Endometrial and ovarian carcinomas with undifferentiated components: clinically aggressive and frequently underrecognized neoplasms. Mod Pathol. 2010;23(6):781–9.
69. McCluggage WG. Ovarian neoplasms composed of small round cells: a review. Adv Anat Pathol. 2004;11(6):288–96.
70. Jin Z, Katayama Y, Fukase M, Yajima M, Motoyama T. Carcinosarcomas (malignant mullerian mixed tumors) of the uterus and ovary: a genetic study with special reference to histogenesis. Int J Gynecol Pathol. 2003;22(4):368–73.
71. Young RH, Oliva E, Scully RE. Small cell carcinoma of the ovary, hypercalcemic type. A clinicopathological analysis of 150 cases. Am J Surg Pathol. 1994;18(11):1102–16.
72. Walt H, Hornung R, Fink D, Dobler-Girdziunaite D, Stallmach T, Spycher MA, et al. Hypercalcemic-type of small cell carcinoma of the ovary: characterization of a new tumor line. Anticancer Res. 2001;21(5):3253–9.

Pathology of Non-epithelial Malignancies of the Ovary

5

Eleni Ieremia and Naveena Singh

Introduction

The pathological diagnosis of ovarian tumours and their diagnostic pitfalls are primarily the concern of the gynaecological pathologist. However, it is vital that all members of the gynaecological oncology multidisciplinary team appreciate the diversity in their pathological features and often vast morphological differential diagnostic considerations as well as immunohistochemical findings in order to promote accuracy in interpretation of imaging and intraoperative findings and details contained within histopathology reports and scientific publications. Although tumours of epithelial origin account for the overwhelming majority of ovarian malignancies, the ovary can also give rise to a variety of non-epithelial tumours. Non-epithelial ovarian malignancies present unique clinical challenges, both diagnostic and therapeutic. Their clinical presentation, behaviour, response to treatment and prognosis differ significantly from those of epithelial malignancies. Broadly these include the two large groups of germ cell and sex cord-stromal tumours. Minor categories such as miscellaneous mesenchymal and haematolymphoid malignancies also exist and will be considered briefly.

Classification of Non-epithelial Ovarian Tumours

Table 5.1 represents a classification of non-epithelial ovarian tumours derived from the 2003 World Health Organization (WHO) classification and incorporating suggestions from the AFIP and ISGYP [1].

Germ Cell Tumours

Germ cell tumours are a group of gonadal, and rarely extragonadal, neoplasms with identical counterparts in the ovary and the testis, albeit with biological and clinical diversity [2, 3]. Ovarian germ cell tumours are classified by the WHO into primitive germ cell tumours and teratomas [4]. The primitive germ cell tumours are dysgerminoma, yolk sac tumour, embryonal carcinoma and choriocarcinoma. The prognostic significance of each tumour type has altered significantly after the introduction of combination chemotherapy, improving survival rates to almost comparable levels [5–7]. Teratomas are neoplasms containing components from the three germ cell layers (endoderm, mesoderm and ectoderm) and can contain derivatives from one, two or all three layers. Hence, they are subclassified

E. Ieremia, FRCPath
Department of Cellular Pathology,
Barts Health NHS Trust, 2nd Floor, 80 Newark Street,
London E11 1LT, England, UK

N. Singh, MBBS, FRCPath (✉)
Department of Cellular Pathology,
Barts Health NHS Trust, 2nd Floor, 80 Newark Street,
London E1 2ES, England, UK
e-mail: n.singh@bartshealth.nhs.uk

S.A. Farghaly (ed.), *Advances in Diagnosis and Management of Ovarian Cancer*,
DOI 10.1007/978-1-4614-8271-0_5, © Springer Science+Business Media New York 2014

Table 5.1 Histological classification of primary ovarian non-epithelial tumours

Germ cell tumours
Dysgerminoma
Variant
With syncytiotrophoblastic cells
Yolk sac tumours
Variants
Polyvesicular vitelline
Hepatoid
Glandular
Embryonal carcinoma
Polyembryoma
Choriocarcinoma, non-gestational
Teratoma
Immature
Mature
Solid
Cystic (dermoid cyst):
With secondary tumour (specify type)
Fetiform
Monodermal
Struma ovarii
With secondary tumour (specify type)
Carcinoid
Insular
Trabecular
Strumal carcinoid
Mucinous carcinoid
Neuroectodermal tumour (specify type)
Sebaceous tumour
Mixed germ cell tumour (specify types)
Sex cord-stromal tumours
Granulosa-stromal cell tumours
Granulosa cell tumour
Adult
Juvenile
Tumours in thecoma-fibroma group
Thecoma
Typical
Luteinised
Malignant
Fibrothecoma
Fibroma
Typical
Cellular
With sex cord elements
Fibrosarcoma
Sclerosing stromal tumour
Sertoli–stromal cell tumours
Well differentiated
Sertoli cell tumour
Sertoli–Leydig cell tumour
Sertoli–Leydig cell tumour of intermediate differentiation
Variant: With heterologous elements
Sertoli–Leydig cell tumour, poorly differentiated
Variant: With heterologous elements
Retiform
Variant: With heterologous elements
Sex cord tumour with annular tubules
Gynandroblastoma
Steroid cell tumours
Leydig cell tumour, hilus and stromal variants
Adrenal rest tumour
Steroid cell tumour, not otherwise specified
Mixed germ cell and sex cord-stromal tumours
Gonadoblastoma
Variant: With dysgerminoma or other germ cell tumour
Germ cell sex cord tumour on non-gonadoblastoma type
Variant: With dysgerminoma or other germ cell tumour
Tumours of rete ovarii
Adenoma and cystadenoma
Adenocarcinoma
Mesothelial tumours
Adenomatoid tumour
Mesothelioma
Tumours of uncertain origin and miscellaneous tumours
Small cell carcinomas
Tumour of probable Wolffian origin
Hepatoid carcinoma
Myxoma
Gestational trophoblastic diseases
Soft tissue tumours not specific to ovary
Malignant lymphomas and leukaemia

as biphasic/triphasic teratomas, the most common being the dermoid cyst, and monodermal teratomas, represented by struma ovarii and ovarian carcinoid. Biphasic and triphasic teratomas are further categorised as mature or immature teratomas, a distinction based on the presence of immature neuroepithelium. Mature teratomas are benign while immature teratomas behave in a malignant fashion.

Germ cell tumours constitute the second largest group of ovarian tumours after surface epithelial tumours and comprise 30 % of all ovarian neoplasms. The vast majority (95 %) are benign mature cystic teratomas (dermoid cysts) [8]. Malignant germ cell tumours are rare, representing 3–5 % of ovarian cancers in Europe and America, while in Asia and Africa, and especially in Japanese women, where surface epithelial tumours are less common, their relative incidence is higher, up to 20 % [9, 10]. Malignant germ cell tumours are almost always encountered in children, adolescents and young women, in which group of patients maintenance of fertility is an important clinical issue. In this age group, they represent the most common ovarian cancer, with 60 % of ovarian tumours up to the age of 21 being germ cell tumours, and one-third of them being malignant [11]. Overall, malignant germ cell tumours are rare beyond the fourth decade of life. In older adults, the majority of germ cell neoplasms are mature cystic teratomas, although case reports of primitive germ cell tumours in postmenopausal women have been published where they appear to arise from surface epithelial tumours [12].

Germ cell tumours originate from the primitive germ cells, which migrate to the gonadal anlage from the yolk sac endoderm. They reach the genital ridge during the fifth and sixth week of embryonic life. During embryogenesis, these primordial germ cells will ultimately form the primary oocytes through developmental stages of mitosis, atresia and meiosis. Different germ cell tumours are considered to arise from germ cells at different stages of development in the ovarian gonad. A widely held hypothetical model of histogenesis by Teilum regards seminoma (and thereby dysgerminoma) as immediately arising from germ cells without any further differentiation [13–15]. Embryonal carcinoma, on the other hand, is regarded to arise from germ cells with pluripotential dynamics of differentiation, and in this context 'embryonal carcinoma' has a dual meaning: a conceptual term of tumourigenesis and an actual tumour type. According to Telium's model, tumourigenesis can then follow two pathways. One is the embryonic pathway, producing endoderm, ectoderm and mesoderm, thereby producing teratomas. The second follows the extraembryonic pathway of differentiation towards endodermal sinus tumour (yolk sac tumour) and choriocarcinoma (tumour recapitulating trophoblast). This dynamic process of differentiation explains why some of these components can coexist in mixed germ cell tumours [16].

Germ cell tumours usually present with abdominal pain, most likely from ovarian torsion, the presence of a mass and/or abdominal distension [17, 18]. Although they are hormonally inert tumours, unusual presentations include pregnancy-like presentation due to human chorionic gonadotropin (HCG) secretion and hyperandrogenaemia [19]. Very rarely, germ cell tumours present during pregnancy, raising management issues of treatment and pregnancy salvation [20]. Tumour markers such as alpha-fetoprotein (AFP) and beta-HCG (bHCG), produced by the tumour cells, are useful clinical tools for diagnosis and follow-up after treatment. Radiological diagnostic differentiation of germ cell tumour types is difficult, with the exception of computed tomography (CT) identification of Rokitansky protuberances and fatty cyst contents in mature cystic teratomas.

Dysgerminoma

Dysgerminoma, the ovarian counterpart of testicular seminoma, is the most common malignant germ cell tumour of the ovaries, accounting for 3–5 % of ovarian cancer and 1–2 % of primary ovarian neoplasia [21, 22]. The median age at diagnosis is 22 years, although it has been reported in infants and in women of up to 70 years of age [23, 24]. The clinical symptoms are similar to those of most ovarian neoplasms, i.e. abdominal pain due to ovarian torsion, presence of a mass and abdominal distension. It is a rapidly growing mass presenting as a large tumour within a short period of time. Dysgerminomas with syncytiotrophoblasts or with luteinised

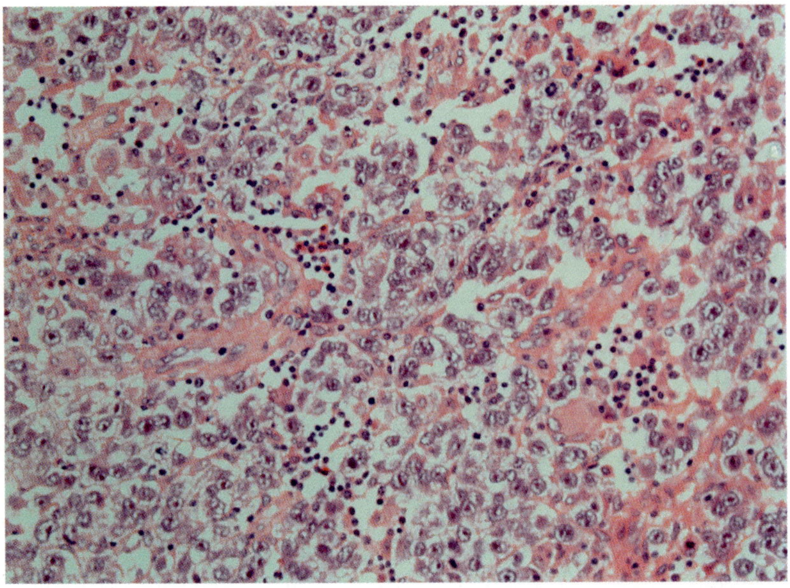

Fig. 5.1 Dysgerminoma is composed of solid sheets of cells with abundant clear to pale cytoplasm and atypical vesicular nucleoli with prominent nucleoli. Infiltration of fibrous septa by mature lymphocytes is a characteristic feature

stromal cells may present with endocrine symptomatology [25]. Rare cases present with hypercalcaemia due to parathormone-related peptide or 1,25-dihydroxyvitamin D secretion [26, 27]. On imaging, the ultrasound finding of a highly vascularised, large, solid, lobulated adnexal mass with irregular internal echogenicity, in a woman 20–30 years old, raises the suspicion of ovarian dysgerminoma [25]. It is important to note that the traditional tumour markers for germ cell tumours are not raised: AFP is never elevated except in cases with an additional germ cell component (i.e. as a mixed germ cell tumour) and HCG only in 3–5 % of cases [28]. Serum lactate dehydrogenase is usually raised and useful for monitoring treatment and recurrence [29].

Dysgerminoma is most commonly unilateral but it may also be bilateral, with gross or microscopic evidence of contralateral ovarian involvement. It is a well-circumscribed, encapsulated tumour with a solid, uniform, lobular cut surface, approximately 15 cm in size, although larger masses up to 50 cm have been recorded in the literature [30]. They may show areas of necrosis, cystic change and calcification. When the tumours are bilateral and calcification is sandy and pinpoint, the presence of concurrent gonadoblastoma may be considered. Cystic change suggests the presence of a second germ cell tumour component, especially a teratoma. The recommended sampling of ovarian tumours dictates one section per centimetre of maximum dimension, with additional sampling of heterogenous areas, to exclude the presence of other germ cell tumour components.

The typical histological appearances of dysgerminoma (Fig. 5.1) resemble those of seminoma. The architectural pattern is that of a nodular, lobulated tumour or of tumour cells arranged in islands, cords and strands, depending on the amount of stroma present, which may vary from scanty to abundant. The tumour cells are large cells with distinct cell membranes, high nuclear cytoplasmic ratio (almost 50 %), showing round nuclei with a prominent nuclear membrane, uneven granular chromatin and one or two nucleoli. Mitotic activity may be scanty or brisk and does not correlate with behaviour [31]. The cytoplasm is slightly granular and eosinophilic to clear and contains glycogen and fat. The stroma is composed of fibrous tissue forming septa separating the tumour into lobules, to hyalinised or oedematous areas or abundant dense fibrous tissue, causing variable cellularity within the same tumour and between tumours. It characteristically contains a lymphocytic infiltrate, which is a diagnostic pointer towards dysgerminoma, and although it is mostly composed of T lymphocytes, it may also include follicles with germinal centres. Foreign body giant cell reaction and granuloma formation may also be seen within the stroma. The tumours contain thin-walled vessels within the stroma. Syncytiotrophoblastic cells form an inconspicuous to prominent component of the tumour. Their presence is associated with raised levels of bHCG in the serum, but at levels much lower than those seen in choriocarcinoma, which can be used for tumour monitoring. Syncytiotrophoblastic cells are sometimes seen in close proximity to areas of haemorrhage within the tumour, and care should be taken to exclude the presence of choriocarcinoma by making sure there is no cytotrophoblast component intermixed with the syncytiotrophoblastic cells, which is the diagnostic hallmark of choriocarcinoma. Areas of haemorrhage with or without syncytiotrophoblast can be encountered in pure dysgerminomas without any choriocarcinomatous component. Also, luteinised stromal cells can rarely be seen and their presence may be related to symptoms of virilisation or feminisation.

In similarity to their testicular counterparts, molecular analysis in dysgerminomas has shown chromosome 12p abnormalities, including i12p and 12p over-representation. Fluorescence in situ hybridisation (FISH) analysis for chromosome 12p abnormalities may be a useful diagnostic adjunct for confirming the diagnosis of dysgerminoma, but i12p has also been reported in non-dysgerminomatous germ cell tumours [32, 33]. C-KIT mutations have also been identified in ovarian dysgerminomas similar to testicular seminomas. They tend to occur in advanced stage tumours and may pose a target for therapeutic treatment for those dysgerminomas that carry the mutation [21].

Dysgerminoma is positive for seminoma markers placental alkaline phosphatase (PLAP) (membranous), OCT3/4 (nuclear), CD117, SALL4 and D2-40. It should be noted that occasional cells are positive for low molecular weight keratins (e.g. CAM 5.2). PLAP is positive in all malignant germ cell tumours and its use does not offer any differential diagnostic value between germ cell tumours, but it does aid in the differential diagnosis from non-germ cell tumours (lymphoma, carcinoma). OCT3/4 is positive in dysgerminomas and embryonal carcinomas only, and therefore offers some specificity. CD117 is positive in nearly all dysgerminomas, although this does not indicate an underlying mutation which is only seen in a minority of cases [21, 34]. SALL4 is expressed in primitive germ cell tumours and it is also encountered in gastric carcinomas with hepatoid differentiation [35]. D2-40 is not specific for dysgerminoma as it is expressed in a variety of human tumours; however, dysgerminoma is the only germ cell tumour in which D2-40 is expressed. Low molecular weight keratin helps in the differential diagnosis from embryonal carcinoma and yolk sac tumour, which are both diffusely positive, in comparison with occasional cell positivity in dysgerminoma.

Dysgerminoma must be differentiated from lymphoma, clear cell carcinoma, granulosa cell tumour, embryonal carcinoma, yolk sac tumour and steroid cell tumours. Characteristic features of dysgerminoma are the nodularity of the tumour, tumour cells with more or less uniform cytological atypia and closely intermixed lymphoid infiltrate, as well as immunohistochemical expression of PLAP, OCT3/4 and CD117. Clear cell carcinoma, embryonal carcinoma and yolk sac tumour, even if predominantly solid, show areas of papillary and glandular architecture which can be identified as minor components following careful examination and thorough sampling. Also, embryonal carcinoma shows greater nuclear pleomorphism. Steroid cell tumours are encountered in older patients than dysgerminomas and they show finely vacuolated cytoplasm with positive staining for inhibin and calretinin.

Dysgerminoma is a rapidly growing tumour with metastatic potential, more often through the lymphatic than the haematogenous route, but with less aggressive behaviour than the rest of the malignant germ cell tumours. This tumour responds well to chemotherapy, even in the presence of disseminated disease, as well as radiotherapy. Its prognosis is excellent for stage I and stage III retroperitoneal disease with worsening outcome in the presence of peritoneal spread

[22, 36]. When disease is confined to one ovary without rupture, treatment may consist of unilateral oophorectomy or salpingo-oophorectomy alone for preservation of fertility. The role of adjuvant chemotherapy in these cases is controversial [7, 30, 31, 37].

Yolk Sac Tumour

Yolk sac tumours constitute a multifaceted group of malignant neoplasms for which the term primitive endodermal tumours may be more suitable, as they differentiate towards various extraembryonal and somatic directions. The endodermal sinus is actually an exceptional pattern of differentiation in these tumours but the name has prevailed. During embryogenesis, yolk sac first develops in its primary form made of primitive endoderm cells which form the lining epithelium of the sac, while on day 13 it evolves to a secondary embryonal sac composed of a combination of primitive endodermal cells and mesoblast. In the 13th week, the primitive endoderm is replaced by the embryonic endoderm. From this the three somatic germ layers will emerge. This embryological development may explain the diversity in the morphological patterns encountered in these tumours [38].

Of the ovarian primitive germ cell tumours, yolk sac tumours are second in frequency after dysgerminomas. These occur in children and young adults while exceedingly rare case reports of presentation in postmenopausal women exist [12]. They present with similar symptoms to other germ cell tumours. These can present in pregnancy but are not associated with endocrine manifestations as are some other types of malignant germ cell tumours. High levels of serum AFP are almost pathognomonic of the tumour, although raised levels of AFP at a lower concentration are seen in other tumours, such as hepatoid carcinoma, embryonal carcinoma and Sertoli–Leydig tumours [39–41].

Yolk sac tumours are commonly unilateral. If there is a concurrent tumour in the contralateral ovary it is often a mature teratoma [42] and bilateral yolk sac tumours signify metastatic disease. Yolk sac tumours are usually encapsulated, large tumours which have a characteristic grey yellow micro- or macrocystic cut surface or may show areas of necrosis, haemorrhage and liquefaction.

Histologically there is a diversity of architectural patterns encountered in these tumours which can make tumour typing rather difficult. The characteristic reticular pattern should be sought, and its presence makes the diagnosis easier. The reticular/microcystic pattern is composed of a loose myxoid stroma associated with lacunar spaces lined by attenuated epithelium of variable degrees of atypia (Fig. 5.2) with or without periodic acid–Schiff (PAS)-positive hyaline globules, reminiscent of the mesodermal/endodermal tissue pattern encountered in yolk sac. Schiller–Duval bodies (Fig. 5.3) are papillaroid structures with a fibrovascular core lined by a layer of cuboidal to columnar cells showing vesicular nuclei, prominent nucleoli and eosinophilic to clear cytoplasm. These papillae project into spaces which are lined by a monolayer of cells with hyperchromatic nuclei. These structures have been identified in murine placentas and they recapitulate endodermal sinuses, constituting the hallmark of these tumours. Histological variants are polyvesicular vitelline, solid, parietal, hepatoid and glandular (e.g. intestinal, pulmonary).

On immunohistochemistry, yolk sac tumour cells are positive for AFP, glypican-3 and SALL4 [43–45]. They are positive for pancytokeratin markers but usually negative for CK7 and EMA [46]. Yolk sac tumours may be positive for PLAP but are negative for OCT3/4 and CD117 [2].

Yolk sac tumours usually have characteristic morphological features but may need to be differentiated from dysgerminomas, embryonal carcinomas, endometrioid carcinomas and clear cell carcinoma of the ovary and rarely from juvenile granulosa cell tumours. Typical features of dysgerminoma, such as a lymphocytic infiltrate closely intermixed with tumour cells and expression of CD117 and OCT3/4, aid in the differential. Solid forms of yolk sac tumour may be mistaken for embryonal carcinomas. The nuclear pleomorphism in the latter is greater, and even when it is better differentiated, it does not form the structures encountered in yolk sac

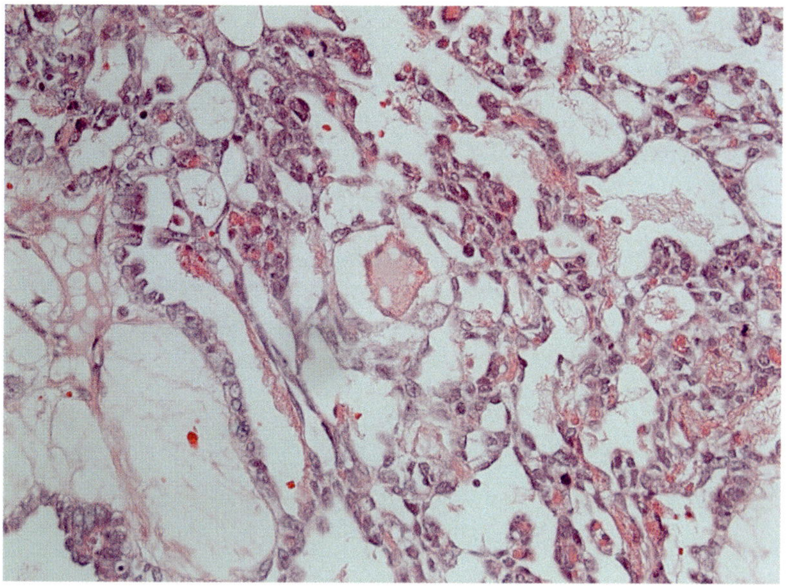

Fig. 5.2 Yolk sac tumour: tumour arranged in a reticular/microcystic pattern, composed of a loose myxoid stroma associated with lacunar spaces lined by attenuated epithelium showing variable atypia

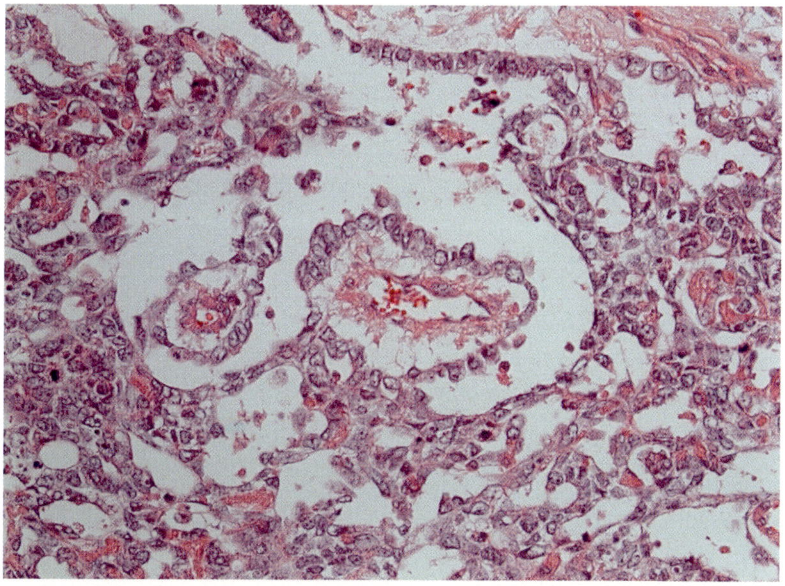

Fig. 5.3 Schiller–Duval body in a yolk sac tumour, papillaroid structure with a fibrovascular core lined by a layer of cuboidal to columnar cells projecting into a space lined by a monolayer of flattened cells with hyperchromatic nuclei

tumour. Finally, yolk sac tumours are much more common than embryonal carcinomas as ovarian malignant germ cell tumours. The glandular variant of yolk sac tumour occasionally mimics endometrial secretory pattern with subnuclear vacuolation, in which case it needs to be differentiated from endometrioid ovarian adenocarcinoma. Oestrogen (ER) and progesterone (PR) positivity and squamous differentiation favour endometrioid adenocarcinoma. When clear cell carcinoma of the ovary is predominantly composed of a tubular architectural pattern, its tubules show a typical hobnail pattern of their epithelial lining and they are not lined partly by cuboidal and partly by flattened mesothelial-like epithelium, as is yolk sac tumour, especially the perivitelline variant. Inhibin helps in the differential diagnosis between yolk sac tumour and sex cord-stromal tumours such as granulosa cell tumour with macrofollicular pattern resembling yolk sac tumour and Sertoli–Leydig cell tumours with raised AFP.

With the advent of multiagent chemotherapy, an overall 80 % complete cure rate for all stages of this tumour has been achieved, transforming the previous poor prognosis of this highly malignant tumour, which metastasises to lymph nodes and organs and also spreads by direct extension [47].

Teratoma

Teratomas are broadly classified into mature and immature, immature teratomas being the malignant representatives of this group. They are the only tumours within the group of malignant germ cell tumours which are graded, as grading has prognostic significance and determines the use or not of adjuvant chemotherapy. Mature (cystic) teratomas (dermoid cysts) are the most common germ cell tumours of the ovary. These are benign but rarely may be associated with somatic transformations of one of their components into malignant tumours, the most common being squamous cell carcinoma, adenocarcinoma or adenosquamous carcinoma. Another feature of clinical significance regarding mature teratomas is the fact that they can be associated with autoimmune haemolytic anaemia [48]. This dictates pelvic and lower abdominal investigation for a mature teratoma in the workup of autoimmune haemolytic anaemia in a female child or young woman to avoid inappropriate splenectomy. Although very rare, solid mature teratomas may contain immature components which, if present, lead to tumour recurrence. Monophasic teratoma is a mature teratoma deriving from a single germ cell layer. The most common is struma ovarii, which consists entirely of normal or hyperplastic thyroid tissue. Rarely thyroid tissue in struma ovarii may show neoplastic change towards benign or malignant thyroid tumours such as follicular adenoma, follicular carcinoma and papillary carcinoma, with the latter being the most common neoplasm. Histogenetically, all teratomas appear to be the product of parthenogenesis, arising from a primordial germ cell after implantation in the ovarian gonad, post first meiotic division.

Immature Teratoma

Immature teratomas have an age range of presentation in the first two to three decades of life, being almost unheard of in postmenopausal women [49, 50]. They present as most other germ cell tumours and they grow much more rapidly than mature teratomas, although when the latter have reached a significant size at the time of diagnosis this feature is no longer helpful.

Immature teratomas are usually unilateral solid or less commonly solid and cystic masses, which are often associated with capsular rupture and peritoneal spread. They have a grey white to haemorrhagic and necrotic cut surface, while areas resembling cartilage or bone may be present.

Immature teratomas contain embryonal type and immature tissues of all three germ cell layers, endoderm, mesoderm and ectoderm. It is essentially the presence of immature neuroepithelium that is not only diagnostic but also of prognostic value in being the basis for grading. Other forms of immature tissue may be present but in the absence of immature neuroepithelium, or rarely immature glial tissue, are in themselves insufficient for a diagnosis of immature teratoma [2]. Less mature tissue may be present in mature teratomas as well, but in immature teratomas these are more disorganised with no organoid appearance. A grading system devised by AFIP and incorporated by WHO is applied in both the primary ovarian tumour and any peritoneal deposits (Tables 5.2 and 5.3 [50, 51]). Immature neuroepithelium is formed of small blue cells

Table 5.2 Grading of ovarian immature teratomas [50, 51]

Grade 1	Immature neuroepithelium <1 low power field (X4 objective) in one slide
Grade 2	Immature neuroepithelium 1–3 low power fields (X4 objective) in one slide
Grade 3	Immature neuroepithelium >3 low power fields (X4 objective) in one slide

with formation of rosettes and brisk mitotic activity (Fig. 5.4) [50]. Immature mesoderm presents as loose myxoid stroma containing immature mesenchymal components such as immature cartilage and rhabdomyoblasts. Less common are immature endodermal structures, which may be glands with basal vacuolation or embryonic renal tissue resembling Wilms tumour.

Immunohistochemistry does not have such a useful place in the diagnosis of immature teratoma and the diagnosis is essentially morphological, although some markers have recently been suggested to have prognostic value [52]. Immature teratomas should be differentiated from carcinosarcomas or malignant mixed Müllerian tumours of the ovary, also tumours with a mixture of epithelial and mesenchymal components which occur in older women rather than the younger target group of immature teratomas. The presence of adenocarcinoma and malignant stromal elements versus the immature elements of teratoma aids the differential diagnosis.

Table 5.3 Management of immature teratomas according to grade of primary tumours and/or implants [50, 51]

Three-tier grading	Combination chemotherapy
Grade 1 ovarian tumour	Not required
Grade 2 or 3 ovarian tumour	Required
Grade 2 or 3 implants	Required
Grade 0 implants regardless of ovarian tumour grade	Not required

Grade 0 refers to implants of mature glial tissue (gliomatosis peritonei)

Unilateral salpingo-oophorectomy with or without triple chemotherapy is the treatment of choice. The use of chemotherapy is determined by grading and the presence of metastatic disease. Immature teratomas may metastasise to lymph nodes and other organs and the phenomenon of chemotherapy retroversion may lead to the presence of mature teratoma in metastatic foci [53].

Mature Teratoma

Mature teratomas are almost always cystic but 1 % may be solid. Mature cystic teratomas, also called dermoid cysts, are the most common germ cell tumours of the ovary [8], more common in young but also seen in older women. Histogenetically, they arise from a single germ cell after the first meiotic division and develop a diploid karyotype, which points to a parthenogenetic mechanism of histogenesis. They have a benign clinical course, in comparison to testicular mature teratomas which are aneuploid and malignant, although very rarely they may undergo

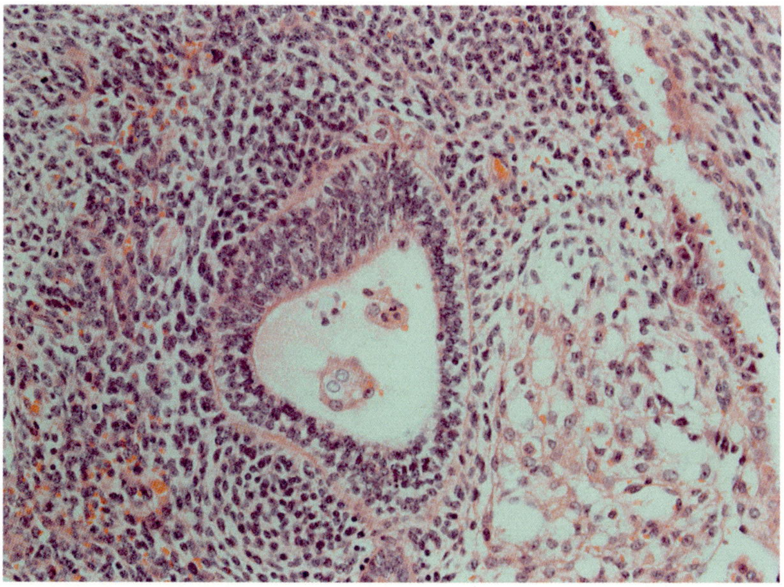

Fig. 5.4 Immature teratoma is characterised by variable amounts of immature neuroepithelium and neuroblastoma-like areas

malignant somatic mutation of one of their components. They present with the symptoms of most germ cell tumours or they may be asymptomatic, presenting as an incidental finding during other investigations. Rokitansky protuberances, the presence of fat and teeth, are diagnostic features on imaging.

Mature cystic teratoma is composed of a thin-walled cyst that usually contains hair and sebum. It may show focal thickening of the wall with calcification (Rokitansky protuberance), which should be sampled thoroughly as it may harbour different types of tissues. The cyst wall is usually lined by skin and its adnexa. Often, there is a foreign body giant cell reaction with cholesterol clefts. Other ectodermal derivatives present are mature neuroglial tissue and ocular structures including retina. Mesoderm may be represented by islands of mature cartilage, fat and smooth and skeletal muscle. Endoderm derivatives may be encountered in the form of respiratory or intestinal epithelium among others [4]. Immature tissue may be present, but if this is limited (less than 21 mm^2) the prognosis is still excellent. Rarely, well-formed embryonal structures may be seen within a teratoma and this is termed teratoma with fetiform features (homunculus). It should be differentiated from fetus in fetu, which is retroperitoneal and derives from a monozygotic diamniotic twin.

Mature Cystic Teratoma with Malignant Transformation

Malignant transformation in a mature cystic teratoma occurs in up to 2 % of cases and this makes the prognosis unfavourable. It is more often encountered in older women. The most common tumour type is squamous cell carcinoma, but other malignancies have also been reported such as mucinous carcinoma, neuroendocrine tumours (carcinoid), thyroid carcinoma, basal cell carcinoma, malignant melanoma and sarcomas [2, 54–56]. Of interest, somatic transformation in testicular teratomas usually leads to a sarcomatous rather than carcinomatous malignancy [2]. These malignancies are characterised by wide local spread rather than metastatic nodal disease, contrary to the rest of the malignant germ cell tumours. The best prognostic scenario is squamous cell carcinoma within a mature cystic teratoma without any capsular breach. Treatment is total abdominal hysterectomy and bilateral salpingo-oophorectomy. Somatic transformations in teratomas are more often seen in older women, at an age where fertility issues are less commonly relevant. These tumours do not respond well to chemotherapy [54].

When tumours with mucinous features arise within a teratoma, these are likely to be of germ cell and not surface epithelial origin. They can have a spectrum of appearances ranging from cystadenomas, borderline tumours, to adenocarcinomas with intestinal phenotype. The presence of a teratomatous component excludes the possibility of metastatic spread from a gastrointestinal primary [57]. Only a small number of such cases have been reported and the prognosis has been good for cystadenomas and borderline tumours and variable for adenocarcinomas. Occasional tumours present with features of pseudomyxoma peritonei [58].

Monophasic Teratoma

Struma Ovarii

Monophasic teratomas are those which are entirely or almost entirely composed of derivatives of one germ cell layer. The most common is thyroid tissue in the ovary, known as struma ovarii (Fig. 5.5). It may be entirely composed of benign thyroid tissue and it may present as a palpable abdominal mass or rarely with features of Meigs syndrome simulating ovarian carcinoma [59]. Struma ovarii may show features of a follicular adenoma or carcinoma [60], and the distinction is difficult because usually the lesion is not encapsulated and the diagnostic criteria of capsular invasion cannot be applied. The diagnosis of follicular carcinoma is made when there is lymphovascular invasion or infiltration of normal ovarian parenchyma present. Papillary thyroid carcinoma may also arise in the background of struma ovarii and constitutes the most common malignant change.

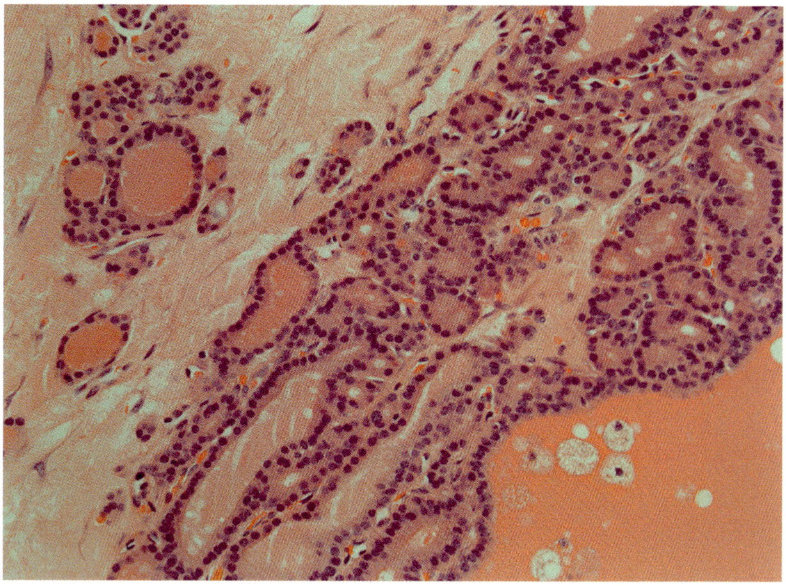

Fig. 5.5 Struma ovarii is composed of a sole, predominant or nodule-forming component of mature thyroid tissue characterised by colloid-filled follicles lined by cuboidal cells

Occasionally, benign thyroid tissue peritoneal implants may be present (struma peritonei) and this does not have any clinical significance with regard to prognosis, although this is controversial owing to the rarity of such cases [61].

Carcinoid

In other parts of the body, the term carcinoid is tending towards becoming obsolete in favour of the broader term neuroendocrine tumour and further qualifiers describing its biological behaviour, as exemplified by terminology used in lung and gastrointestinal pathology. However, a broad consensus has not been established and the term is retained in the WHO classification of tumours of the female genital tract [4]. Ovarian carcinoids may be pure or part of a dermoid cyst. They are rare and may present with carcinoid syndrome. A diagnostic feature is elevated serum 5-hydroxy-indolacetic-acid (5-HIAA) levels. These are tan to yellow firm nodules grossly and they resemble gastrointestinal carcinoids microscopically. The tumour cells show neuroendocrine features which consist in round central nuclei with a granular ('salt and pepper') chromatin pattern and eosinophilic granular cytoplasm due to the presence of neurosecretory granules (Fig. 5.6). They are distinguished into insular or trabecular types [62–64], depending on how the tumour cells are arranged, strumal carcinoids if they are associated with struma ovarii and mucinous (goblet cell carcinoid, a distinct type of tumour classified traditionally as a carcinoid, which is much more aggressive than a common carcinoid). Insular carcinoid is the most common primary ovarian carcinoid and is considered to be malignant [62]. It is usually seen in older women, and total abdominal hysterectomy and bilateral salpingo-oophorectomy is the treatment of choice. There is little experience with chemotherapy in the treatment of these tumours. Trabecular carcinoids of the ovary should be distinguished from metastases. They are called trabecular because of a ribbon-like architectural pattern. They are not associated with metastases and they are treated surgically with follow-up and no further treatment [63]. Strumal carcinoid usually behaves in a benign fashion [65]. Goblet cell carcinoid is much more aggressive, similar to its appendiceal counterpart, it is associated with lymph node spread and it is preferentially treated with hysterectomy and bilateral salpingo-oophorectomy when maintenance of fertility is not a relevant issue [66].

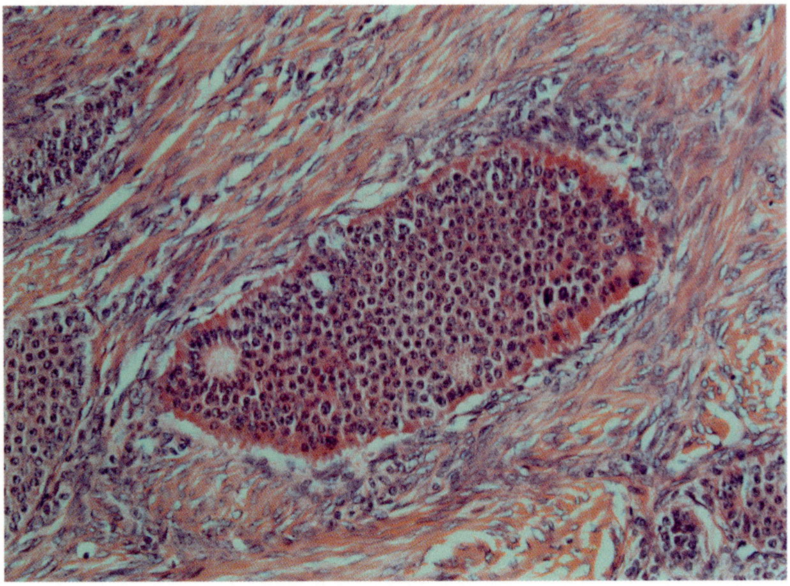

Fig. 5.6 Carcinoid in its characteristic insular pattern is characterised by islands of cells with monomorphic nuclei. The cells at the periphery in the islands illustrated show eosinophilic granular cytoplasm

Embryonal Carcinoma and Polyembryoma

Pure embryonal carcinoma is the rarest germ cell tumour type of the ovaries with the teratomas being the most common and the reverse pertaining to testicular germ cell tumours [2]. Embryonal carcinoma arises from totipotential germ cells with the capability to differentiate towards various somatic or extraembryonal structures, and although it is the least differentiated malignant germ cell neoplasm, it is more often a part of a mixed germ cell tumour rather than a pure embryonal carcinoma. It presents similarly to other germ cell tumours. It may contain syncytiotrophoblasts, in which case it is associated with a rise in bHCG in the serum, although at levels much lower than a choriocarcinoma, and seemingly, it may express AFP without the presence of a yolk sac tumour component [67].

An embryonal carcinoma tumour component is grey white solid tumour with slightly granular focally necrotic or haemorrhagic appearance. The morphological appearances of embryonal carcinoma depend on the degree of primitive or more differentiated forms of the tumour. The primitive features consist of sheets of cells with epithelioid appearance and indistinct cell borders showing highly anaplastic nuclear features, with horseshoe nuclei among other nuclear shapes and sizes, vesicular to coarse chromatin pattern and prominent one or more nucleoli. The cytoplasm is usually basophilic. Mitoses are frequent. The more differentiated forms of the tumour have a pseudoglandular appearance, with tumour cells lining clefts and spaces rather than forming true glands. They may show a pseudopapillary appearance, with no core or with tumour cells around a thin-walled vessel. Multinucleated cells may be present. Areas of necrosis and haemorrhage may be present, and these should be differentiated from choriocarcinoma.

Embryonal carcinoma is positive for keratins and CD30 and focally positive for AFP. The solid component of embryonal carcinoma should be differentiated from dysgerminoma because of the prognostic implications. The degree of nuclear pleomorphism and the presence of pseudoglandular spaces are in favour of embryonal carcinoma. The nuclear membrane of dysgerminoma cells is much more pronounced than that of embryonal carcinoma. Positivity for keratins and even focal positivity for AFP exclude dysgerminoma. The latter may be focally positive for CD30. Embryonal carcinoma is negative for CD117. OCT3/4 does not help in the differential diagnosis between embryonal carcinoma and dysgerminoma as it is positive in both, but it aids in the differential between embryonal carcinoma and non-germ cell poorly differentiated carcinoma [2]. Embryonal carcinoma is highly aggressive as it is associated with early lymphatogenous and potentially haematogenous spread, local invasion and recurrence. It has a favourable response to chemotherapy. The presence of differentiated tumour components versus the more primitive morphology is considered to predict a more indolent course.

Polyembryoma represents an organoid form of embryonal carcinoma with features resembling early embryos (embryonic bodies). The embryonic bodies are composed of blastocyst-like formations, formed by embryonic discs, amniotic sacs and primary yolk sac cavities with focal AFP positivity, which are surrounded by mesoblastic loose connective tissue. It is a highly malignant neoplasm which is primarily treated surgically and responds well to combination chemotherapy.

Choriocarcinoma

Primary choriocarcinoma of the ovary is an exceedingly rare neoplasm with an incidence of less than 0.6 % of all ovarian neoplasms; therefore, its characteristics have not been widely studied. Pure primary ovarian choriocarcinoma is much less common than mixed germ cell tumour with choriocarcinoma [68, 69].

The distinction between gestational and non-gestational choriocarcinoma is considered to be crucial as non-gestational choriocarcinoma is much more aggressive, although current treatment options have ameliorated prognosis comparable to the rest of the malignant germ cell tumours. The presence of paternal DNA in the tumour is in favour of a gestational type, while the presence of other germ cell tumour components is in favour of a non-gestational type. It is more common in children and younger patients than it is in postmenopausal women, but rare incidents have been reported in postmenarcheal (and postmenopausal) women where the distinction between gestational and non-gestational choriocarcinoma (metastatic uterine choriocarcinoma to the ovary or in association with ovarian ectopic pregnancy) may be impossible to make [70, 71]. The clinical symptoms are similar to those of other germ cell tumours, including precocious puberty, vaginal bleeding and rarely thyrotoxicosis. Serum levels of bHCG produced by tumour cells are a useful diagnostic and follow-up tool.

Choriocarcinomas are typically large, solid, grey white, necrotic and haemorrhagic tumours and may be associated with other cystic or nodular lesions in the ovary, which are the result of progesterone effect induced by the production of HCG. They may be part of a mixed germ cell neoplasm, hence the importance of thorough sampling of ovarian tumours, especially focusing on areas of heterogeneity, with haemorrhagic or necrotic appearance, to exclude the presence of a choriocarcinomatous component. Choriocarcinomas are formed by closely intermixed cytotrophoblasts and syncytiotrophoblasts with very rare, if at all, presence of intermediate trophoblasts. The architectural pattern is predominantly composed of solid sheets of cytotrophoblasts with a plexiform, pseudopapillary or fenestrated appearance, surrounded by layers of syncytiotrophoblasts, almost always in areas of haemorrhage and necrosis. The cytotrophoblasts show well-defined cytoplasmic borders, with variable nuclei ranging from central round, hyperchromatic nuclei to vesicular nuclei with prominent nucleoli. Mitotic activity may be brisk. The cytoplasm is usually clear. Syncytiotrophoblasts are large, usually elongated, multinucleated cells with basophilic and vacuolated cytoplasm with irregular borders. The nuclei vary in shape and size with dense hyperchromatic chromatin pattern. Choriocarcinoma is characteristically positive for bHCG, expressed by the terminally differentiated syncytiotrophoblast. Cytokeratin and human placental lactogen are also expressed. When typical features are present, the differential diagnosis is straightforward. Occasionally, solid type embryonal carcinoma may be difficult to differentiate but CD30 positivity of the latter may be helpful.

Choriocarcinoma has had a notoriously aggressive behaviour before the introduction of chemotherapy which revolutionised the management of germ cell neoplasia. Its malignant behaviour is due to its excessive propensity to metastasise widely through the haematogenous route, often at the time of diagnosis. In comparison to gestational choriocarcinoma, the non-gestational form spreads more often through lymphatic and local invasion, and haematogenous spread may be less prominent. It has been suggested that there are two options for treatment: treatment as for gestational tumours using single-agent or multiagent chemotherapy or with a germ cell tumour protocol, such as vincristine/actinomycin D/cyclophosphamide (VAC) or bleomycin/etoposide/cisplatinum (BEP) [72], the last considered the more favourable combination.

Mixed Germ Cell Tumours

Up to one-fifth of malignant germ cell tumours are composed of more than one type, defined as having a mixture of two, three or more malignant, i.e. not mature teratomatous, components [73, 74]. These occur in children and young women and present with non-specific features or hormonal manifestations. Serum markers depend on the elements present; AFP is raised in the presence of yolk sac tumour and HCG when choriocarcinomatous or embryonal carcinoma components occur. These patients can be managed with conservative surgery and effective chemotherapy which has blurred the survival differences seen previously with different components [17, 75]. Histologically, dysgerminoma, yolk sac tumour and immature teratoma in diminishing frequency are the most commonly encountered components. Embryonal carcinoma, choriocarcinoma and polyembryoma are less frequent but are seen more often as mixed tumours than in pure form in the ovary. Immunohistochemical results are as described for the different malignant germ cell tumours [44, 76].

Sex Cord-Stromal Tumours

The term sex cord-stromal encompasses derivatives of the specialist steroid hormone-secreting cells of the gonadal stroma. These encompass the gonadal stroma-derived fibroblasts, theca cells, lutein cells and Leydig cells and the sex cord-derived Sertoli cells and their ovarian counterparts, albeit of less certain embryological origin, the granulosa cells. Although individual entities show characteristic features, these tumours are broadly characterised by occurrence at a younger age than epithelial malignancies and by their propensity for hormonal manifestations as part of the clinical picture as a result of oestrogen, progesterone or androgen secretion. The malignant entities, and those that can clinically or morphologically simulate malignancy, in each of these groups are described below.

Granulosa-Stromal Cell Tumours

This term encompasses granulosa cell tumours of adult and juvenile types and tumours of the thecoma-fibroma group.

Adult Granulosa Cell Tumour

Granulosa cell tumour of adult type (AGCT) most commonly occurs in the perimenopausal age group but can be seen at all ages. This is the most common malignant sex cord-stromal tumour [77–80]. Clinical presentation is often with signs or symptoms attributable to hormone, usually oestrogen, production by the tumour cells, a pelvic mass or both. Oestrogenic manifestations are generally in the form of abnormal uterine bleeding resulting from endometrial hyperplasia, and rarely endometrial carcinoma. Rarely the tumours cause progestogenic or virilising features resulting from secretion of progesterone or androgens. Serum markers useful in diagnosis and monitoring recurrence are therefore serum oestradiol or alpha-inhibin, a polypeptide hormone secreted by granulosa cells with a role in regulating follicle-stimulating hormone (FSH) secretion [81].

Macroscopically, these tumours have a variable size with an average diameter of 13 cm at clinical presentation. These tumours are unilateral and most are confined to the ovary. They typically show a smooth outer surface and a solid and cystic cut surface. Solid areas have variable consistency and may be hard and white or soft and yellow depending on the amount of the

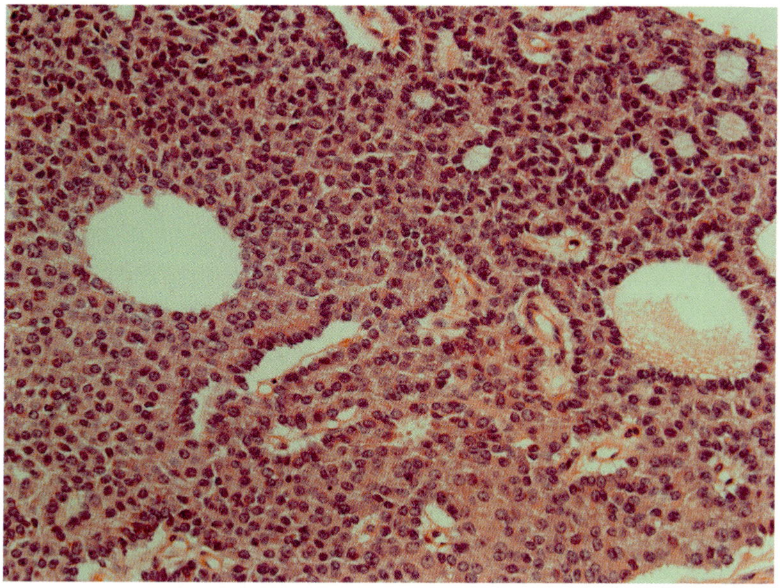

Fig. 5.7 Granulosa cell tumour is characterised by a monotonous cell population; a typical arrangement if in the form of follicle-like structures known as Call-Exner bodies

stromal component and extent of luteinisation. Cystic areas may be filled with blood and necrosis may be present. Some tumours occur as thin-walled cysts—these are the most likely to show androgenic manifestations.

Microscopically, these tumours are typically composed of a monotonous population of cells with scanty cytoplasm and uniform ovoid nuclei. Nuclei are pale and characteristically show longitudinal grooves. Mitotic activity is very variable but typically low. The most characteristic arrangement is in the form of microfollicular structures, recapitulating the appearances seen in the developing Graafian follicle. In these the tumour cells are arranged around a central space filled with pale eosinophilic material, the Call-Exner body (Fig. 5.7). These, however, are not always seen, as tumour cells in AGCT may be arranged in a variety of patterns: macrofollicular, diffuse (or 'sarcomatoid'), watered silk, trabecular, insular or gyriform. It is usual for a number of patterns to coexist. Very occasional tumours show bizarre tumour cells with marked cytological atypia. When accompanied by increased mitotic activity, this may indicate true sarcomatous differentiation, which is a poor prognostic sign. Variable degrees of luteinisation may be present. The neoplastic cells are separated by spindle cell stroma. This in turn can vary in amount and cellularity. When excessive the features border on those of fibroma with minor sex cord elements—by definition the granulosa cell component should account for 10 % or more of the tumour for a diagnosis of granulosa cell tumour. A variety of minor variations on this basic morphology may occur.

The tumour has a wide differential diagnosis with other epithelial and non-epithelial malignancies. Principal among these are the small cell carcinoma of hypercalcaemic type and endometrioid carcinoma, mimics with potential for serious misdiagnosis. Granulosa cell tumour also resembles Brenner tumour and carcinoid, as well as endometrial stromal sarcoma and Sertoli–Leydig cell tumour. The overlap with tumours of the fibroma-thecoma group with sex cord elements is mentioned above. Granulosa cell tumours have recently been demonstrated to harbour missense somatic mutations in the gene *FOXL2*, a gene encoding a transcription factor involved in ovarian development and particularly granulosa cell function and follicular development. This has potential use in diagnosis as it appears to be relatively unique to granulosa cell tumour of adult type [82, 83]. Immunohistochemical reactivity for sex cord-stromal markers inhibin, calretinin, steroidogenic factor 1 (SF1) and *FOXL2* are helpful in diagnosis although all markers may not be positive in an individual case [84, 85]. It is important to remember that cytokeratins are expressed in granulosa cells, and indeed in other sex cord-stromal tumours, and are therefore not useful in the differential diagnosis with epithelial tumours. Granulosa cell tumours are negative for epithelial membrane antigen (EMA) and CK7, and these are the two markers useful in this context [86, 87]. Similarly, granulosa cell tumours are positive for CD 56 and CD 10 markers, which are therefore not useful in distinguishing carcinoid and endometrial stromal sarcomas, respectively [88, 89].

In terms of behaviour, AGCT are low-grade malignancies with potential for local and distant recurrence. Typically these recurrences occur some years following removal of the primary tumour and survival therefore varies with length of follow-up, averaging around 90 % at 5 years, 80 % at 10 years and 50–60 % at 20 years. The most significant adverse prognostic factors are extra-ovarian involvement at presentation, tumour rupture and age over 50 years. Pathological features are disappointingly poor predictors of adverse behaviour but size greater than 5 cm and the presence of high mitotic activity (≥5/10 high-power field [hpf]) are reported to be significant [77–80, 90].

Juvenile Granulosa Cell Tumour

Around 5 % of granulosa tumours occur in prepubertal girls and young women. The vast majority of juvenile granulosa cell tumours (JGCT) are seen in the first three decades although occasional cases are reported in older women [91, 92]. Tumours in childhood usually present with clinical features of isosexual pseudoprecocity. These tumours differ morphologically and clinically from adult granulosa cell tumours in being more atypical in their histological appearance but usually clinically benign. The vast majority are diagnosed at stage I. Recurrences and metastases are much less frequent, and when they do occur, unlike adult granulosa cell tumours, this is in the first few years after treatment.

JGCT are almost always unilateral, ranging from 3 to 32 cm in diameter. These are solid or solid and cystic massive with a grey or yellow cut surface that includes areas of haemorrhage and necrosis. Histologically, these are composed of cells with abundant eosinophilic cytoplasm and hyperchromatic, mitotically active nuclei that lack nuclear grooves. The cells are arranged in solid and macrocystic patterns, the latter comprising cystic spaces of varying size and shape, filled with eosinophilic or basophilic material. Call-Exner bodies are not seen. Widespread luteinisation is typical in both granulosa cells and stromal cells and lipid droplets are readily identified on oil red O staining.

JGCT must be distinguished from AGCT because of their different clinical behaviour. Because of its more atypical appearance and occurrence at a younger age group, JGCT may be confused with germ cell tumours such as yolk sac tumour and embryonal carcinoma. Another potential pitfall is the similarity of this tumour to a variant small cell carcinoma of hypercalcaemic type which can occasionally be composed of a larger, rhabdoid appearing cells. Clear cell carcinoma and metastatic malignant melanoma should also be excluded. Immunohistochemistry is usually characteristic with positive staining for inhibin, calretinin and SF1. The most important prognostic factors are stage and tumour size. Recurrences are rare and tend to be early, within 3 years of diagnosis, and potentially fatal.

Fibroma

Fibroma is the most common sex cord-stromal tumour. These are benign tumours, which can occasionally present with ascites or ascites and pleural effusion (Meigs syndrome) and elevated CA-125, clinically simulating malignancy. These features disappear on removal of the mass. Fibromas occur in the fourth and fifth decades and do not show hormonal manifestations [93].

Macroscopically, these are unilateral, solid, firm white masses though cystic degeneration is common and may be widespread within the tumour. Histological diagnosis is straightforward as the tumours are composed of bland spindle cells arranged in a storiform or whorled arrangement in a collagenous background. Dystrophic calcification may be present.

The differential diagnosis is with cellular fibroma and fibrosarcoma, discussed below [94].

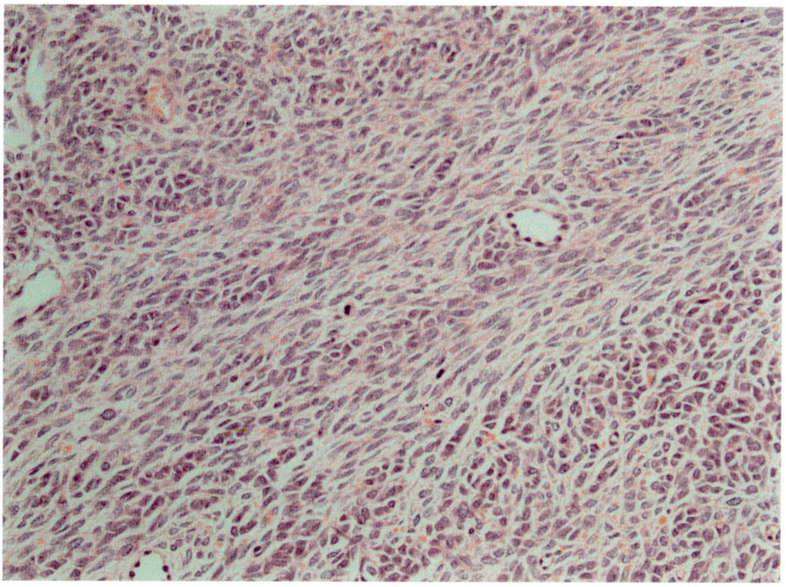

Fig. 5.8 Mitotically active cellular fibroma: spindle cells with high mitotic activity but no severe cytological atypia in a young woman

Fibromas sometimes harbour sex cord elements which by definition must not exceed 10 % of the tumour area examined [95]. An important pitfall is distinction from a metastatic signet ring carcinoma (Krukenberg tumour) with a prominent cellular stromal component and inconspicuous malignant epithelial cells.

Cellular Fibroma Including Mitotically Active Cellular Fibroma

A small proportion of fibromas exhibit strikingly greater cellularity than is usually present. By definition this should not be accompanied by diffuse cytological atypia. These show greater nuclear density with less collagenisation and hyalinisation, imparting an overall blue appearance to the sections. In the presence of mitotic activity which is reported to be as high as 19 per 10 hpfs, the lesion is referred to as a mitotically active cellular fibroma, to distinguish from the more sinister fibrosarcoma (Fig. 5.8). Both cellular fibroma and mitotically active cellular fibroma are benign, but the latter is less well studied and clinical follow-up is recommended [96].

Fibrosarcoma

This is an exceedingly rare clinically aggressive tumour which occurs in elderly women. The tumour shows a malignant proliferation of fibroblastic cells showing diffuse moderate to severe nuclear atypia and high mitotic activity [96, 97]. It is possible that many cases diagnosed as fibrosarcoma previously represent examples of mitotically active cellular fibroma. These tumours are unilateral, soft haemorrhagic masses. Apart from mitotically active cellular fibroma, they should be distinguished from the more common carcinosarcomas (malignant mixed Müllerian tumour) with a predominant sarcomatous component. Similarly, adenosarcomas with sarcomatous overgrowth, leiomyosarcoma, gastrointestinal stromal tumours, sarcomatoid Sertoli–Leydig cell tumours and carcinomas with spindle cells form the differential diagnosis of this rare malignancy.

Thecoma

Thecomas are clinically benign tumours that occur in the sixth decade. These are clinically distinguished from fibromas by their presentation with hormonal manifestations in the majority of cases [98]. The tumour cells in thecomas have a less fibroblastic and more polygonal appearance. As with fibromas, cellular and mitotically active

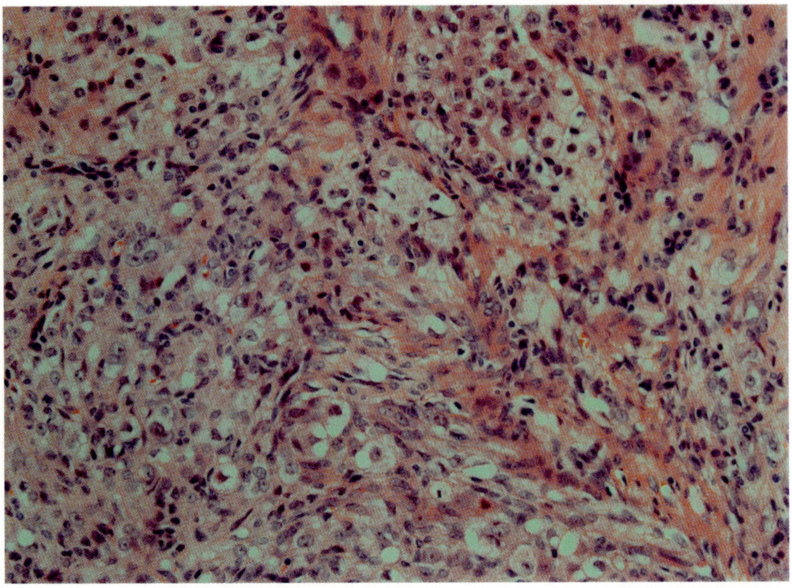

Fig. 5.9 Luteinised thecoma: large round cells with pale cytoplasm interspersed among the spindle cells of a thecoma

counterparts exist as do those with minor sex cord elements.

Luteinised thecomas are clinically benign tumours that occur in younger women (Fig. 5.9). These include significant collections of luteinised cells in the stromal addition to the spindle cell population. A rare subtype of luteinised thecoma is bilateral, hormonally inactive, occurs in the third decade and is associated with sclerosing peritonitis; this is now believed to represent a reactive proliferation. This entity may be associated with abdominal complications as a result of the peritonitis though the ovarian tumours are benign [99, 100].

Sertoli–Stromal Tumours

This group of tumours includes tumours arising from or differentiating into Sertoli and Leydig cells.

Sertoli Cell Tumour

This is a rare and generally nonfunctioning category of Sertoli–stromal tumours which occurs in young women [101, 102]. The tumours are unilateral, yellow brown masses that histologically are composed solely of tubules. The differential diagnosis is therefore with epithelial tumours from which they can be distinguished by positive staining for sex cord-stromal markers and negative staining for epithelial membrane antigen. Behaviour is benign the vast majority of cases. An oxyphilic variant exists which is associated with Peutz–Jeghers syndrome.

Sertoli–Leydig Cell Tumours

Sertoli–Leydig cell tumours are rare ovarian sex cord-stromal tumours, which occur in young women (average age, 25 years) [4]. These may present with features of virilisation, in addition to a pelvic mass. Some cases, especially those with heterologous elements, may present with increased serum alpha-fetoprotein raising suspicion for a germ cell tumour, although these elevations are usually modest. These are divided into well, intermediate, and poorly differentiated forms. Behaviour is dependent on stage, as well as differentiation with intermediate and poorly differentiated cases showing a potential for recurrence and metastasis. When recurrence occurs, it is usually early, within 1–2 years of diagnosis.

Macroscopically, these tumours show a variable appearance and range from being completely solid to unilocular cysts, with an average diameter of 13 cm. Haemorrhage and necrosis may be

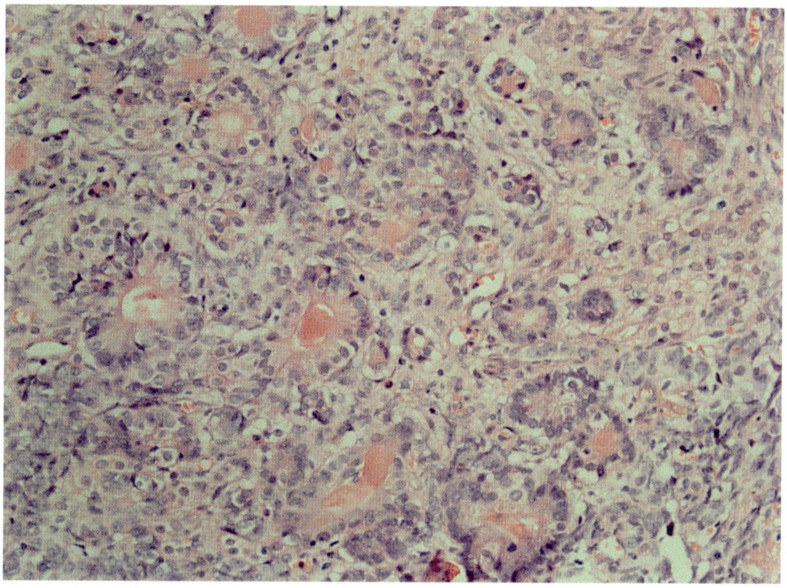

Fig. 5.10 Sertoli–Leydig cell tumour showing tubular structures typical of a well-differentiated Sertoli cell component

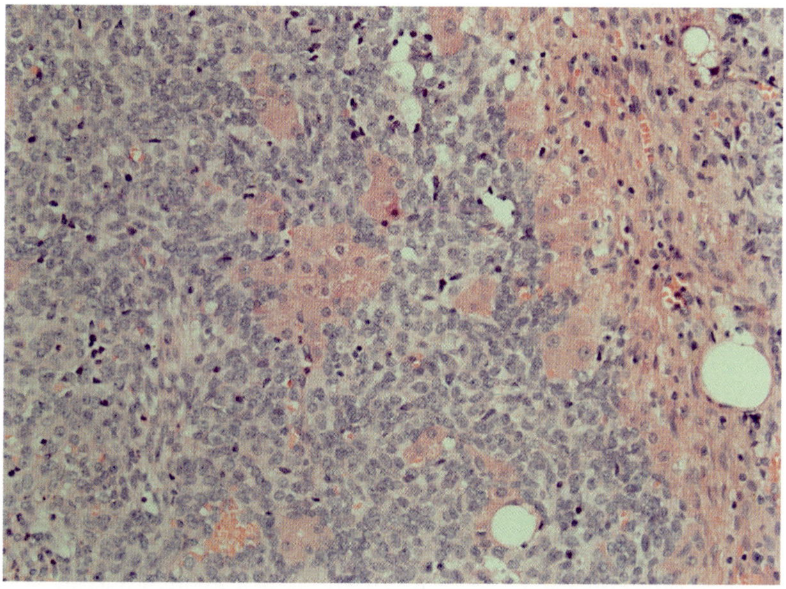

Fig. 5.11 Leydig cell aggregates in a poorly differentiated Sertoli–Leydig cell

seen in poorly differentiated tumours. The solid component may be white to yellow depending on the extent of luteinisation.

Histologically, well-differentiated tumours show a relatively uniform appearance with a mixture of tubular (Sertoli cell) elements (Fig. 5.10) and stromal components, the latter including aggregates of Leydig cells (Fig. 5.11), characterised by central round nuclei, abundant eosinophilic granular cytoplasm in which typical Reinke crystalloids may be identified. Tumours of intermediate and poor differentiation tend to have a more heterogenous appearance. The Sertoli component exists as cords or solid trabeculae which may be seen only focally. The stromal component is represented by a proliferation of spindle cells. Leydig cells may be seen very focally and are generally difficult to find. About one-fifth of tumours contain heterologous elements in the form of cystic and glandular structures lined by mucinous epithelium or islands of cartilage, skeletal muscle and other elements [103, 104]. The retiform variant can mimic an epithelial tumour grossly and microscopically. This subset, accounting for about 15 % of all tumours, tends to occur in younger women and is usually nonfunctioning [105].

The differential diagnosis of these heterogenous tumours is with malignant epithelial tumours, especially endometrioid carcinoma, as well as others [106]. Immunohistochemically, the tumour cells are positive for inhibin, calretinin and SF1. It is important to remember that cytokeratin is expressed and CK7 and EMA are therefore preferable to broad-spectrum cytokeratins in distinguishing these tumours from epithelial malignancies.

Prognosis of Sertoli–Leydig tumours is stage and differentiation dependent. Malignant cases almost invariably show poor differentiation or mesenchymal heterologous elements. The retiform variants appear to have a worse prognosis. Recurrence is characteristically early and localised to the pelvis.

Steroid Cell Tumours

Steroid cell tumours of the ovary are of three types: stromal luteoma, Leydig cell tumour and steroid cell tumour, not otherwise specified. The first two are clinically benign while about one-third of steroid cell tumours, not otherwise specified (NOS), are reported to show malignant behaviour in the form of local recurrence or distant spread. These are rare tumours and there are few data on prognostic factors [107, 108]. These tumours are seen in the third or fourth decade and often present with hormonal manifestations, either androgenic or cushingoid. The tumours are unilateral, multilobulated yellow or orange masses measuring on average 10 cm. Histologically, the tumours are composed of large round or polygonal with abundant vacuolated or granular cytoplasm and uniform round nuclei. Tumour size greater than 8 cm, mitotic activity more than 2/10 hpf, necrosis, haemorrhage and nuclear atypia are reported to be associated with adverse outcome.

Miscellaneous Non-epithelial Malignant Ovarian Tumours

A variety of malignant non-epithelial tumours can arise in the ovary that are unrelated to either germ cell or sex cord-stromal elements.

Leiomyosarcoma

Smooth muscle tumours rarely occur as primaries in the ovary [94]. These are believed to arise in areas of stromal smooth muscle metaplasia. Pathological criteria for malignancy used in uterine smooth muscle tumours apply. Primary ovarian leiomyosarcoma occurs in the fifth and sixth decades as solid firm white masses, which may show necrosis and haemorrhage. Histologically, these show diffuse cytological atypia and high mitotic activity. Behaviour is usually aggressive.

Endometrial Stromal Sarcoma

Rare examples of low-grade endometrial stromal sarcomas arise in the ovary where they are presumed to originate in a background of endometriosis [109]. These can occur at any age. They are unilateral, solid, tan-coloured masses composed of bland spindle cells arranged in a basketweave pattern and with a rich arteriolar network. Immunohistochemical confirmation is essential as these mimic sex cord-stromal tumours closely. In addition to diffuse CD10 positivity, which may be seen in sex cord-stromal tumours, these should be negative for sex cord-stromal markers. These tumours are low-grade sarcomas with high potential for local and metastatic spread via vascular channels.

Intra-abdominal Desmoplastic Small Round Cell Tumour

This is a rare tumour of unknown origin that occurs in young persons with a high male predilection (4:1). Cases in women can involve the ovary and/or mimic ovarian carcinoma by their presentation as multiple peritoneal nodules, characteristically including omental involvement, and raised serum CA-125. Macroscopically, the tumour shows multiple large tumour nodules of variable consistency and areas of haemorrhage and necrosis. Histologically, this tumour consists of small round monomorphic cells with hyperchromatic nuclei and scanty cytoplasm within an abundance of desmoplastic stroma [110]. The cells show high mitotic activity. Many variations in the appearance and arrangement of the cells are described. On immunohistochemistry, the tumour cells stain with epithelial and mesenchymal markers including cytokeratin, epithelial membrane antigen, WT1, desmin and neuron-specific enolase (NSE), the combination of WT1 and desmin positivity being characteristic. There is also a diagnostic molecular abnormality, t(11;22)(p13:q12). The tumour is aggressive and rapidly fatal.

Primitive Neuroectodermal Tumour

The ovary is a rare site of tumours of the Ewing's sarcoma family of peripheral primitive neuroectodermal tumours [110]. These tumours are composed of small round blue cells which are typically positive for CD99 (MIC2). There is a wide differential diagnosis and a panel of markers should be used. The tumour cells typically show the t(11;22)(q24:q12) translocation.

Haematological Malignancies

All types of leukaemias and lymphomas can involve the ovary secondarily. Rarely lymphomas can arise as primary or apparently primary ovarian masses. Most commonly these are Burkitt's lymphoma, especially in endemic areas where this is one of the most common causes of childhood ovarian masses, and diffuse large B cell lymphomas [110–113]. The tumours present as solid unilateral or bilateral masses. Burkitt's lymphoma shows a characteristic proliferation of intermediate-sized atypical lymphocytes in a starry sky pattern. Diffuse large B cell lymphoma is the most common malignancy in adults and is composed of large atypical lymphocytes. Immunohistochemistry varies with subtype. The differential diagnosis includes dysgerminoma, melanoma and small cell carcinoma as well as other primary and metastatic tumours. Survival is over 50 % with chemotherapy.

References

1. Appendix B Histologic classification of tumors and precursor conditions of the female genital tract. In: Robboy SJ, et al., editors. Robboy's pathology of the female genital tract. Edinburgh: Churchill Livingstone Elsevier; 2009.
2. Ulbright TM. Germ cell tumors of the gonads: a selective review emphasizing problems in differential diagnosis, newly appreciated, and controversial issues. Mod Pathol. 2005;18 Suppl 2:S61–79.
3. Ulbright TM. Gonadal teratomas: a review and speculation. Adv Anat Pathol. 2004;11(1):10–23.
4. Tavassoli FA, Devilee P. Pathology and genetics of tumours of the breast and female genital tract, World Health Organization classification of tumours. Lyons: IARC Press; 2003.
5. Lee KH, Lee IH, Kim BG, Nam JH, Kim WK, Kang SB, et al. Clinicopathologic characteristics of malignant germ cell tumors in the ovaries of Korean women: a Korean Gynecologic Oncology Group Study. Int J Gynecol Cancer. 2009;19(1):84–7.
6. Topuz S, Iyibozkurt AC, Akhan SE, Keskin N, Yavuz E, Salihoglu Y, et al. Malignant germ cell tumors of the ovary: a review of 41 cases and risk factors for recurrence. Eur J Gynaecol Oncol. 2008;29(6): 635–7.
7. Pectasides D, Pectasides E, Kassanos D. Germ cell tumors of the ovary. Cancer Treat Rev. 2008; 34(5):427–41.
8. Koonings PP, Campbell K, Mishell Jr DR, Grimes DA. Relative frequency of primary ovarian neoplasms: a 10-year review. Obstet Gynecol. 1989; 74(6):921–6.
9. Nakashima N, Nagasaka T, Fukata S, Oiwa N, Nara Y, Fukatsu T, Takeuchi J. Study of ovarian tumors treated at Nagoya University Hospital, 1965-1988. Gynecol Oncol. 1990;37(1):103–11.
10. Guillem V, Poveda A. Germ cell tumours of the ovary. Clin Transl Oncol. 2007;9(4):237–43.
11. Norris HJ, Jensen RD. Relative frequency of ovarian neoplasms in children and adolescents. Cancer. 1972;30(3):713–9.
12. Nogales FF, Bergeron C, Carvia RE, Alvaro T, Fulwood HR. Ovarian endometrioid tumors with yolk sac tumor component, an unusual form of ovarian neoplasm. Analysis of six cases. Am J Surg Pathol. 1996;20(9):1056–66.

13. Czaja JT, Ulbright TM. Evidence for the transformation of seminoma to yolk sac tumor, with histogenetic considerations. Am J Clin Pathol. 1992;97(4):468–77.
14. Young RH. Dusting off another shelf: further comments on classic gynecologic pathology books of yesteryear. Int J Gynecol Pathol. 2005;24(1):100–10.
15. Parkash V, Carcangiu ML. Transformation of ovarian dysgerminoma to yolk sac tumor: evidence for a histogenetic continuum. Mod Pathol. 1995;8(8):881–7.
16. Teilum G. Classification of endodermal sinus tumour (mesoblatoma vitellinum) and so-called "embryonal carcinoma" of the ovary. Acta Pathol Microbiol Scand. 1965;64(4):407–29.
17. Tewari K, Cappuccini F, Disaia PJ, Berman ML, Manetta A, Kohler MF. Malignant germ cell tumors of the ovary. Obstet Gynecol. 2000;95(1):128–33.
18. Schwartz PE. Surgery of germ cell tumours of the ovary. Forum (Genova). 2000;10(4):355–65.
19. Dennedy MC, Smith D, O'Shea D, McKenna TJ. Investigation of patients with atypical or severe hyperandrogenaemia including androgen-secreting ovarian teratoma. Eur J Endocrinol. 2010;162(2):213–20.
20. Shimizu Y, Komiyama S, Kobayashi T, Nakata K, Iida T. Successful management of endodermal sinus tumor of the ovary associated with pregnancy. Gynecol Oncol. 2003;88(3):447–50.
21. Cheng L, Roth LM, Zhang S, Wang M, Morton MJ, Zheng W, Abdul Karim FW, Montironi R, Lopez-Beltran A. KIT gene mutation and amplification in dysgerminoma of the ovary. Cancer. 2011;117(10):2096–103.
22. De Palo G, Lattuada A, Kenda R, Musumeci R, Zanini M, Pilotti S, et al. Germ cell tumors of the ovary: the experience of the National Cancer Institute of Milan. I. Dysgerminoma. Int J Radiat Oncol Biol Phys. 1987;13(6):853–60.
23. Vicus D, Beiner ME, Klachook S, Le LW, Laframboise S, Mackay H. Pure dysgerminoma of the ovary 35 years on: a single institutional experience. Gynecol Oncol. 2010;117(1):23–6.
24. Mueller CW, Topkins P, Lapp WA. Dysgerminoma of the ovary; an analysis of 427 cases. Am J Obstet Gynecol. 1950;60(1):153–9.
25. Guerriero S, Van Holsbeke C, Ajossa S, Fischerova D. Imaging of gynecological disease (6): clinical and ultrasound characteristics of ovarian dysgerminoma. Ultrasound Obstet Gynecol. 2011;37(5):596–602.
26. Inoue H, Kikuchi Y, Hirata J, Wada S, Seki K, Nagata I. Dysgerminoma of the ovary with hypercalcemia associated with elevated parathyroid hormone-related protein. Jpn J Clin Oncol. 1995;25(3):113–7.
27. Hibi M, Hara F, Tomishige H, Nishida Y, Kato T, Okumura N, et al. 1,25-dihydroxyvitamin D-mediated hypercalcemia in ovarian dysgerminoma. Pediatr Hematol Oncol. 2008;25(1):73–8.
28. Zaloudek CJ, Tavassoli FA, Norris HJ. Dysgerminoma with syncytiotrophoblastic giant cells. A histologically and clinically distinctive subtype of dysgerminoma. Am J Surg Pathol. 1981;5(4):361–7.
29. Pressley RH, Muntz HG, Falkenberry S, Rice LW. Serum lactic dehydrogenase as a tumor marker in dysgerminoma. Gynecol Oncol. 1992;44(3):281–3.
30. Asadourian LA, Taylor HB. Dysgerminoma. An analysis of 105 cases. Obstet Gynecol. 1969;33(3):370–9.
31. Bjorkholm E, Lundell M, Gyftodimos A, Silfverswärd C. Dysgerminoma. The Radiumhemmet series 1927-1984. Cancer. 1990;65(1):38–44.
32. Cossu-Rocca P, Zhang S, Roth LM, Eble JN, Zheng W, Karim FW, et al. Chromosome 12p abnormalities in dysgerminoma of the ovary: a FISH analysis. Mod Pathol. 2006;19(4):611–5.
33. Poulos C, Cheng L, Zhang S, Gersell DJ, Ulbright TM. Analysis of ovarian teratomas for isochromosome 12p: evidence supporting a dual histogenetic pathway for teratomatous elements. Mod Pathol. 2006;19(6):766–71.
34. Sever M, Jones TD, Roth LM, Karim FW, Zheng W, Michael H, et al. Expression of CD117 (c-kit) receptor in dysgerminoma of the ovary: diagnostic and therapeutic implications. Mod Pathol. 2005;18(11):1411–6.
35. Ushiku T, Shinozaki A, Shibahara J, Iwasaki Y, Tateishi Y, Funata N, Fukayama M. SALL4 represents fetal gut differentiation of gastric cancer, and is diagnostically useful in distinguishing hepatoid gastric carcinoma from hepatocellular carcinoma. Am J Surg Pathol. 2010;34(4):533–40.
36. De Palo G, Pilotti S, Kenda R, Ratti E, Musumeci R, Mangioni C, et al. Natural history of dysgerminoma. Am J Obstet Gynecol. 1982;143(7):799–807.
37. Patterson DM, Murugaesu N, Holden L, Seckl MJ, Rustin GJ. A review of the close surveillance policy for stage I female germ cell tumors of the ovary and other sites. Int J Gynecol Cancer. 2008;18(1):43–50.
38. Nogales FF, Preda O, Nicolae A. Yolk sac tumours revisited. A review of their many faces and names. Histopathology. 2012;60:1023–33.
39. Talerman A, Haije WG, Baggerman L. Serum alpha fetoprotein (AFP) in diagnosis and management of endodermal sinus (yolk sac) tumor and mixed germ cell tumor of the ovary. Cancer. 1978;41(1):272–8.
40. Talerman A. Ovarian Sertoli-Leydig cell tumor (androblastoma) with retiform pattern. A clinicopathologic study. Cancer. 1987;60(12):3056–64.
41. Talerman A, Haije WG. Ovarian Sertoli cell tumor with retiform and heterologous elements. Am J Surg Pathol. 1985;9(6):459–60.
42. Vos A, Oosterhuis JW, de Jong B, Castedo SM, Hollema H, Buist J, Aalders JG. Karyotyping and DNA flow cytometry of metastatic ovarian yolk sac tumor. Cancer Genet Cytogenet. 1990;44(2):223–8.
43. Cao D, Humphrey PA, Allan RW. SALL4 is a novel sensitive and specific marker for metastatic germ cell tumors, with particular utility in detection of metastatic yolk sac tumors. Cancer. 2009;115(12):2640–51.
44. Chang MC, Vargas SO, Hornick JL, Hirsch MS, Crum CP, Nucci MR. Embryonic stem cell transcription

factors and D2-40 (podoplanin) as diagnostic immunohistochemical markers in ovarian germ cell tumors. Int J Gynecol Pathol. 2009;28(4):347–55.
45. Esheba GE, Pate LL, Longacre TA. Oncofetal protein glypican-3 distinguishes yolk sac tumor from clear cell carcinoma of the ovary. Am J Surg Pathol. 2008;32(4):600–7.
46. Ramalingam P, Malpica A, Silva EG, Gershenson DM, Liu JL, Deavers MT. The use of cytokeratin 7 and EMA in differentiating ovarian yolk sac tumors from endometrioid and clear cell carcinomas. Am J Surg Pathol. 2004;28(11):1499–505.
47. Lu KH, Gershenson DM. Update on the management of ovarian germ cell tumors. J Reprod Med. 2005;50(6):417–25.
48. Glorieux I, Chabbert V, Rubie H, Baunin C, Gaspard MH, Guitard J, et al. [Autoimmune hemolytic anemia associated with a mature ovarian teratoma]. Arch Pediatr. 1998;5(1):41–4.
49. Gershenson DM, del Junco G, Silva EG, Copeland LJ, Wharton JT, Rutledge FN. Immature teratoma of the ovary. Obstet Gynecol. 1986;68(5):624–9.
50. Norris HJ, Zirkin HJ, Benson WL. Immature (malignant) teratoma of the ovary: a clinical and pathologic study of 58 cases. Cancer. 1976;37(5):2359–72.
51. O'Connor DM, Norris HJ. The influence of grade on the outcome of stage I ovarian immature (malignant) teratomas and the reproducibility of grading. Int J Gynecol Pathol. 1994;13(4):283–9.
52. Abiko K, Mandai M, Hamanishi J, Matsumura N, Baba T, Horiuchi A, et al. Oct4 expression in immature teratoma of the ovary: relevance to histologic grade and degree of differentiation. Am J Surg Pathol. 2010;34(12):1842–8.
53. Djordjevic B, Euscher ED, Malpica A. Growing teratoma syndrome of the ovary: review of literature and first report of a carcinoid tumor arising in a growing teratoma of the ovary. Am J Surg Pathol. 2007;31(12):1913–8.
54. Chiang AJ, La V, Peng J, Yu KJ, Teng NN. Squamous cell carcinoma arising from mature cystic teratoma of the ovary. Int J Gynecol Cancer. 2011;21(3):466–74.
55. Sakuma M, Utsunomiya H, Nagase S, Takano T, et al. Malignant transformation arising from mature cystic teratoma of the ovary: a retrospective study of 20 cases. Int J Gynecol Cancer. 2010;20(5):766–71.
56. Park JY, Kim DY, Kim JH, Kim YM, Kim YT, Nam JH. Malignant transformation of mature cystic teratoma of the ovary: experience at a single institution. Eur J Obstet Gynecol Reprod Biol. 2008;141(2):173–8.
57. Vang R, Gown AM, Zhao C, Barry TS, Isacson C, Richardson MS, Ronnett BM. Ovarian mucinous tumors associated with mature cystic teratomas: morphologic and immunohistochemical analysis identifies a subset of potential teratomatous origin that shares features of lower gastrointestinal tract mucinous tumors more commonly encountered as secondary tumors in the ovary. Am J Surg Pathol. 2007;31(6):854–69.
58. Hwang JH, So KA, Modi G, Lee JK, Lee NW, Lee KW, Kim I. Borderline-like mucinous tumor arising in mature cystic teratoma of the ovary associated with pseudomyxoma peritonei. Int J Gynecol Pathol. 2009;28(4):376–80.
59. Simkin PH, Ramirez LA, Zweizig SL, Afonso SA, Fraire AE, Khan A, et al. Monomorphic teratoma of the ovary: a rare cause of triiodothyronine toxicosis. Thyroid. 1999;9(9):949–54.
60. Devaney K, Snyder R, Norris HJ, Tavassoli FA. Proliferative and histologically malignant struma ovarii: a clinicopathologic study of 54 cases. Int J Gynecol Pathol. 1993;12(4):333–43.
61. Robboy SJ, Shaco-Levy R, Peng RY, Snyder MJ, Donahue J, Bentley RC, et al. Malignant struma ovarii: an analysis of 88 cases, including 27 with extraovarian spread. Int J Gynecol Pathol. 2009;28(5):405–22.
62. Robboy SJ, Norris HJ, Scully RE. Insular carcinoid primary in the ovary. A clinicopathologic analysis of 48 cases. Cancer. 1975;36(2):404–18.
63. Talerman A, Evans MI. Primary trabecular carcinoid tumor of the ovary. Cancer. 1982;50(7):1403–7.
64. Talerman A. Carcinoid tumors of the ovary. J Cancer Res Clin Oncol. 1984;107(2):125–35.
65. Robboy SJ, Scully RE. Strumal carcinoid of the ovary: an analysis of 50 cases of a distinctive tumor composed of thyroid tissue and carcinoid. Cancer. 1980;46(9):2019–34.
66. Baker PM, Oliva E, Young RH, Talerman A, Scully RE. Ovarian mucinous carcinoids including some with a carcinomatous component: a report of 17 cases. Am J Surg Pathol. 2001;25(5):557–68.
67. Kurman RJ, Norris HJ. Embryonal carcinoma of the ovary: a clinicopathologic entity distinct from endodermal sinus tumor resembling embryonal carcinoma of the adult testis. Cancer. 1976;38(6):2420–33.
68. Jacobs AJ, Newland JR, Green RK. Pure choriocarcinoma of the ovary. Obstet Gynecol Surv. 1982;37(10):603–9.
69. Goswami D, Sharma K, Zutshi V, Tempe A, Nigam S. Nongestational pure ovarian choriocarcinoma with contralateral teratoma. Gynecol Oncol. 2001;80(2):262–6.
70. Tsujioka H, Hamada H, Miyakawa T, Hachisuga T, Kawarabayashi T. A pure nongestational choriocarcinoma of the ovary diagnosed with DNA polymorphism analysis. Gynecol Oncol. 2003;89(3):540–2.
71. Yamamoto E, Ino K, Yamamoto T, Sumigama S, Nawa A, Nomura S, Kikkawa F. A pure nongestational choriocarcinoma of the ovary diagnosed with short tandem repeat analysis: case report and review of the literature. Int J Gynecol Cancer. 2007;17(1):254–8.
72. Weiss S, Amit A, Schwartz MR, Kaplan AL. Primary choriocarcinoma of the vulva. Int J Gynecol Cancer. 2001;11(3):251–4.
73. Gershenson DM, Del Junco G, Copeland LJ, Rutledge FN. Mixed germ cell tumors of the ovary. Obstet Gynecol. 1984;64(2):200–6.

74. Kurman RJ, Norris HJ. Malignant mixed germ cell tumors of the ovary. A clinical and pathologic analysis of 30 cases. Obstet Gynecol. 1976;48(5):579–89.
75. Smith HO, Berwick M, Verschraegen CF, Wiggins C, Lansing L, Muller CY, Qualls CR. Incidence and survival rates for female malignant germ cell tumors. Obstet Gynecol. 2006;107(5):1075–85.
76. Cheng L, Zhang S, Talerman A, Roth LM. Morphologic, immunohistochemical, and fluorescence in situ hybridization study of ovarian embryonal carcinoma with comparison to solid variant of yolk sac tumor and immature teratoma. Hum Pathol. 2010;41(5):716–23.
77. Fox H, Agrawal K, Langley FA. A clinicopathologic study of 92 cases of granulosa cell tumor of the ovary with special reference to the factors influencing prognosis. Cancer. 1975;35(1):231–41.
78. Stenwig JT, Hazekamp JT, Beecham JB. Granulosa cell tumors of the ovary. A clinicopathological study of 118 cases with long-term follow-up. Gynecol Oncol. 1979;7(2):136–52.
79. Bjorkholm E, Silfversward C. Prognostic factors in granulosa-cell tumors. Gynecol Oncol. 1981;11(3): 261–74.
80. Malmstrom H, Högberg T, Risberg B, Simonsen E. Granulosa cell tumors of the ovary: prognostic factors and outcome. Gynecol Oncol. 1994;52(1):50–5.
81. Boggess JF, Soules MR, Goff BA, Greer BE, Cain JM, Tamimi HK. Serum inhibin and disease status in women with ovarian granulosa cell tumors. Gynecol Oncol. 1997;64(1):64–9.
82. Kim MS, Hur SY, Yoo NJ, Lee SH. Mutational analysis of FOXL2 codon 134 in granulosa cell tumour of ovary and other human cancers. J Pathol. 2010;221(2): 147–52.
83. Schrader KA, Gorbatcheva B, Senz J, Heravi-Moussavi A, Melnyk N, Salamanca C, et al. The specificity of the FOXL2 c.402C>G somatic mutation: a survey of solid tumors. PLoS One. 2009;4(11):e7988.
84. Al-Agha OM, Huwait HF, Chow C, Yang W, Senz J, Kalloger SE, et al. FOXL2 is a sensitive and specific marker for sex cord-stromal tumors of the ovary. Am J Surg Pathol. 2011;35(4):484–94.
85. Zhao C, Vinh TN, McManus K, Dabbs D, Barner R, Vang R. Identification of the most sensitive and robust immunohistochemical markers in different categories of ovarian sex cord-stromal tumors. Am J Surg Pathol. 2009;33(3):354–66.
86. Costa MJ, DeRose PB, Roth LM, Brescia RJ, Zaloudek CJ, Cohen C. Immunohistochemical phenotype of ovarian granulosa cell tumors: absence of epithelial membrane antigen has diagnostic value. Hum Pathol. 1994;25(1):60–6.
87. Baker PM, Oliva E. Immunohistochemistry as a tool in the differential diagnosis of ovarian tumors: an update. Int J Gynecol Pathol. 2005;24(1):39–55.
88. McCluggage WG, McKenna M, McBride HA. CD56 is a sensitive and diagnostically useful immunohistochemical marker of ovarian sex cord-stromal tumors. Int J Gynecol Pathol. 2007;26(3):322–7.
89. Oliva E, Garcia-Miralles N, Vu Q, Young RH. CD10 expression in pure stromal and sex cord-stromal tumors of the ovary: an immunohistochemical analysis of 101 cases. Int J Gynecol Pathol. 2007;26(4): 359–67.
90. Fox H. Pathologic prognostic factors in early stage adult-type granulosa cell tumors of the ovary. Int J Gynecol Cancer. 2003;13(1):1–4.
91. Biscotti CV, Hart WR. Juvenile granulosa cell tumors of the ovary. Arch Pathol Lab Med. 1989;113(1):40–6.
92. Young RH, Dickersin GR, Scully RE. Juvenile granulosa cell tumor of the ovary. A clinicopathological analysis of 125 cases. Am J Surg Pathol. 1984;8(8): 575–96.
93. Leung SW, Yuen PM. Ovarian fibroma: a review on the clinical characteristics, diagnostic difficulties, and management options of 23 cases. Gynecol Obstet Invest. 2006;62(1):1–6.
94. Irving JA, McCluggage WG. Ovarian spindle cell lesions: a review with emphasis on recent developments and differential diagnosis. Adv Anat Pathol. 2007;14(5):305–19.
95. Young RH, Scully RE. Ovarian stromal tumors with minor sex cord elements: a report of seven cases. Int J Gynecol Pathol. 1983;2(3):227–34.
96. Irving JA, Alkushi A, Young RH, Clement PB. Cellular fibromas of the ovary: a study of 75 cases including 40 mitotically active tumors emphasizing their distinction from fibrosarcoma. Am J Surg Pathol. 2006;30(8):929–38.
97. Prat J, Scully RE. Cellular fibromas and fibrosarcomas of the ovary: a comparative clinicopathologic analysis of seventeen cases. Cancer. 1981;47(11): 2663–70.
98. Roth LM, Czernobilsky B. Perspectives on pure ovarian stromal neoplasms and tumor-like proliferations of the ovarian stroma. Am J Surg Pathol. 2011;35(3):e15–33.
99. Mellembakken JR, Engh V, Tanbo T, Czernobilsky B, Edelstein E, Lunde O, Roth LM. Mitotically active cellular luteinized thecoma of the ovary and luteinized thecomatosis associated with sclerosing peritonitis: case studies, comparison, and review of the literature. Pathol Res Pract. 2010;206(11):744–8.
100. Staats PN, McCluggage WG, Clement PB, Young RH. Luteinized thecomas (thecomatosis) of the type typically associated with sclerosing peritonitis: a clinical, histopathologic, and immunohistochemical analysis of 27 cases. Am J Surg Pathol. 2008; 32(9):1273–90.
101. Tavassoli FA, Norris NJ. Sertoli tumors of the ovary. A clinicopathologic study of 28 cases with ultrastructural observations. Cancer. 1980;46(10): 2281–97.
102. Young RH, Scully RE. Ovarian Sertoli cell tumors: a report of 10 cases. Int J Gynecol Pathol. 1984;2(4): 349–63.
103. Dicker D, Dekel A, Feldberg D, Goldman JA, Kessler E. Bilateral Sertoli-Leydig cell tumor with

heterologous elements: report of an unusual case and review of the literature. Eur J Obstet Gynecol Reprod Biol. 1986;22(3):175–81.
104. Prat J, Young RH, Scully RE. Ovarian Sertoli-Leydig cell tumors with heterologous elements. II. Cartilage and skeletal muscle: a clinicopathologic analysis of twelve cases. Cancer. 1982;50(11):2465–75.
105. Mooney EE, Nogales FF, Bergeron C, Tavassoli FA. Retiform Sertoli-Leydig cell tumours: clinical, morphological and immunohistochemical findings. Histopathology. 2002;41(2):110–7.
106. McCluggage WG, Young RH. Ovarian sertoli-leydig cell tumors with pseudoendometrioid tubules (pseudoendometrioid sertoli-leydig cell tumors). Am J Surg Pathol. 2007;31(4):592–7.
107. Hayes MC, Scully RE. Ovarian steroid cell tumors (not otherwise specified). A clinicopathological analysis of 63 cases. Am J Surg Pathol. 1987;11(11):835–45.
108. Seidman JD, Abbondanzo SL, Bratthauer GL. Lipid cell (steroid cell) tumor of the ovary: immunophenotype with analysis of potential pitfall due to endogenous biotin-like activity. Int J Gynecol Pathol. 1995;14(4):331–8.
109. Young RH, Prat J, Scully RE. Endometrioid stromal sarcomas of the ovary. A clinicopathologic analysis of 23 cases. Cancer. 1984;53(5):1143–55.
110. McCluggage WG. Ovarian neoplasms composed of small round cells: a review. Adv Anat Pathol. 2004;11(6):288–96.
111. Abell MR, Holtz F. Ovarian neoplasms in childhood and adolescence. II. Tumors of non-germ cell origin. Am J Obstet Gynecol. 1965;93(6):850–66.
112. Linden MD, Tubbs RR, Fishleder AJ, Hart WR. Immunotypic and genotypic characterization of non-Hodgkin's lymphomas of the ovary. Am J Clin Pathol. 1988;90(2):156–62.
113. Osborne BM, Robboy SJ. Lymphomas or leukemia presenting as ovarian tumors. An analysis of 42 cases. Cancer. 1983;52(10):1933–43.

Strategies for the Management of Ovarian Cancer

6

Tim Mould

Introduction

Chapters 9 and 10 are separate chapters on the treatment of early-stage ovarian and advanced-stage ovarian cancer. This chapter comprises an overview of the management of ovarian cancer with a focus on the contentious aspects that need to be considered when considering a strategy for individual patient management.

Early-Stage Ovarian Cancer

Staging

In presumed early-stage ovarian cancer, the rationale for full staging is strong, as 25 % of cases will be upstaged, usually to stage III, due to disease in the omentum or lymph glands. This will determine the need for chemotherapy. Although there are no randomised studies showing increased survival in patients who have been staged versus those who were unstaged, unrandomised studies support this logic [1].

T. Mould, MD, FRCOG, MBBS, MA, DM, FRCOG
Department of Gynaecological Oncology,
University College London, London, UK
e-mail: tim.mould@uclh.nhs.uk

Fertility Preservation

In younger patients who require fertility, the issue of preservation of the contralateral ovary and uterus needs to be discussed carefully. There is a presumed risk that microscopic disease may be present, particularly in the contralateral ovary. A case series of 118 patients showed a 2.5 % involvement of the contralateral ovary with microscopic disease [2]. Consequently, it is not surprising that recurrent disease presenting in the preserved ovary is seen in 4–6 % of cases [3, 4]. The limited historical case control evidence shows that survival is not compromised. Thus, low risk cases such as stage I grade 1,2 may treated conservatively, assuming that the preserved ovary is monitored carefully with ultrasound [5]. A 10.3 % chance of recurrence and 5.5 % chance of death have been quoted in a review paper of 507 women treated with fertility-sparing surgery for early ovarian cancer [6].

Adjuvant Chemotherapy

In patients with higher risk stage I ovarian cancer, such as grade III tumours or tumours with adverse histology such as clear cell carcinoma, they are advised to have adjuvant single-agent carboplatin due to a significant advantage for survival being shown [7]. Any uncertainty about staging would also be included as a category for which chemotherapy may add additional survival.

S.A. Farghaly (ed.), *Advances in Diagnosis and Management of Ovarian Cancer*,
DOI 10.1007/978-1-4614-8271-0_6, © Springer Science+Business Media New York 2014

Late-Stage Ovarian Cancer

Surgical Debulking Principles

In late-stage ovarian cancer, the importance of surgery continues to be shown in numerous publications. However, the definition of optimal debulking surgery has changed from the initial trial by Griffiths in 1975, where optimal was described as residual deposits of not more than 1.5 cm [8]. The most recent definition is no residual visible disease is optimal. In order to achieve this, the strategy of surgery may require extended or supraradical surgery. Case series have shown that resection of areas of the abdomen previously regarded as inoperable will improve the proportion of patients with no residual disease from 30 to 70 % [9, 10]. These areas will include diaphragm, liver, spleen and coeliac axis. In order to achieve such surgical results, the patient should be treated in specialist centres where there is a high volume of patients with advanced ovarian cancer. The centre would require a specific strategy to involve different surgical specialities to train the gynaecological oncology team to operate in areas where they have previously been unable to resect the disease. The gynaecological oncology surgical team would need to ensure that the respective surgeons were unified in the aim of achieving full resection. The intensive care team and nurse specialist team should all be in line with this approach. The case series show an increase in overall survival as a result of this systematic approach to surgery [10].

Supporters of extended or aggressive surgery recommend that primary surgery is undertaken before the commencement of chemotherapy. However, there are situations where the patient is too frail to survive extended supraradical surgery or where the disease may be judged to be too extensive on preoperative computed tomography (CT) scans to achieve no residual disease despite maximal surgical effort. Careful analysis of the CT images in the specialist multidisciplinary team meeting setting is essential. The position of disease should no longer be regarded as a measure of inoperability. More important is the overall amount of disease in the relevant parts of the abdomen in relation to the performance measure and co-morbidity of the patient.

In these situations, neoadjuvant chemotherapy may be considered. The only randomised trial as to whether primary surgery is more effective than neoadjuvant chemotherapy with delayed surgery showed no difference in survival between the two strategies [11]. Furthermore, the neoadjuvant chemotherapy group had less morbidity from the surgery. An important feature seen in this study shows that the achievement of no residual disease at surgery produced increased survival in both arms of the study. Of interest, recruiting centres demonstrated very different rates of primary surgery and rates of achieving no residual disease.

Chemotherapy Options

Adjuvant or neoadjuvant chemotherapy strategies must be compared against the gold standard of intravenous carboplatin and paclitaxel combination chemotherapy.

Different strategies to be considered are whether dose-dense paclitaxel should be used, intraperitoneal chemotherapy should be advised and maintenance treatment should be recommended.

Dose-dense paclitaxel using weekly paclitaxel plus 3-weekly carboplatin has been shown to have a survival advantage in a Japanese trial [12]. A further randomised study, ICON8, has started in order to corroborate this finding.

Intraperitoneal chemotherapy is strongly advised in those centres that have adopted it. Numerous trials have looked into intraperitoneal administration of chemotherapy. A significant survival advantage has been demonstrated, but the variety of regimes and dosage used and the amount of crossover in the trials have meant that the results have been difficult to interpret [13]. Thus many institutions do not use intraperitoneal chemotherapy due to these concerns over the data and the potential for increased complications from the treatment. However, the strategy must be considered in view of the possible survival advantage.

The strategy of maintenance treatment has been investigated at some length due to the recurrent nature of advanced ovarian cancer. Conventional agents have not shown survival advantages. New biological agents have been proposed more recently, and bevacizumab has shown progression-free survival advantage in maintenance therapy [14, 15]. We await the results of further trials to see an overall survival benefit is present. The strategy is frequently used across Europe and North America already.

Recurrent Ovarian Cancer

The chemotherapy strategy used in recurrent disease is dependent on the length of time to relapse. Relapse less than 6 months from the end of first-line chemotherapy is deemed platinum-resistant disease, which will respond to further platinum in less than 10 % of cases. Relapse between 6 and 12 months is partially sensitive disease with a response rate to platinum of 25–30 %. Relapse after 12 months is deemed platinum sensitive, with a response rate between 30 and 60 %.

Combination chemotherapy has been shown to be advantageous over single-agent platinum in platinum-sensitive disease [16–18]. In platinum-resistant disease, the response to chemotherapy is poor, and there is no consensus on management. The choice of agent will depend on the patient's ability to tolerate treatment as judged by toxicity and patient wishes. Novel therapy should be offered in the context of clinical trials.

The use of surgery in relapsed disease is gaining increasing attention. Where a patient has had a significant interval between end of treatment and disease relapse, surgical debulking to no residual disease may offer prolonged survival in a similar manner as case series show in primary disease. Thus careful assessment of individual patients and the pattern of disease recurrence on their CT should be undertaken in order to determine whether surgery should be undertaken. Desktop 2 has identified patients who may benefit from surgery [19]. Desktop 3 is a randomised trial of this being undertaken to provide further evidence to possible survival benefit from surgery and recurrent disease.

References

1. Le T, Adolph A, Krepart GV, Lotocki R, Heywood MS. The benefits of comprehensive surgical staging in the management of early-stage epithelial ovarian carcinoma. Gynecol Oncol. 2002;85(2):351–5.
2. Benjamin I, Morgan MA, Rubin SC. Occult bilateral involvement in stage I epithelial ovarian cancer. Gynecol Oncol. 1999;72(3):288–91.
3. Kajiyama H, Shibata K, Suzuki S, Ino K, Nawa A, Kawai M, Nagasaka T, Kikkawa F. Fertility-sparing surgery in young women with invasive epithelial ovarian cancer. Eur J Surg Oncol. 2010;36(4):404–8.
4. Schilder JM, Thompson AM, DePriest PD, Ueland FR, Cibull ML, Kryscio RJ, et al. Outcome of reproductive age women with stage IA or IC invasive epithelial ovarian cancer treated with fertility-sparing therapy. Gynecol Oncol. 2002;87(1):1–7.
5. Morice P, Denschlag D, Rodolakis A, Reed N, Schneider A, Kesic V, Colombo N, Fertility Task Force of the European Society of Gynecologic Oncology. Recommendations of the Fertility Task Force of the European Society of Gynecologic Oncology about the conservative management of ovarian malignant tumors. Int J Gynecol Cancer. 2011;21(5):951–63.
6. Vitobello D, Siesto G, Bulletti C, Accardi A, Levi Setti PE. Gynecological fertility-sparing surgery. Placenta. 2011;32 Suppl 3:S224–31.
7. Trimbos JB, Parmar M, Vergote I, Guthrie D, Bolis G, Colombo N, International Collaborative Ovarian Neoplasm 1, European Organisation for Research and Treatment of Cancer Collaborators-Adjuvant ChemoTherapy un Ovarian Neoplasm, et al. International Collaborative Ovarian Neoplasm trial 1 and Adjuvant ChemoTherapy In Ovarian Neoplasm trial: two parallel randomized phase III trials of adjuvant chemotherapy in patients with early-stage ovarian carcinoma. J Natl Cancer Inst. 2003;95(2):105–12.
8. Griffiths CT. Surgical resection of tumor bulk in the primary treatment of ovarian carcinoma. J Natl Cancer Inst Monogr. 1975;42:101–4.
9. Eisenhauer EL, Abu-Rustum NR, Sonoda Y, Levine DA, Poynor EA, Aghajanian C, et al. The addition of extensive upper abdominal surgery to achieve optimal cytoreduction improves survival in patients with stages IIIC-IV epithelial ovarian cancer. Gynecol Oncol. 2006;103(3):1083–90.
10. Chi DS, Eisenhauer EL, Zivanovic O, Sonoda Y, Abu-Rustum NR, Levine DA, et al. Improved progression-free and overall survival in advanced ovarian cancer as a result of a change in surgical paradigm. Gynecol Oncol. 2009;114(1):26–31.
11. Vergote I, Tropé CG, Amant F, Kristensen GB, Ehlen T, Johnson N, European Organization for Research and Treatment of Cancer-Gynaecological Cancer Group, NCIC Clinical Trials Group, et al. Neoadjuvant chemotherapy or primary surgery in stage IIIC or IV ovarian cancer. N Engl J Med. 2010;363(10):943–53.

12. Katsumata N, Yasuda M, Takahashi F, Isonishi S, Jobo T, Aoki D, Japanese Gynecologic Oncology Group, et al. Dose-dense paclitaxel once a week in combination with carboplatin every 3 weeks for advanced ovarian cancer: a phase 3, open-label, randomised controlled trial. Lancet. 2009;374(9698):1331–8.
13. Armstrong DK, Bundy B, Wenzel L, Huang HQ, Baergen R, Lele S, Gynecologic Oncology Group, et al. Intraperitoneal cisplatin and paclitaxel in ovarian cancer. N Engl J Med. 2006;354(1):34–43.
14. Perren TJ, Swart AM, Pfisterer J, Ledermann JA, Pujade-Lauraine E, Kristensen G, ICON7 Investigators, et al. A phase 3 trial of bevacizumab in ovarian cancer. N Engl J Med. 2011;365(26):2484–96.
15. Burger RA, Brady MF, Bookman MA, Fleming GF, Monk BJ, Huang H, Gynecologic Oncology Group, et al. Incorporation of bevacizumab in the primary treatment of ovarian cancer. N Engl J Med. 2011;365(26):2473–83.
16. Parmar MK, Ledermann JA, Colombo N, du Bois A, Delaloye JF, Kristensen GB, et al. Paclitaxel plus platinum-based chemotherapy versus conventional platinum-based chemotherapy in women with relapsed ovarian cancer: the ICON4/AGO-OVAR-2.2 trial. The ICON and AGO Collaborators. Lancet. 2003;361(9375):2099–106.
17. Pfisterer J, Plante M, Vergote I, du Bois A, Hirte H, Lacave AJ, AGO-OVAR, NCIC CTG, EORTC GCG, et al. Gemcitabine plus carboplatin compared with carboplatin in patients with platinum-sensitive recurrent ovarian cancer: an intergroup trial of the AGO-OVAR, the NCIC CTG, and the EORTC GCG. J Clin Oncol. 2006;24(29):4699–707.
18. Wagner U, Marth C, Largillier R, Kaern J, Brown C, Heywood M, et al. Final overall survival results of phase III GCIG CALYPSO trial of pegylated liposomal doxorubicin and carboplatin vs paclitaxel and carboplatin in platinum-sensitive ovarian cancer patients. Br J Cancer. 2012;107(4):588–91.
19. Harter P, Sehouli J, Reuss A, Hasenburg A, Scambia G, Cibula D, et al. Prospective validation study of a predictive score for operability of rec urrent ovarian cancer: the Multicenter Intergroup Study DESKTOP II. A project of the AGO Kommission OVAR, AGO Study Group, NOGGO, AGO-Austria, and MITO. Int J Gynecol Cancer. 2011;21(2):289–95.

Management of Hereditary Ovarian–Breast Cancer

7

Andrea Tinelli, Sarah Gustapane, Antonio Malvasi, Daniele Vergara, Michele Maffia, Marilena Greco, Caterina Accettura, Marianna Giampaglia, Silvana Leo, and Vito Lorusso

A. Tinelli, MD (✉)
Department of Obstetrics and Gynecology, Vito Fazzi Hospital, Lecce 73100, Italy
e-mail: andreatinelli@gmail.com

S. Gustapane, MD
Department of Obstetrics and Gynecology, SS. Annunziata Hospital, Chieti, Italy
e-mail: sarahgustapane@gmail.com

A. Malvasi, MD
Department of Obstetrics and Gynecology, Santa Maria Hospital, Bari, Italy
e-mail: antoniomalvasi@gmail.com

D. Vergara, BSc, PhD • M. Maffia, PhD
Department of Biological and Environmental Sciences and Technologies, University of Salento, Lecce, Italy
e-mail: danielevergara@libero.it; michele.maffia@unisalento.it

M. Greco, PhD, BSc
Laboratory of Medical Genetics, Giovanni Paolo II Oncological Centre, Lecce Hospital, Lecce, Italy
e-mail: grecomarilena@gmail.com

C. Accettura, MD • M. Giampaglia, MD
S. Leo, MD
Department of Oncology, Vito Fazzi Hospital, Lecce 73100, Italy
e-mail: caterinaaccettura@libero.it; mariannagiampaglia@yahoo.it; silvileo@libero.it

V. Lorusso, MD
Department of Medical Oncology, National Institute for Cancer Research, Istituto Tumori Giovanni Paolo II, Bari, Italy
e-mail: vitolorusso@me.com

Introduction

Ovarian cancer represents the sixth most commonly diagnosed cancer among women in the world; it is the second most common gynaecologic malignancy, varies widely in frequency among different geographic regions and ethnic groups, with a high incidence in Northern Europe and the United States, and a low incidence in Japan; and results in approximately 14,500 deaths annually. In fact, more than 50 % of the 21,650 women diagnosed with ovarian cancer die annually of this disease [1].

The majority of cases are sporadic, and only 5–10 % of ovarian cancers are familial. Unfortunately, the aetiology of this disease remains poorly understood. Numerous reproductive, environmental and genetic risk factors have been identified. The most important is a family history of breast or ovarian cancer as up to 10 % of ovarian cancer patients may have inherited a germline mutation from their mother or father that places them at increased risk for the disease. The most significant risk factor is a family history of the disease. Infertility may contribute to ovarian cancer risk among nulliparous women, and other possible risk factors for ovarian cancer include: postmenopausal hormone-replacement therapy and lifestyle factors, such as cigarette smoking and alcohol consumption. Many of the causes of ovarian cancer are yet to be identified, even if established risk factors for ovarian cancer include age and having a family history of the disease. In contrast, protective factors from ovarian cancer include: increasing parity, oral

S.A. Farghaly (ed.), *Advances in Diagnosis and Management of Ovarian Cancer*,
DOI 10.1007/978-1-4614-8271-0_7, © Springer Science+Business Media New York 2014

Table 7.1 Risk factors for ovarian cancer by evidences

Established risk factors	Possible risk factors	Suspected risk factors
Age	Early age at menarche	Hormonal replacement therapy
Family history – genetics	Late age at menopause	Dietary fat
Nulliparity	Infertility	Obesity
Oral contraceptive use (protective)	Lactation (protective)	Sedentary lifestyle
Oophorectomy (protective)	Tubal ligation (protective)	Cigarette smoking
	Hysterectomy (protective)	Alcohol consumption
	Low vegetable intake	

Adapted from Tinelli et al. [1]

contraceptive use and oophorectomy; nevertheless, the lactation, the incomplete pregnancies and surgeries. Hysterectomy and tubal legation have, in fact, a weak protective effect ranging from 30 to 40 %, for each of these procedures, against ovarian cancer [1].

All the risk factors for ovarian cancer development are visualized in Table 7.1.

Furthermore, approximately 10 % of ovarian cancers may be due to an inherited genetic predisposition, since familial predisposition to cancer has been recognized for many years [2].

Other, rarer hereditary gene mutations are associated with increased risk of breast cancer, such as Li–Fraumeni syndrome, Cowden syndrome, Peutz–Jeghers syndrome and hereditary diffuse gastric cancer syndrome [3].

The History of Hereditary Ovarian Cancer (HOC) Discovery

The discovery 15 years ago of some of the genes that are involved in the heritance of very common malignant diseases, like breast and ovarian cancers, has represented a substantial improvement in the understanding of hereditary ovarian cancer and a challenge for cancer prevention [3].

Over the last four decades, Henry Lynch has collected pedigrees and samples from high-risk breast and/or ovarian cancer families, showing autosomal-dominant inheritance patterns for breast cancer in the late 1960s; Henry Lynch was the first to hypothesize forward a probable genetic etiologic association between carcinoma of the breast and ovary [5].

These families allowed the discovery of a genetic association between breast and ovarian cancer predisposition, contributing to the mapping of the *BRCA1* and *BRCA2* genes. They advanced the idea of the existence of other breast cancer susceptibility genes, allowing the evaluation of BRCA-associated cancer risks and psychosocial aspects of BRCA testing and so on [1–4].

In 1990, Mary-Claire King followed in demonstrating the first convincing linkage data in early onset breast cancer families which mapped the susceptibility gene, subsequently named *BRCA1* for breast cancer 1 [5].

A particular aspect of this collection was the predominance of families with both breast and ovarian cancers and broad availability of biological samples [6].

The two genes involved in breast and ovarian cancer, called *BRCA1* and *BRCA2*, belong to the group of tumour-suppressor genes, are transmitted in an autosomal-dominant way and encode proteins that are involved in DNA repair pathways [7].

So far, hundreds of different mutations have been reported in *BRCA1* and *BRCA2*, with deleterious frameshift and missense mutations from variants of unknown functional significance and polymorphisms [8].

Epidemiology of Ovarian Cancer and of *BRCA* Mutations in Hereditary Ovarian Cancer

A large amount of epidemiologic research focusing on hereditary ovarian cancers (HOC) target on epithelial ovarian cancers because they are the predominant subtype; the highest age-adjusted incidence rates are detected in developed parts of the world, including North America and Western and Northern Europe, with rates in these areas exceeding 10 per 100,000 [9].

Practically, all benign and malignant ovarian tumours derive from one of three cell types: epithelial cells, stromal cells and germ cells;

in developed countries, more than 90 % of malignant ovarian tumours are epithelial in origin, 5–6 % of tumours constitute sex cord-stromal tumours and 2–3 % are germ cell tumours [10, 11].

The incidence of ovarian cancer increases with age, with a median age at diagnosis of 63 years; more than 80 % of ovarian cancers occur after age 45 years [12].

One of the most considerable risk factors for ovarian cancer is a family history of the disease: it is estimated that approximately 7 % of women with ovarian cancer have a positive family history of this disease. The first-degree relatives of ovarian cancer probands have a threefold to sevenfold increased risk, particularly if multiple relatives are affected and at an early age at onset [13].

Three clinical manifestations of hereditary ovarian cancer have been identified: site-specific ovarian cancer, hereditary breast and/or ovarian cancer (HBOC) mostly due to *BRCA1* and *BRCA2* gene mutations and Lynch syndrome, formerly known as hereditary nonpolyposis colorectal cancer (HNPCC) syndrome.

On these data, a subset of ovarian cancers occurs as part of a hereditary cancer syndrome that is inherited in an autosomal-dominant pattern. The majority of hereditary ovarian cancers can be attributed to mutations in the *BRCA1* and *BRCA2* genes, located on chromosomes 17 and 13, respectively [14].

The prevalence of *BRCA* mutations in the general population is assessed to be approximately 0.1 %. Generally, mutations in highly penetrant genes account for 10–15 % of epithelial ovarian cancers; in various populations over the world, founder mutations have been found [13, 14].

Women with a *BRCA1* mutation have an 85 % risk of developing breast cancer, a 60 % risk of ovarian cancer by age 70 and an increased risk of colon cancer. Those with mutations of the *BRCA2* gene have a lower cancer risk, but, in addition to being a causal gene of familial breast and ovarian cancer, the *BRCA2* gene is also involved in Fanconi anaemia, subtype B and familial pancreatic cancer [15].

In every case, it is important to identify population founder mutations and other recurrent mutations in each geographical area because they simplify genetic testing and facilitates counselling due to a better knowledge of the risk associated to mutation. The reported frequency of *BRCA* mutations in high-risk HOC families is approximately 50 % [15].

On the other hand, when unselected families are tested in the context of clinical practice, the frequency of *BRCA* mutations is lower, ranging between 15 and 30 % depending on selection criteria and diagnostic methods [8].

Genomic of *BRCA1* Genes

The *BRCA1* (*BR*east *CA*ncer*1*) gene is located on 17q21 and has a total length of about 100 kb. It was isolated in 1994 by Wiseman, Skolnick and their co-workers.

This gene consists of 24 exons, and the coding region starts at the middle of exon 2; the size of the molecular RNA (mRNA) is 7.8 kb, and *BRCA1* expression depends on the cell cycle and increases during the G1 to S phase.

The gene product of *BRCA1* is a nuclear phosphorylated protein that consists of 1,863 amino acids with a molecular weight of 220 kDa; the protein is phosphorylated in a cell cycle-dependent manner, it undergoes hyperphosphorylation during the S phase and is dephosphorylated after the M phase [16, 17]. These observations suggest a role of *BRCA1* in cell cycle regulation as experimentally demonstrated in vivo and in vitro [18].

A RING-finger domain is present in the N-terminal region; two *BRCA1* C-terminal (BRCT) domains, also found in cell cycle checkpoint DNA repair proteins, are present in the C-terminal region. BRCT domain was found to interact with phosphorylated peptides with a role in cell cycle control [19, 20].

BRCA1 is believed to contribute to the maintenance of chromosomal stability, since *BRCA1-deficient* cultured cells show decreased cell growth and hypersensitivity to ionizing radiation, resulting in DNA damage associated with chromosomal abnormalities such as breaks and aneuploidy [21].

BRCA1 has also a role in the regulation of gene expression. It acts as a coactivator in *p53*-dependent transcription and as a ligand-dependent and independent transcriptional repressor of the oestrogen receptor alpha (ERalpha) [22–24].

Genomic of *BRCA2* Genes

The *BRCA2* gene is located on 13q12.3; it has a total length of 70 kb and was isolated in 1995. It consists of 27 exons with a translational start sites in exon 2. The size of the transcription product is approximately 11.5 kb.

The expression of *BRCA2* is high in thymus and testis and relatively high in mammary gland and ovary. The expression of *BRCA2* is cell cycle dependent.

BRCA2 is a nuclear protein that has a molecular weight of 384 kDa; it consists of 3,418 amino acids with eight repetitive units (BRC motifs).

The sequence of *BRCA2* protein shares no homology with that of *BRCA1* protein; however, the *BRCA2* gene is similar to the *BRCA1* gene in terms of structure and expression, suggesting for both genes a common role in the control of cell proliferation and differentiation [25].

BRCA2-deficient cell lines are hypersensitive to drugs causing DNA double-strand breaks and to DNA cross-linking agents; these cell lines are considered to have abnormalities in the DNA repair of double-strand breaks.

BRCA2 binds to the DNA repair protein Rad51 at the BRC repeat regions and contributes to the maintenance of chromosomal stability and to homologous recombination [26].

Another function of *BRCA2* is transcriptional regulation; Marmorstein et al. demonstrated that *BRCA2* interacts with *p53* in vivo and inhibits its transcriptional activity [27].

Carcinogenesis in *BRCA2*-mutated cells appears to be similar to that in *BRCA1*-mutated cells [21].

The Role of Genetics in Hereditary Ovarian Cancer

For ovarian cancer it is estimated that approximately 10 % of cases seem to be related to germline *BRCA1* and *BRCA2* genes; the risk of cancer related to *BRCA* germline mutations is variable and it derives on the type of mutation and also on the population where the risk has been studied.

The risk of ovarian cancer is slightly higher for *BRCA1* than for *BRCA2*, of 40 and of 25 %, respectively [28].

Families with clear autosomal-dominant inheritance of ovarian cancer, but without apparent excess of breast cancer are defined at risk for HOC [12].

Three distinct clinical patterns of cancer have been noted in the families of women with ovarian cancer [14, 15]:

- Ovarian cancer in association with breast cancer
- Ovarian cancer alone
- Ovarian cancer in association with cancers of the colon, rectum, endometrium, stomach, urothelium and pancreas, the HNPCC syndrome or "Lynch II" syndrome.

The identification of the genes that predispose to ovarian cancer has gone a long way towards explaining the patterns of cancers seen in families. Nevertheless, various tumours are related with *BRCA* mutations: colorectal cancer in *BRCA1* mutation carriers (relative risk of 4) and prostate cancer in both *BRCA1* and *BRCA2* mutation carriers (relative risk 3). Other types of tumours are mainly associated to *BRCA2* mutation: male breast cancer, melanoma, laryngeal and pancreatic tumours [28, 29].

The ovarian cancers in families with *BRCA* mutations are mainly serous adenocarcinomas, often showing papillary changes. Epithelial ovarian adenocarcinomas that occur in a hereditary setting due to transmitted germline *BRCA1* mutations are predominantly of the serious type, with under presentation of mucinous and border line tumours [10, 11].

When prevention measures are to be discussed with patients or otherwise healthy women, authors have to consider the individual risk and take special care with new *BRCA* mutations discovered in families with a very low number of breast cancer cases [30].

Basing on the expensive costs of genetic testing, who also creates expectations in the families, when BRCA testing is planned, a prior calculation of probability of finding a mutation should be done [20].

Full sequencing is considered the standard technique for diagnosis, in view that in about 15 % of these families, rearrangements have been described. Direct sequencing is currently the main technique used for sequence analysis. A set of primers is designed for the amplification by polymerase chain reaction (PCR) of the DNA extracted from lymphocytes or cancer tissues; the complete nucleotide sequence is then performed on a DNA auto sequencer [32].

Multiple Genes Involved in Ovarian Cancer

Ovarian cancer shows a high mortality rate because it is often only diagnosed when it is in an advanced stage. Great effort is to identify screening and diagnostic strategies that improve the likelihood of early diagnosis. In the last few years, there has been an improvement of the knowledge base relating to the molecular biology of ovarian cancer.

Genes such as *BRCA1*, *BRCA2*, *TP53*, *ATM*, *SKT11*, *PTEN*, *PTCH*, *MLH1*, *MSH2*, *KRAS/BRAF*, *HER2/neu* and many others have been associated with increased risk of breast and ovarian cancer as part of other cancer syndromes [33].

Upregulation or downregulation of these genes can be determined on the basis of a statistically significant increase or decrease in level of the biomarker.

The morphologic and molecular genetic data support different pathways of development for each of the major histological types of ovarian carcinoma [34]:

1. Low- and high-grade serous carcinoma most probably arise via different pathways, the former progressing along an adenoma–borderline tumour–carcinoma sequence involving mutations in *KRAS* and *BRAF* and the latter from alterations in surface epithelial inclusion glands involving mutations of *TP53* and dysfunction of *BRCA1* and/or *BRCA2*.
2. Mucinous carcinomas most probably arise via an adenoma–borderline tumour–carcinoma sequence with mutations of *KRAS*.
3. Endometrioid carcinomas arise from endometriosis with mutations of *CTNNB1* (the gene encoding b-catenin) and *PTEN*.
4. The genetic alterations in clear cell carcinoma are the least investigated but also support an origin from endometriosis.

The Role of Epigenetics and of Cancer Genetic Counselling Units

Mutations in *BRCA1* and *BRCA2* genes explain the greatest part of hereditary breast and ovarian cancers; epigenetic events, such as methylation of the promoter region, but not mutations, are considered to cause inactivation of *BRCA1*. Abnormalities of *BRCA1/2*, caused by epigenetic influencing factors, can often be implicated in carcinogenesis not only in hereditary breast and ovarian cancer but also in its sporadic forms [32].

There are several models that calculate the risk of cancer based on personal conditions or familial history; one of these is indicated in Table 7.2.

Testing for genes related to hereditary cancer allows the selection of individuals who will really benefit of prevention measures in such high prevalent diseases. The majority of these genes belong to the category of tumour-suppressor genes, so a second genetic hit is always needed for cancer developing [15].

Epigenetics, described as the factors that modulate the penetrance of a genetic disease, play an important role in hereditary cancer predisposition. Due to the complexity of genetics and clinical management of the hereditary cancers, all individuals with risk should be seen at

Table 7.2 The common indications to test potential patients with suspicion of hereditary ovarian cancer (HOC)

A family with two or more ovarian cancer, at least two between first-degree relatives
Two first-degree relatives affected by breast cancer and ovarian cancer, respectively
Breast cancer and ovarian cancer in the same patient

Adapted from Tinelli et al. [1]

specialized group of researchers, so-called Cancer Genetic Counselling Units: the clinicians that work in these units should have special training in genetic counselling, cancer genetics and hereditary cancer management [35].

Cancer genetic counselling is a communication process in which genetics, medical and psychological questions related to hereditary cancer risk development and prevention options are discussed with the individuals and families [36].

A collaborative model between counsellor and patient is preferred, and all the following points should be included in the informed consent process: options for risk estimation if genetic testing is not done, information on the specific test (accuracy, limitations), interpretation of all possible test results, implications of results for the individual and family, confidentiality issues, risk of psychological distress, options for care after testing and limitations [36].

Some ethical and legal issues arise in the global processes of cancer genetic counselling that must be recognized and taken in account. Several questions still do not have answers in this field [35–37].

Indications for testing for *BRCA* mutations should be based, in every case, on the prevalence in the own population, previous reported frequencies in unselected families from the same geographical and also in cost-effectiveness criteria. Nonetheless, it would be inappropriate to dismiss the potential benefits of genetic counselling as a reaction to sporadic uncritical application of genetic testing [38].

Genetic Tests in High-Risk Subject for Hereditary Ovarian Cancer

The recent progress of research into the molecular basis of cancer in general and hereditary cancer particularly has provided more insight into the aetiology of hereditary cancer; regarding the methods of genetic risk calculation, there are several models that can be used to do that [39].

Mutation analysis of the *BRCA* genes should always be performed through the Regional Clinical Genetics departments, after appropriate counselling about the implications of a positive result for the individual and their family [38].

Diagnostic genetic testing can be offered in the following circumstances:

- The pedigree falls into the high-risk category.
- A living, affected member is available to give a blood sample for analysis.

A computer program, called BRCAPRO, is available to test positive women to risk assessment primarily based on the family history of ovarian cancers.

It applies Bayesian analysis to calculate the probability of mutation carrier for a given individual based on family history (number of breast or ovarian cancers, or age at diagnosis of cancer, presence of bilateral or male cancer and Ashkenazi origin) [40].

Since a mutation cannot be always found, the false-negative rate of the test should be considered. A large variety of methods is currently available for the detection of mutations [41].

As stated before, there is no one technique that is ideally suited to a complete analysis of *BRCA1* and/or *BRCA2*. Some techniques are simple to perform but not very sensitive, whereas others may be very sensitive but laborious and, therefore, usually expensive [42].

The most commonly used techniques include:

- Direct (semiautomated) sequencing (DS); this is generally considered the gold standard for mutation detection because of its high sensitivity, but the disadvantages are the time consuming and laborious procedures involved, although the availability of semiautomated, fluorescent sequencing systems has increased the feasibility of this method for large-scale (clinical) use.
- Allele-specific oligonucleotide analysis (ASO).
- Single-strand conformation polymorphism analysis (SSCP/SSCA) and heteroduplex analysis (HA); both techniques are easy to perform and relatively quick. Compared to DS, the sensitivity is much lower at a reputed 60–80 %.
- Conformational sensitive gel electrophoresis (CSGE); this method has an increased sensitivity compared to HA and SSCP, but is more labour intensive.

- (Constant) denaturing gradient gel electrophoresis (DGGE/CDGE); this technique, which is based on the melting behaviour of the DNA double helix, is more sensitive than SSCP; however, the technique only detects differences between both alleles; therefore, additional techniques are required to identify the precise nature of the mutation. Another disadvantage of all techniques mentioned thus far is that it may be difficult to distinguish between benign polymorphisms and pathogenic mutations.
- The protein truncation test (PTT) overcomes the previous problem by detecting nonsense and frameshift mutations that result in a stop codon by visualizing a truncated protein in an in vitro transcription–translation assay.
- Southern analysis (for genomic deletions); recently, specific founder mutations have been identified that consist of the loss of large fragments of coding sequence. Such genomic alterations can be detected by Southern analysis in specific populations, which have a high-expected frequency of such alterations [39–42].

Diagnostic genetic testing is still far from straightforward and the reasons for this are the following [43]:

- There are more than hundreds of different mutations within the *BRCA* genes and each family will have its own mutation.
- It is still not possible to look through the whole of these genes with current technology; therefore, the mutation cannot be found in every family whose cancer is linked to a *BRCA* gene.
- Testing is time consuming and expensive.

Even in research laboratories undertaking extensive screening, mutations are found in less than 50 % of families with two or more women with ovarian cancer [40–43].

Genetic testing offers the following benefits: identification of high-risk individuals who will benefit from the initiation of recommended cancer risk management; identification of noncarriers in families with a known mutation, who do not need to have rigorous cancer screening and would be considered at "general population risk"; education in early detection and prevention strategies; and perhaps relief of anxiety through increasing the understanding of medical options. However, it also has its risks and limitations, including its inability to detect all mutations, the continued risk of sporadic cancer, the unproven efficacy of some interventions and the possibility of psychosocial or economic harm [44].

The goal of genetic counselling is to ensure that women have been sufficiently educated regarding inherited breast/ovarian cancer to make informed decisions concerning genetic testing and available preventive and treatment options. The majority of published studies have found that genetic counselling is effective in increasing knowledge and awareness of cancer risk and of the consequences of genetic testing [45–47].

Pedigree Information in Family with Hereditary Ovarian Cancer

As extensive, a family tree as possible should be taken including all second-degree relatives (grandparents, aunts and uncles) and third-degree relatives (cousins). It is important to take the history from the paternal side, as well as the maternal side as the genes involved are equally likely to be inherited from the paternal side of the family [48].

High-risk families are those which fulfil the following criteria [30]:

- The family contains two or more individuals with ovarian cancer at any age who are first-degree relatives.
- The family contains one individual with ovarian cancer at any age and one individual with breast cancer diagnosed under 50 years who are first-degree relatives.
- The family contains one individual with ovarian cancer at any age and two individuals with breast cancer diagnosed under 60 years who are connected by first-degree relationships.
- The family contains an affected individual with one of the known ovarian cancer predisposing genes.
- The family contains three individuals with colorectal cancer with at least one case diagnosed before 50 years and one case of ovarian cancer connected by first-degree relationships.

There are problems associated with using pedigree information to assess risk.

Many families nowadays are not large enough to reach the above criteria, and families with a preponderance of males may also not reach the criteria, despite carrying an ovarian cancer susceptibility gene. However, it still remains the most useful tool for assessing risk [49]. Armel et al. evaluated the demographics of the nonresponder population to assess genetic risk estimates for mutations in the *BRCA1* and *BRCA2* genes and genetic testing eligibility as compared to a responder population of patients who completed a mailed family history questionnaire. A total of 430 pedigrees were obtained, 215 from nonresponders and 215 from responders. Results of this study indicate that 69 % of nonresponders were either unreachable by telephone (42 %), declined an appointment (19 %) or were previously seen in another centre for a genetic counselling visit (8 %). Additionally, results indicate that nonresponders are less likely to be eligible for genetic testing (40 %) as compared to responders (57 %) ($p=0.0004$). Together these data shed light on a population of patients for which limited information exists and suggest that we question how and to what extent clinics should pursue nonresponders, particularly in light of global reductions in health care funding [50].

The Risk Management of Hereditary Ovarian Cancer

An accurate estimation of the risk of ovarian cancer is important in counselling these women, since important decisions have to be made during a crucial phase of life, the childbearing years. Risk assessment and counselling are based on penetrance estimates of ovarian cancer at certain ages, which have been investigated by many studies worldwide [51]. Unfortunately, those penetrance studies show varying results, due to the choice of the population studied and the cancer incidence. Estimates of the average penetrance up to 70 years of age are 40 % (95 % CI, 35–46 %) for *BRCA1* and 18 % (95 % CI, 13–23 %) for *BRCA2* mutations carriers [52].

Mortality for ovarian cancer is generally high because women typically present with late-stage disease, when the overall 5-year relative survival rate is 45 % [53].

Despite success in pinpointing precursor lesions in cervical and uterine malignancies, little progress has been made in identifying premalignant conditions in the ovary: they rest in ultrasonography and in cancer antigen 125 (CA-125) serum level and in the majority of ovarian cancers; no transition area from normal to dysplastic to malignant epithelium can be identified [54].

Difficulties involved in monitoring the ovaries in high-risk subjects are complicated: biopsy is hampered by the ovaries' location deep in the pelvis and imaging; via ultrasound and computed tomography is helpful for determining ovarian size and morphology, but cannot distinguish more subtle lesions such as ovarian dysplasia or inclusion cysts [55].

Even in high-risk populations, traditional approaches to screening such as pelvic exam, ultrasound and CA-125 are hampered by their poor ability to detect early stage disease and to distinguish benign from malignant neoplasm [56].

Genetic consultation and testing are currently mainstream components of a multidisciplinary, individualized medical evaluation aimed at identification of individuals at risk for hereditary ovarian cancer syndromes [44].

Various options for risk management of hereditary ovarian cancer are available: surveillance, prophylactic surgeries and chemoprevention [57].

Lifestyle factors might be important in reducing penetrance or delaying the onset of disease. Although there is not enough scientific evidence for unequivocal recommendations, they should be included for discussion in the counselling process. All of them should be discussed for each woman at risk for HOC, including those that refused BRCA testing or families with uninformative result [58].

It is not possible to make strong recommendations for each option because their effectiveness is not always well known and depends of many factors, such the risk of cancer in each family and a variety of women/patient conditions. Acceptance also

Table 7.3 Clinical and instrumental surveillance for high-risk patients in our department

Surveillance for BRCA1/2 mutation carriers for ovarian cancer/peritoneal tumour at gynaecological examination
Examination interval, every 3 months
Gynaecological examination
Transvaginal ultrasonography
CA 125
Optional examinations and treatments proposed to patients
Pelvic computerized tomography or magnetic resonance imaging (annual)
Positron emission tomography (annual)
Laparoscopic prophylactic oophorectomy

Adapted from Tinelli et al. [1]

depends on factors like patient age, reproductive desire and personal beliefs [43].

Women that assist to a process of genetic counselling for HOC make their decisions based more on personal conditions than in the risk concept, and that must be taken in account for clinicians and counsellors [42].

Surveillance recommendations have been based on expert opinion or by singular institute recommendation (see Table 7.3); surveillance in high-risk patients is critical, both for patients with a family history or personal history of cancer, who have negative genetic test results and for mutation carriers with positive genetic results [59].

However, preliminary data from ongoing observational studies do support, in part, the current clinical practice, even if the surveillance for ovarian cancer is difficult, owing to the difficulty in detecting early stage tumours. Because the ovary faces the abdominal cavity, peritoneal dissemination can occur even at an early stage [56].

Despite enormous effort, there is no proof that routine screening for ovarian cancer in either the high-risk or general populations with serum markers, sonograms or pelvic examinations decreases mortality. Further evaluation is needed to determine whether any novel biomarkers, or panels of markers, have clinical utility in early detection. Prospective clinical trials have to be designed and completed prior to offering of any of these new diagnostic tests. CA-125 is currently the only biomarker recommended for monitoring of therapy as well as detection of recurrence [60].

Annual rectovaginal pelvic examination, measurement of serum carbohydrate antigen CA-125 levels and transvaginal ultrasound (TVU) are recommended for women with a high risk of ovarian cancer. However, data demonstrating that the screening of high-risk women reduces mortality from ovarian cancers are lacking [61].

One study has recommended that TVU with colour Doppler studies and the monitoring of serum CA-125 levels should be performed in *BRCA1* mutation carriers aged 25–35 years or older, but the benefits of such a programme remain to be established [62].

Chemoprevention for women with *BRCA* mutations is still controversial, since hormonal agents, such as progestins and selective oestrogen receptor modulators, have differing effects on breast, uterine and ovarian tissues.

Critical requirement for successful chemoprevention trials is identification of a high-risk population for ovarian cancer. Assessments of lifetime ovarian cancer risk for women who carry the mutations are still being defined: currently they range from 16 to 60 % *for BRCA1* and 10 to 27 % for *BRCA2* [30, 53, 57].

This pool of potential subjects is generally highly motivated to enrol in chemoprevention trials and to remain compliant with a given preventive therapy to identify methods that reduce cancer risk for themselves and their families. The most popular chemopreventive agents are discussed in the following section.

Women diagnosed with a *BRCA1/2* mutation are given several options to reduce their risk of dying of ovarian cancer. One is to choose screening, with the main objective of identifying ovarian cancer in early stage, to improve the prognosis and reduce morbidity and mortality. Available screening tests for ovarian cancer include bimanual pelvic examination, TVU and measurements of serum CA-125 [51].

There are several criteria for the definition of an abnormal TVU to predict ovarian malignancy. According to the Sassone criteria, in premenopausal women only simple cysts of more than 6 cm need further investigation. The main limitation to the use of TVU as a screening tool is the high false-positive rate, mainly in premenopausal women. Due to frequent follicle cyst formation and persist follicles in premenopausal ovaries, criteria for further investigation need to be described carefully and have a large effect on numbers needed to operate to find one ovarian cancer.

In postmenopausal women, the specificity of TVU is higher than in premenopausal women due to the absence of follicle cyst formation. However, even in postmenopausal women adnexal lesions are frequently found. Altered blood vessels resistance in malignant compared to benign ovarian cysts visualized by Doppler imaging was hoped to improve the identification of malignant ovarian tumours; its role in ovarian cancer screening has not been firmly established [51].

CA-125 is expressed by coelomic and Mullerian epithelia, but the surface epithelium of normal ovaries does not express CA-125. The finding that CA-125 is a serum marker for ovarian cancer gave the promise of a biomarker for monitoring of (early) ovarian cancer. However, as ovarian cancer presents late and spreads early, the sensitivity of serum CA-125 is very low for the early detection of ovarian cancer, since only 25–50 % of the women with a stage I ovarian tumour have an elevated serum CA-125 level at the time of diagnosis. In addition, especially in premenopausal women, an elevated CA-125 level is not very specific for the diagnosis of ovarian cancer, including menstruation, pregnancy, endometriosis, uterine leiomyomas, infectious disease as well as in other malignancies. The application of algorithms for calculating the risk of ovarian cancer algorithm in healthy postmenopausal women as well as in women at increased risk may be useful in aiding the interpretation of CA-125 and ultrasound results. However, the endpoint of these studies should not be the detection of ovarian cancer but deaths attributed to ovarian cancer [63–66].

It is therefore of the utmost importance to develop new circulating (panels of) biomarkers which are specific for (early) ovarian cancer and specifically in mutation carriers to improve traditional screening results. More than 30 serum markers have been evaluated alone and in combination with CA-125, and mathematical techniques are being developed to analyse combinations of marker levels to improve sensitivity and specificity [51].

Chemopreventive Agents in Hereditary Ovarian Cancer Population Trials

The oral contraceptive pill (OCP) is one agent that has already emerged as an effective means of reducing epithelial ovarian cancer risk: abundant evidence supports a 50 % reduction in epithelial ovarian cancer risk with 5 years of OCP use and a 30 % reduction with ever use and reduced risk persists for at least 10 years after cessation of OCP use [67, 68]. Use of oral contraceptives (OCs) is associated with a reduction in ovarian cancer risk of 40–50 % after 3 years' cumulative use. Long-term use of OCs has been associated with a slight increase in risk of breast cancer among *BRCA1* mutation carriers; however, there is no measurable increased risk of breast cancer with OC use (in other high-risk women) of 5 or fewer years.

Advantages of chemoprevention of ovarian cancer with OC use are that it is well tolerated and inexpensive, does not affect future fertility and leaves other options open.

Disadvantages include the adverse effects of OCs, including thromboembolic risk, the continued need to screen for ovarian cancer and the possible increased risk of breast cancer with use exceeding 5 years [44].

Retinoids, the natural and synthetic analogue of vitamin A, represent another class of agents with potential application as chemopreventive agents for ovarian cancer. Toxicity associated with natural retinoids frequently limits their use; consequently, synthetic vitamin A analogues have been developed [69].

Fenretinide has emerged as one of the most promising alternatives to natural retinoids, even if fenretinide's protective effect did not persist after discontinuation of therapy [70].

Retinoid derivatives containing heteroatoms in a cyclic ring, termed heteroarotenoids, are emerging as a class of compounds with structural similarity to fenretinide but a higher therapeutic index [71].

Heteroarotenoids effectively induced cellular differentiation, growth inhibition and apoptosis in organotypic ovarian cancer cultures; while new retinoid derivatives such as heteroarotenoids are being characterized, the mechanism of fenretinide activity in ovarian cancer cells is still unclear. Thus, data are accumulating to suggest that retinoids may be effective chemopreventive agents for ovarian cancer, but larger clinical trials are required to effectively evaluate fenretinide as a chemopreventive agent [72].

Ovarian cancer mortality has been shown to be inversely proportional to sunlight exposure, a primary source of vitamin D; receptors for 1,25-dihydroxyvitamin D3 (calcitriol) are documented in ovarian cancer tumour specimens and cell lines, and, further, calcitriol causes a decrease in proto-oncogene c-*myc* expression and leads to ovarian cancer cell growth inhibition [73].

Vitamin D therefore requires further investigation, as it may represent a useful chemopreventive strategy for ovarian cancer [74].

Anti-inflammatory agents, such as salicylate analgesics, may be an effective option for ovarian cancer chemoprevention [75].

Large epidemiologic cohorts have demonstrated that local inflammatory processes, including talc and/or asbestos exposures, endometriosis and pelvic inflammatory disease, are risk factors for ovarian cancer [76].

In contrast, several case–control studies failed to show a statistical association between use of anti-inflammatory agents and ovarian cancer risk [77]; however, they reported a decreased risk of ovarian cancer with acetaminophen, another over-the-counter analgesic [78].

Molecular studies indicate that one group of anti-inflammatory agents, cyclooxygenase (COX)-2 inhibitors, represent a primary candidate for ovarian cancer chemoprevention [79, 80].

While COX-1 is ubiquitously expressed, COX-2 is an early response gene that generally maintains low-level expression until induced by growth factors and carcinogens [79].

Preliminary work demonstrates that COX-2 is over expressed in ovarian cancer specimens and in ovarian cancer cell lines; notably, COX-2 inhibitors inhibit ovarian cancer cell growth and induce apoptosis [80].

Thus, clinically available COX-2 inhibitors represent a promising chemopreventive candidate for several epithelial malignancies, including ovarian carcinoma [81].

Peroxisome proliferator-activated receptor (PPAR)γ ligands represent another clinically available class of compounds with potential application to ovarian cancer chemoprevention [82].

The combination of several clinically available agents, as retinoids, COX-2 inhibitors, PPAR ligands and calcitriol, potentially in combination with OCPs, offers exciting potential for reducing ovarian cancer mortality through chemoprevention [83, 84].

All these agents are reassumed in Table 7.4.

Unfortunately, the design of any trial evaluating chemopreventive effects of pharmacological agents against ovarian cancer must recognize the significant role that gynaecologic prophylactic surgery plays in reducing ovarian cancer risk [85].

The Promising Role of PARP Inhibitors in the Treatment of Epithelial Ovarian Cancer

Poly(ADP-ribose) polymerase-1 (PARP-1) is an important novel target in cancer therapy. This enzyme is central in the repair of single-stranded breaks in DNA via the base excision repair pathway. Drugs which inhibit PARP are emerging as a promising new class of anticancer agents mainly effective against tumours which have lost homologous recombination (HR) through loss of functional *BRCA1* and *BRCA2*. PARP inhibitors potentially represent a major breakthrough for patients with hereditary *BRCA*-associated cancers [86].

Although the with efficacy of platinum-based chemotherapy, over 75 % of women with stage III/IV epithelial ovarian cancer (EOC) at last relapse and die from their disease.

Table 7.4 Chemopreventive agents in high-risk patients for hereditary ovarian cancers

Agent	Potential mechanisms	Advantages
Oral contraceptive pill (OCP)	Ovulation suppression Reduction of LH, FSH levels Progestin-mediated apoptosis	Largely prescribed in the general population Substantial ovarian cancer risk reduction, already demonstrated in scientific evidences
Retinoids and heteroarotenoids	Alter expression and/or activate retinoid receptors Increase production of reactive oxygen species	Currently used in treatment of leukaemia and head and neck
1,25-dihydroxyvitamin D3	Activate vitamin D receptors Decrease c-myc expression	A vitamin derivative frequently taken in the general population
COX-2 inhibitors	Reduce activity of COX-2 enzyme Induce apoptosis and reduce angiogenesis	Currently used in the treatment of arthritis
Peroxisome proliferator-activated receptor (PPARγ)	Activate transcription factor PPARγ Affect target genes involved in cellular differentiation Increase production of reactive oxygen species	Currently used in the treatment of Type II DM

Adapted from Tinelli et al. [1]

Traditional cytotoxics topotecan and liposomal doxorubicin prove limited efficacy in women with platinum-resistant EOC and are associated with considerable toxicity. Over the last few years, it has become evident that in cells which have lost *BRCA1* or *BRCA2*, components of a second DNA repair pathway, HR, are particularly sensitive to PARP inhibition.

At present, the treatment of patients with *BRCA*-associated EOC is the same to those with sporadic EOC. However, even prior to the emergence of the PARP inhibitors, data suggested that cancers associated with *BRCA* mutations responded differently to chemotherapy. Tan et al. compared 22 *BRCA*-positive patients with EOC to 44 nonhereditary EOC controls in a matched case–control study. They found that *BRCA-positive* patients have higher response rates to first-line platinum-based treatment (81.8 % versus 43.2 %, $P=.004$), subsequent lines of platinum-based treatments (second line, 91.7 % versus 40.9 %, $P=.004$), longer tumour-free intervals between relapses and improved overall survival (8.4 versus 2.9 years, $P<.002$) [87]. This data suggests that different strategies may be required in this group of women.

PARP inhibitors appear to be particularly potent in patients who have defects in DNA repair. As most *BRCA1/2* carriers have one normal allele, the hope was that inhibition of PARP would be selective for tumour cells.

Two preclinical papers demonstrated the sensitivity of *BRCA1*- and *BRCA2*-deficient cell lines to PARP inhibition [88, 89]. They concluded that *BRCA2*-deficient cells were sensitive to PARP inhibition and that monotherapy with one of these agents could selectively kill cancer cells. A number of PARP inhibitors have entered the clinic in both intravenous and oral formulations. The four which are furthest along in terms of development are AGO14699 (Pfizer), AZD2281 (AstraZeneca), ABT-888 (Abbott) and BSI-201 (BI Par), and all four of these compounds demonstrate profound inhibition of PARP-1 [86].

Prophylactic Surgery in Hereditary Ovarian Cancer

Several gynaecologic procedures appear to influence the risk for ovarian cancer; it is well established that among high-risk women, bilateral prophylactic oophorectomy reduces ovarian cancer risk by at least 90 % [90].

The preferred method for preventing the HOC in high-risk patients is performing a prophylactic oophorectomy by using video laparoscopy [91].

Miller et al. reviewed factors associated with uptake of risk-reducing salpingo-oophorectomy (RRSO) by women at increased hereditary risk for ovarian cancer, as well as quality-of-life issues following surgery [92]. A number of factors have been identified that are positively associated with RRSO uptake; these include demographic variables (older age, having had children, lower educational level) and medical variables (*BRCA* mutation carrier status, family history of ovarian cancer, personal history of breast cancer-related distress). Postsurgery, the majority of women are satisfied with their decision to undergo RRSO and report positive quality of life (QOL)-related changes, including reduced perceived ovarian cancer risk, reduced cancer-related distress and an increased sense of control. Women who report the most surgery-related problems (e.g. impact of surgery on sexual activity and hot flashes) were, for the most part, premenopausal at the time of the surgery and did not take hormone-replacement therapy (HRT).

Women at increased putative hereditary risk for ovarian cancer are faced with complex information that needs to be cognitively and emotionally processed, in order to make a high-quality decision about their risk management options [92].

The guidelines for ovarian cancer risk management now recommend RRSO at the completion of childbearing or by age 35–40 [93].

For premenopausal women who test *BRCA1/2* positive, RRSO has been associated with an 85–90 % reduction in breast cancer risk, provided the surgery is done before the age of 50 [92].

The characteristics of *BRCA1* gene therapy may have the potential to prevent the progression of ovarian cancer, and enzyme/prodrug gene therapy is the efficient approach to do so. Both the efficacy and technique of prophylactic oophorectomy and gene therapy protocol for developed cancer will be presented since, at present, there is no evidence for a reduction in the mortality rate as a result of early cancer detection [94].

The opinion of genetic counsellor or the clinician will of course influence patient choices. In all cases the patient's decision must be respected, even if prophylactic surgery must be discussed as a first option; however, to perform such surgeries at early ages is not easily accepted for at-risk women [91].

For ovarian cancer, the surveillance protocols are less effective, so oophorectomy has become a strong prevention option for women with *BRCA1* and some *BRCA2* mutations, especially in families with a high ovarian cancer penetrance [95].

Table 7.5 Proposed criteria for prophylactic bilateral salpingo-oophorectomy (PBSO) in our department

Age >40 years, almost one son/daughter
BRCA1 (BRCA2) mutation carriers (>25 % lifetime risk for ovarian cancer)
Life expectancy not significantly reduced by the presence of severe illness
Surgical option discussed in a multidisciplinary setting (included psychological consultation)
Information about incomplete protection from subsequent cancer development
Laparoscopic approach
HRT proposed in premenopausal women (to age 50 years, then consider a SERM)
Postsurgical psychological support offered

Adapted from Tinelli et al. [1]

There is also a lack of detailed guidelines on surveillance protocols in high-risk subjects. The National Institutes of Health (NIH) Consensus Development Panel on Ovarian Cancer recommends TVU and CA-125 assessments for the screening of *BRCA* mutation carriers every 6–12 months, starting at the age of 35 years. In interdisciplinary genetics clinics in Germany, biannual TVU and pelvic examination are recommended starting at the age of 25 years [96].

So, minimally invasive prophylactic surgeries, such as laparoscopic oophorectomy, should be always discussed with HOC high-risk women, and they must be always followed by an informed personal decision on proposed criteria for its consideration, as proposed in our department in Table 7.5. In general, oophorectomy reduces the risk of ovarian cancer, although peritoneal recurrences can be observed in 0.5–2 % of the patients who underwent this procedure [30].

Taking into account the lethality of ovarian cancer even in early stage disease, oophorectomy must be always discussed with women with *BRCA* mutations, also in patients and families with an unclassified variant of the *BRCA1* and/or *BRCA2* (numbers 113705 and 600185, respectively), a prominent issue for genetic counsellors and oncologists.

In fact, about one third of the genetic variants in *BRCA1* and 50 % of those found in *BRCA2* are considered genetic variants of unknown clinical significance, also known as unclassified variants, because of the uncertainty about their cancer risks; presymptomatic testing is not possible in families with an unknown clinical significant variants, and surveillance can only be based upon the severity of the cancer family history [97].

The greatest gain is obtained if surgery is performed at early ages; however, this benefit has to be balanced with the reproductive desire and the hormonal deprivation consequences [98].

Furthermore, studies have demonstrated that RRSO is strongly associated with reductions in the risk of breast, ovarian and fallopian tube cancers and should provide guidance to women in planning cancer risk-reduction strategies [99]; the risk reduction from these surgical procedures seems to last for at least 10–15 years, which goes against the hypothesis that screening bias (due to selective removal of sub clinical ovarian tumours) can explain the protective effect against ovarian cancer [100].

A Probable Alternative: Bilateral Salpingectomy with Ovarian Retention

For women who have completed childbearing but who are not ready for RRSO, bilateral salpingectomy with ovarian retention (BSOR) might be a temporary measure while definitive risk-reducing surgery is being contemplated [101].

This procedure is based on the risk reduction of both sporadic and hereditary ovarian cancer observed after bilateral tubal ligation.

However, this risk reduction has not been observed consistently. Although Narod et al. [102] showed that bilateral tubal ligation was associated with a 61 % reduction in ovarian cancer risk among *BRCA1* mutation carriers; this observation was not replicated in a larger study.

Tubal ligation rarely is presented as a treatment option among young women who are mutation carriers.

Potential benefits to BSOR as a short-term, intermediate bridge to risk-reducing bilateral oophorectomy (RRBO) include: (1) A proportion of the pelvic serous carcinoma (PSC) risk that would otherwise be experienced by a *BRCA1/2* mutation carrier who declines/defers RRSO might be eliminated for the period before undergoing definitive ovarian cancer risk-reducing surgery by removing the fallopian tubes. Even if we do not know the exact proportion, a review of 11 RRSO series that targeted *BRCA1/2* mutation carriers found that 64 of 94 occult cancers (68 %) originated in the fallopian tubes (range, 43–100 %) [14, 17–21, 30–34]. These data suggest that the risk-reducing impact of bilateral salpingectomy could be considerable. (2) Premature menopause would be postponed temporarily, and the need to consider short-term menopausal hormone therapy (MHT) and its uncertain risks would be avoided, thus decreasing the time during which the patient could undergo acute and chronic oestrogen deficiency symptoms and may be reducing the nononcologic morbidity that is associated with premature menopause. BSOR could be done laparoscopically in most women. This procedure would also provide an earlier opportunity to evaluate the tubes histologically, to assess the ovaries and peritoneal space by direct inspection and to collect peritoneal cytologic and biopsy specimens, if indicated. This approach postpones the difficult and irrevocable decision to undergo premature infertility because the option of assisted reproductive technologies would still be available. The simply knowing one could potentially still get pregnant brings significant emotional benefit.

Despite evidence of the clinical benefit for RRSO, a significant fraction of high-risk women are not prepared to undergo this procedure on completion of reproductive planning. For example, 36 % of the 785 women who knew they were *BRCA* mutation positive at the time they enrolled in GOG-199 (the National Ovarian Cancer Prevention and Early Detection Study) elected an investigational ovarian cancer screening option rather than RRSO [100].

For that reason BSOR would represent an active, potentially empowering treatment strategy that might be acceptable to a significant number of these women. Choosing BSOR simultaneously could reduce both their risk of PSC and their psychologic distress that is related to delaying RRSO. If the risk-reducing effect of tubal ligation is mediated through the prevention of some cancers that truly arise in the ovary, BSOR could produce a larger risk reduction than that anticipated by salpingectomy-related elimination of fallopian tube cancer (FTC) risk. Hypothetically, this is an option, given that similar relative magnitude of tubal ligation effect is seen in the sporadic setting, a context in which FTC is rare. However, an alternative explanation for this phenomenon may be that the advanced stage at which most sporadic ovarian cancers are diagnosed prevents our recognizing those that actually originated in the fallopian tube.

A pilot study of BSOR is currently under consideration by the Gynecologic Oncology Group [101].

Effect of Screening on Ovarian Cancer Mortality

Several controversies exist about the effectiveness of screening for ovarian cancer.

Screening for ovarian cancer with CA-125 and TVU has shown unknown effect on mortality. A recent randomized controlled trail of 78,216 women aged 55–74 years assigned to undergo either annual screening or usual care at ten screening centres across the United States between November 1993 and July 2001. They found no statistically significant reduction in mortality from ovarian cancer in a cohort of women derived from the general population who were screened for ovarian cancer with six annual CA-125 tests and four annual TVU examinations. The mortality rate from ovarian cancer were similar in the two trial groups over the entire period of follow-up, with a modestly greater cause-specific mortality in the intervention group (RR, 1.18; 95 % CI, 0.82–1.71). They conclude that the screening intervention was not effective in reducing mortality caused by ovarian cancer. They also established that in this trial, there was a lack of an observed stage shift (i.e. a decrease in the absolute number of late-stage [III or IV] cases in the intervention group compared with the usual care group is considered to be necessary but not sufficient for a mortality benefit to be realized). This lack of a stage shift suggests the possibility that the two screening modalities used (CA-125 and TVU) with the cutoffs used in the Prostate, Lung, Colorectal and Ovarian (PLCO) trial for screening positivity were not effective in detecting ovarian cancers early enough when the cancers were still in a nonadvanced stage. Some evidence from modelling suggests that ovarian tumours need to be found when they are relatively small, considerably smaller than the current threshold used for TVU (10 cm^3 for cysts) to be in an early stage detection [103].

Generally, it is be used the CA-125 as a diagnostic serum markers of ovarian cancer in early stages, which should not exceed the normal value of 35 U/ml; however, this would be at the expense of more false-positive results. Other approaches to ovarian cancer screening with these same modalities, including the risk of ovarian cancer algorithm, which incorporates longitudinal CA-125 and considers changes over time rather than a single cut point, may be able to detect ovarian cancers earlier and at a reasonable costs in terms of increased false-positive results; however, the benefit of this approach has not been demonstrated.

The risk of ovarian cancer algorithm is currently being evaluated in the randomized UK Collaborative Trial of Ovarian Cancer Screening (UKCTOCS), which is a three-group trial comparing two strategies of screening (specifically, annual CA-125 testing interpreted using the risk of ovarian cancer algorithm with TVU as a second-line test [multimodal group] vs. annual TVU only vs. no intervention). To date, only the results of the prevalence screening from the UK CTOCS have been published. The multimodal group had 34 primary invasive epithelial cancers and 16 were stage I or II (47 %); in the TVU group, 50 % of 24 such cancers were stage I or II. Whether these modalities will produce a stage shift and demonstrate a mortality benefit compared with usual care await further findings.

An additional randomized controlled trial of ovarian cancer screening is the Shizuoka Cohort Study of Ovarian Cancer Screening in Japan. This trial randomized women to undergo either five annual screenings with concurrent TVU and CA-125 or to a usual care control group.

They concluded that annual screening for ovarian cancer as performed in the PLCO trial with simultaneous CA-125 and TVU does not reduce disease-specific mortality in women at average risk for ovarian cancer but does increase invasive medical procedures and associated harms [103].

Concerns About Transmitting the Mutation to Children

The possibility of transmitting a mutation to a child may pose a concern to women carrying a *BRCA1/2* or Lynch syndrome mutation because they have a 50 % chance of conceiving a baby with the same mutation. There are different options available to avoid having a child with the same mutation and accessibility of these options differs across countries. Besides avoiding childbearing, options are pregnancy surrogate and DNA analysis of tissue obtained in early pregnancy by chorionic villous biopsy or amniotic fluid assessment, with an abortion if the fetus is affected. Another option is to perform in vitro fertilization with preimplantation genetic diagnosis (PGD) of retrieved embryos, followed by selection of embryo(s) without a mutation and transfer of a selected embryo to the uterus [51, 104].

Clinical Dilemmas

There are several clinical dilemmas patients want to discuss with their doctor:

- Should I go for genetic testing and what are the consequences?
- How can I reduce the risk of breast cancer? What are the pros and cons of prophylactic surgery and breast cancer screening?
- How can I reduce the risk of ovarian cancer? What are the pros and cons of prophylactic bilateral salpingo-oophorectomy and ovarian cancer screening?
- Is it safe to have another child? What are the risks for my new baby and are there possibilities to reduce this risk? [51]

All these questions do not currently have an answer.

Research should improve understanding of this pathology and should aim at finding new molecular markers and new screening strategies for detecting early stage ovarian cancer in women with hereditary ovarian cancer trait.

Conclusion

Ovarian cancer represents a fairly common female malignancy, causes more deaths per year than any other gynaecologic cancers and therefore represents a significant public health problem.

Although most ovarian cancer is sporadic, about 5–10 % is due to the inheritance of an ovarian cancer susceptibility gene; the genes that have currently been identified are the *BRCA* genes, tumour suppressor by regulating homologous recombination: women carrying a mutation in an ovarian cancer susceptibility gene are at relatively high risk of developing the cancer. When clinical gene testing emerged for *BRCA1* and *BRCA2*, little was known about the efficacy of genetic screening, chemoprevention and medical interventions. Although significant gains have been made by annual CA-125 and TVU screening, as in The United Kingdom Collaborative Trial of Ovarian Cancer Screening [105], results of a study at the University of Alabama at Birmingham Comprehensive Cancer Center showed the combo screening caught 70 % of the ovarian cancers in their late stages when effective treatment options are limited. [106]

So major challenges remain in the identification and referral of high-risk patients and families to genetic counselling. Because premonitory physical stigmata are generally absent in most of these high-risk women, an HOC diagnosis may be missed. The only safe method to prevent the HOC in high-risk patients is the prophylactic bilateral oophorectomy. The use of laparoscopy in ovarian cancer treatment is already proved and suggested [107, 108]. This operation should be done between 35 and 40 years in *BRCA1* mutations and between 40 and 45 years for *BRCA2* mutations to reduce HOC in 96 % of cases and, in premenopausal period, it should reduce breast cancer of 53 % [30].

References

1. Tinelli A, Malvasi A, Leo G, Vergara D, Pisanò M, Ciccarese M, et al. Hereditary ovarian cancers: from BRCA mutations to clinical management. A modern appraisal. Cancer Metastasis Rev. 2010;29(2): 339–50.
2. Tinelli A, Vergara D, Martignago R, Leo G, Pisanò M, Malvasi A. An outlook on ovarian cancer and borderline ovarian tumors: focus on genomic and proteomic findings. Curr Genomics. 2009;10(4): 240–9.
3. Lindor NM, McMaster ML, Lindor CJ, Greene MH, National Cancer Institute, Division of Cancer Prevention, Community Oncology and Prevention Trials Research Group. Concise handbook of familial cancer susceptibility syndromes: second edition. J Natl Cancer Inst Monogr. 2008;2008(38):1–93.
4. Lynch HT, Snyder CL, Lynch JF, Riley BD, Rubinstein WS. Hereditary breast-ovarian cancer at the bedside: role of the medical oncologist. J Clin Oncol. 2003;21:740–53.
5. Pisanò M, Mezzolla V, Galante MM, Alemanno G, Manca C, Lorusso V, et al. A new mutation of BRCA2 gene in an Italian healthy woman with familial breast cancer history. Fam Cancer. 2011;10(1):65–71.
6. Nielsen FC, Kruse TA, Gerdes AM. BRCA1 and BRCA2 mutations in Danish families with hereditary breast and/or ovarian cancer. Acta Oncol. 2008;47(4):772–7.
7. Sinilnikova OM, Mazoyer S, Bonnardel C, Lynch HT, Narod SA, Lenoir GM. BRCA1 and BRCA2 mutations in breast and ovarian cancer syndrome: reflection on the Creighton University historical series of high risk families. Fam Cancer. 2006;5:15–20.
8. Brunet J, Pèrez-Segura P. Cancer screening and genetic counselling. Rev Oncol. 2004;6(3):176–83.
9. National Cancer Institute (NCI). http://dcp.cancer.gov/programs-resources/groups/ed/programs/plco/about. Accessed 3 Nov 2008.
10. Kurian AW, Balise RR, McGuire V, Whittemore AS. Histologic types of epithelial ovarian cancer: have they different risk factors? Gynecol Oncol. 2005;96: 520–30.
11. Chiaffarino F, Parazzini F, Bosetti C, Franceschi S, Talamini R, Canzonieri V, et al. Risk factors for ovarian cancer histotypes. Eur J Cancer. 2007;43: 1208–13.
12. Bray F, Loos AH, Tognazzo S, La Vecchia C. Ovarian cancer in Europe: cross-sectional trends in incidence and mortality in 28 countries, 1953–2000. Int J Cancer. 2005;113:977–90.
13. Negri E, Pelucchi C, Franceschi S, Montella M, Conti E, Dal Maso L, et al. Family history of cancer and risk of ovarian cancer. Eur J Cancer. 2003;39:505–10.
14. La Vecchia C. Epidemiology of ovarian cancer: a summary review. Eur J Cancer Prev. 2001; 10:125–9.
15. Simon MS, Petrucelli N. Hereditary breast and ovarian cancer syndrome: the impact of race on uptake of genetic counseling and testing. Methods Mol Biol. 2009;471:487–500.
16. Chen Y, Farmer AA, Chen CF, Jones DC, Chen PL, Lee WH. BRCA1 is a 220-kDa nuclear phosphoprotein that is expressed and phosphorylated in a cell cycle-dependent manner. Cancer Res. 1996;56: 3168–72.
17. Ruffner H, Verma IM. BRCA1 is a cell cycle-regulated nuclear phosphoprotein. Proc Natl Acad Sci U S A. 1997;94:7138–43.
18. Deng CX. BRCA1: cell cycle checkpoint, genetic instability, DNA damage response and cancer evolution. Nucleic Acids Res. 2006;34(5):1416–26.
19. Yu X, Chini CC, He M, Mer G, Chen J. The BRCT domain is a phospho-protein binding domain. Science. 2003;302:639–42.
20. Manke IA, Lowery DM, Nguyen A, Yaffe MB. BRCT repeats as phosphopeptide-binding modules involved in protein targeting. Science. 2003;302:636–9.
21. Arai M, Utsunomiya J, Miki Y. Familial breast and ovarian cancers. Int J Clin Oncol. 2004;9:270–82.
22. Ouchi T, Monteiro AN, August A, Aaronson SA, Hanafusa H. BRCA1 regulates p53-dependent gene expression. Proc Natl Acad Sci U S A. 1998; 95(5):2302–6.
23. Fan S, Yong X, Wang C, Yuan RQ, Meng Q, Wang JA, et al. Role of direct interaction in BRCA1 inhibition of estrogen receptor activity. Oncogene. 2001;20(1):77–87.
24. Zheng L, Annab LA, Afshari CA, Lee WH, Boyer TG. BRCA1 mediates ligand-independent transcriptional repression of the estrogen receptor. Proc Natl Acad Sci U S A. 2001;98(17):9587–92.
25. Rajan JV, Wang M, Marquis ST, Chodosh LA. Brca2 is coordinately regulated with Brca1 during proliferation and differentiation in mammary epithelial cells. Proc Natl Acad Sci U S A. 1996;93:13078–83.
26. Sharan SK, Morimatsu M, Albrecht U, Lim DS, Regel E, Dinh C, et al. Embryonic lethality and radiation hypersensitivity mediated by Rad51 in mice lacking Brca2. Nature. 1997;386:804–10.
27. Marmorstein LY, Ouchi T, Stuart AA. The BRCA2 gene product functionally interacts with p53 and RAD51. Proc Natl Acad Sci U S A. 1998;95(23): 13869–74.
28. Crotser CB, Boehmke M. Survivorship considerations in adults with hereditary breast and ovarian cancer syndrome: state of the science. J Cancer Surviv. 2009;3(1):21–42.
29. Russo A, Calò V, Bruno L, Rizzo S, Bazan V, Di Fede G. Hereditary ovarian cancer. Crit Rev Oncol Hematol. 2009;69(1):28–44.

30. van der Velde NM, Mourits MJ, Arts HJ, de Vries J, Leegte BK, Dijkhuis G, et al. Time to stop ovarian cancer screening in BRCA1/2 mutation carriers? Int J Cancer. 2009;124(4):919–23.
31. Nelson HD, Huffman LH, Fu R, Harris EL, Preventive Services Task Force. Genetic risk assessment and BRCA mutation testing for breast and ovarian cancer susceptibility: systematic evidence review for the U.S. Preventive Services Task Force. Ann Intern Med. 2005;143(5):362–79.
32. Thomassen M, Hansen TV, Borg A, Lianee HT, Wikman F, Pedersen IS, et al. Hereditary ovarian cancer–assessing risk and prevention strategies. Obstet Gynecol Clin North Am. 2007;34(4):651–65.
33. Bell DA. Origin of ovarian carcinoma. Mod Pathol. 2005;18:S19–32.
34. Berliner JL, Fay AM. Risk assessment and genetic counseling for hereditary breast and ovarian cancer: recommendations of the National Society of Genetic Counselors. J Genet Couns. 2007;16:241–60.
35. Skinner CS, Schildkraut JM, Berry D, Calingaert B, Marcom PK, Sugarman J, et al. Pre-counseling education materials for BRCA testing: does tailoring make a difference? Genet Test. 2002;6(2):93–105.
36. Peters N, Domchek SM, Rose A, Polis R, Stopfer J, Armstrong K. Knowledge, attitudes, and utilization of BRCA1/2 testing among women with early-onset breast cancer. Genet Test. 2005;9(1):48–53.
37. Vadaparampil ST, Wey JP, Kinney AY. Psychosocial aspects of genetic counseling and testing. Semin Oncol Nurs. 2004;20(3):186–95.
38. Kehoe SM, Kauff ND. Screening and prevention of hereditary gynecologic cancers. Semin Oncol. 2007; 34(5):406–10.
39. Lux MP, Fasching PA, Beckmann MW. Hereditary breast and ovarian cancer: review and future perspectives. J Mol Med. 2006;84:16–28.
40. De la Hoya M, Diez O, Pérez-Segura P, Godino J, Fernández JM, Sanz J, et al. Pre-test prediction models of BRCA1 or BRCA2 mutation in breast/ovarian families attending familial cancer clinics. J Med Genet. 2003;40:503–10.
41. Myers ER, Havrilesky LJ, Kulasingam SL, Sanders GD, Cline KE, Gray RN, et al. Genomic tests for ovarian cancer detection and management. Evid Rep Technol Assess (Full Rep). 2006;(145):1–100.
42. Low CA, Bower JE, Kwan L, Seldon J. Benefit finding in response to BRCA1/2 testing. Ann Behav Med. 2008;35(1):61–9.
43. Kieran S, Loescher LJ, Lim KH. The role of financial factors in acceptance of clinical BRCA genetic testing. Genet Test. 2007;11(1):101–10.
44. Pruthi S, Gostout BS, Lindor NM. Identification and management of women with BRCA mutations or hereditary predisposition for breast and ovarian cancer. Mayo Clin Proc. 2010;85(12):1111–20.
45. Modugno F, Moslehi R, Ness RB, Nelson DB, Belle S, Kant JA, et al. Reproductive factors and ovarian cancer risk in Jewish BRCA1 and BRCA2 mutation carriers (United States). Cancer Causes Control. 2003;14(5):439–46.
46. Passaperuma K, Warner E, Hill KA, Gunasekara A, Yaffe MJ. Is mammographic breast density a breast cancer risk factor in women with BRCA mutations? J Clin Oncol. 2010;28(23):3779–83.
47. Nkondjock A, Ghadirian P. Epidemiology of breast cancer among BRCA mutation carriers: an overview. Cancer Lett. 2004;205(1):1–8.
48. Herman LM, Clinical and Scientific Affairs Council of the AAPA. Hereditary breast and ovarian cancers. JAAPA. 2008;21(5):18–21.
49. Lacour RA, Daniels MS, Westin SN, Meyer LA, Burke CC, Burns KA, et al. What women with ovarian cancer think and know about genetic testing. Gynecol Oncol. 2008;111(1):132–6.
50. Armel SR, Hitchman K, Millar K, Zahavich L, Demsky R, Murphy J, Rosen B. The use of family history questionnaires: an examination of genetic risk estimates and genetic testing eligibility in the non responder population. J Genet Couns. 2011;20(4): 355–64.
51. Mourits MJ, de Bock GH. Managing hereditary ovarian cancer. Maturitas. 2009;64(3):172–6.
52. Chen S, Parmigiani G. Meta-analysis of BRCA1 and BRCA2 penetrance. J Clin Oncol. 2007;25: 1329–33.
53. Bakos AD, Hutson SP, Loud JT, Peters JA, Giusti RM, Greene MH. BRCA mutation-negative women from hereditary breast and ovarian cancer families: a qualitative study of the BRCA-negative experience. Health Expect. 2008;11(3):220–31.
54. Fields MM, Chevlen E. Ovarian cancer screening: a look at the evidence. Clin J Oncol Nurs. 2006;10(1): 77–81.
55. Wakahara F, Kikkawa F, Nawa A, et al. Diagnostic efficacy of tumor markers, sonography, and intraoperative frozen section for ovarian tumors. Gynecol Obstet Invest. 2001;52:147–52.
56. Woodward ER, Sleightholme HV, Considine AM, Williamson S, McHugo JM, Cruger DG. Annual surveillance by CA125 and transvaginal ultrasound for ovarian cancer in both high-risk and population risk women is ineffective. BJOG. 2007;114(12): 1500–9.
57. Bermejo-Pérez MJ, Márquez-Calderón S, Llanos-Méndez A. Cancer surveillance based on imaging techniques in carriers of BRCA1/2 gene mutations: a systematic review. Br J Radiol. 2008;81(963): 172–9.
58. McInerney-Leo A, Biesecker BB, Hadley DW, Kase RG, Giambarresi TR, Johnson E, Lerman C, Struewing JP. BRCA1/2 testing in hereditary breast and ovarian cancer families II: impact on relationships. Am J Med Genet A. 2005;133A(2): 165–9.
59. Lacey Jr JV, Greene MH, Buys SS, Reding D, Riley TL, Berg CD, Fagerstrom RM, Hartge P. Ovarian cancer screening in women with a family history of breast

or ovarian cancer. Obstet Gynecol. 2006;108(5):1176–84.

60. Schorge JO, Modesitt SC, Coleman RL, Cohn DE, Kauff ND, Duska LR, Herzog TJ. SGO White Paper on ovarian cancer: etiology, screening and surveillance. Gynecol Oncol. 2010;119(1):7–17.
61. Myers ER, Bastian LA, Havrilesky LJ, Kulasingam SL, Terplan MS, Cline KE, et al. Management of adnexal mass. Evid Rep Technol Assess. 2006;130:1–145.
62. Bast Jr RC, Brewer M, Zou C, Hernandez MA, Daley M, Ozols R, et al. Prevention and early detection of ovarian cancer: mission impossible? Recent Results Cancer Res. 2007;174:91–100.
63. Geomini P, Kruiwagen R, Bremer GL, Cnossen J, Mol BW. The accuracy of risk scores in predicting ovarian malignancy: a systematic review. Obstet Gynecol. 2009;113:384–94.
64. Lerner JP, Timor-Tritsch IE, Federman A, Abramovich G. Transvaginal ultrasonographic characterization of ovarian masses with an improved, weighted scoring system. Am J Obstet Gynecol. 1994;170(1 Pt 1):81–5.
65. Oei AL, Massuger LF, Bulten J, Ligtenberg MJ, Hoogerbrugge N, de Hullu JA. Surveillance of women at high risk for hereditary ovarian cancer is inefficient. Br J Cancer. 2006;94(6):814–9.
66. Ueland FR, DePriest PD, Pavlik EJ, Kryscio RJ, Van Nagell Jr JR. Preoperative differentiation of malignant from benign ovarian tumors: the efficacy of morphology indexing and Doppler flow sonography. Gynecol Oncol. 2003;91(1):46–50.
67. Narod SA, Sun P, Risch HA. Ovarian cancer, oral contraceptives, and BRCA mutations. N Engl J Med. 2001;345:1706–7.
68. Modan B, Hartge P, Hirsh-Yechezkel G, Chetrit A, Lubin F, Beller U, National Israel Ovarian Cancer Study Group, et al. Parity, oral contraceptives, and the risk of ovarian cancer among carriers and noncarriers of a BRCA1 or BRCA2 mutation. N Engl J Med. 2001;345:235–40.
69. Sabichi AL, Hendricks DT, Bober MA, Birrer MJ. Retinoic acid receptor beta expression and growth inhibition of gynaecologic cancer cells by the synthetic retinoid N-(4-hydroxyphenyl) retinamide. J Natl Cancer Inst. 1998;90:597–605.
70. Supino R, Crosti M, Clerici M, Warlters A, Cleris L, Zunino F, Formelli F. Induction of apoptosis by fenretinide (4HPR) in human ovarian carcinoma cells and its association with retinoic acid receptor expression. Int J Cancer. 1996;65:491–7.
71. Benbrook DM, Madler MM, Spruce LW, Birckbichler PJ, Nelson EC, Subramanian S, et al. Biologically active heteroarotinoids exhibiting anticancer activity and decreased toxicity. J Med Chem. 1997;40:3567–83.
72. Guruswamy S, Lightfoot S, Gold MA, Hassan R, Berlin KD, Ivey RT, Benbrook DM. Effects of retinoids on cancerous phenotype and apoptosis in organotypic cultures of ovarian carcinoma. J Natl Cancer Inst. 2001;93:516–25.
73. Lefkowitz ES, Garland CF. Sunlight, vitamin D, and ovarian cancer mortality rates in US women. Int J Epidemiol. 1994;23:1133–6.
74. Ahonen MH, Zhuang YH, Aine R, Ylikomi T, Tuohimaa P. Androgen receptor and vitamin D receptor in human ovarian cancer: growth stimulation and inhibition by ligands. Int J Cancer. 2000;86:40–6.
75. Ness RB, Cottreau C. Possible role of ovarian epithelial inflammation in ovarian cancer. J Natl Cancer Inst. 1999;91:1459–67.
76. Moysich KB, Mettlin C, Piver MS, Natarajan N, Menezes RJ, Swede H. Regular use of analgesic drugs and ovarian cancer risk. Cancer Epidemiol Biomarkers Prev. 2001;10:903–6.
77. Rosenberg L, Palmer JR, Rao RS, Coogan PF, Strom BL, Zauber AG, et al. A case–control study of analgesic use and ovarian cancer. Cancer Epidemiol Biomarkers Prev. 2000;9:933–7.
78. Cramer DW, Harlow BL, Titus-Ernstoff L, Bohlke K, Welch WR, Greenberg ER. Over-the-counter analgesics and risk of ovarian cancer. Lancet. 1998;351:104–7.
79. Taketo MM. Cyclooxygenase-2 inhibitors in tumorigenesis (part I). J Natl Cancer Inst. 1998;90:1529–36.
80. Taketo MM. Cyclooxygenase-2 inhibitors in tumorigenesis (Part II). J Natl Cancer Inst. 1998;90:1609–20.
81. Williams CS, Mann M, DuBois RN. The role of cyclooxygenases in inflammation, cancer, and development. Oncogene. 1999;18:7908–16.
82. Murphy GJ, Holder JC. PPAR-gamma agonists: therapeutic role in diabetes, inflammation and cancer. Trends Pharmacol Sci. 2000;21:469–74.
83. Adams M, Montague CT, Prins JB, Holder JC, Smith SA, Sanders L, et al. Activators of peroxisome proliferator-activated receptor gamma have depot-specific effects on human preadipocyte differentiation. J Clin Invest. 1997;100:3149–53.
84. Mueller E, Sarraf P, Tontonoz P, Evans RM, Martin KJ, Zhang M, et al. Terminal differentiation of human breast cancer through PPAR gamma. Mol Cell. 1998;1:465–70.
85. You YN, Lakhani VT, Wells Jr SA. The role of prophylactic surgery in cancer prevention. World J Surg. 2007;31(3):450–64.
86. Gien LT, Mackay HJ. The emerging role of PARP inhibitors in the treatment of epithelial ovarian cancer. J Oncol. 2010;2010:151750.
87. Tan DS, Rothermundt C, Thomas K, Bancroft E, Eeles R, Shanley S, et al. "BRCAness" syndrome in ovarian cancer: a case–control study describing the clinical features and outcome of patients with epithelial ovarian cancer associated with BRCA1 and BRCA2 mutations. J Clin Oncol. 2008;26(34):5530–6.

88. Bryant HE, Schultz N, Thomas HD, Parker KM, Flower D, Lopez E, et al. Specific killing of BRCA2-deficient tumours with inhibitors of poly(ADP-ribose) polymerase. Nature. 2005;434(7035):913–7.
89. Farmer H, McCabe N, Lord CJ, Tutt AN, Johnson DA, Richardson TB, et al. Targeting the DNA repair defect in BRCA mutant cells as a therapeutic strategy. Nature. 2005;434(7035):917–21.
90. Domchek SM, Rebbeck TR. Prophylactic oophorectomy in women at increased cancer risk. Curr Opin Obstet Gynecol. 2007;19(1):27–30.
91. ACOG. ACOG Practice Bulletin No. 89. Elective and risk-reducing salpingo-oophorectomy. Obstet Gynecol. 2008;111(1):231–41.
92. Miller SM, Roussi P, Daly MB, Scarpato J. New strategies in ovarian cancer: uptake and experience of women at high risk of ovarian cancer who are considering risk-reducing salpingo-oophorectomy. Clin Cancer Res. 2010;16(21):5094–106.
93. Daly MB, Axilbund JE, Buys S, Crawford B, Farrell CD, Friedman S, National Comprehensive Cancer Network, et al. Genetic/familial high risk assessment: breast and ovarian. J Natl Compr Canc Netw. 2010;8:562–94.
94. Wood WC, Moley JF, Berchuck A, Karlan BY, Mutch DG, Gagel RF, et al. ASCO/SSO review of current role of risk-reducing surgery in common hereditary cancer syndromes. J Clin Oncol. 2006;24(28):4642–60.
95. Tinelli A, Malvasi A, Casciaro S, Leo G, Vergara D, Pisanò M, et al. Tailoring minimally invasive gynaecological surgery based on biogenomic findings. In: Casciaro S, Gersak B, editors. New technology frontiers in minimally invasive therapies, vol. 6. Lecce: Lupiensis Biomedical Publications; 2007. p. 43–62.
96. Lancaster JM, Powell CB, Kauff ND, Cass I, Chen LM, Lu KH, Society of Gynecologic Oncologists Education Committee, et al. Society of Gynecologic Oncologists Education Committee statement on risk assessment for inherited gynecologic cancer predispositions. Gynecol Oncol. 2007;107(2):159–62.
97. Batista LI, Lu KH, Beahm EK, Arun BK, Bodurka DC, Meric-Bernstam F. Coordinated prophylactic surgical management for women with hereditary breast-ovarian cancer syndrome. BMC Cancer. 2008;8:101.
98. Gómez García EB, Oosterwijk JC, Timmermans M, van Asperen CJ, Hogervorst FBL, Hoogerbrugge N, et al. A method to assess the clinical significance of unclassified variants in the BRCA1 and BRCA2 genes based on cancer family history. Breast Cancer Res. 2009;11(1):R8.
99. Rebbeck TR, Kauff ND, Domchek SM. Meta-analysis of risk reduction estimates associated with risk-reducing salpingo-oophorectomy in BRCA1 or BRCA2 mutation carriers. J Natl Cancer Inst. 2009;101(2):80–7.
100. Greene MH, Piedmonte M, Alberts D, Gail M, Hensley M, Miner Z, et al. A prospective study of risk-reducing salpingo-oophorectomy and longitudinal CA-125 screening among women at increased genetic risk of ovarian cancer: design and baseline characteristics: a Gynecologic Oncology Group study. Cancer Epidemiol Biomarkers Prev. 2008;17(3):594–604.
101. Greene MH, Mai PL, Schwartz PE. Does bilateral salpingectomy with ovarian retention warrant consideration as a temporary bridge to risk-reducing bilateral oophorectomy in BRCA1/2 mutation carriers? Am J Obstet Gynecol. 2011;204(1):19.e1–6.
102. Narod SA, Sun P, Ghadirian P, Lynch H, Isaacs C, Garber J, et al. Tubal ligation and risk of ovarian cancer in carriers of BRCA1 or BRCA2 mutations: a case–control study. Lancet. 2001;357:1467–70.
103. Buys SS, Partridge E, Black A, Johnson CC, Lamerato L, Isaacs C, PLCO Project Team, et al. Effect of screening on ovarian cancer mortality: the Prostate, Lung, Colorectal and Ovarian (PLCO) Cancer Screening Randomized Controlled Trial. JAMA. 2011;305(22):2295–303.
104. Kuliev A, Verlinsky Y. Place of preimplantation diagnosis in genetic practice. Am J Med Genet A. 2005;134A:105–10.
105. Menon U, Gentry-Maharaj A, Hallett R, Ryan A, Burnell M, Sharma A, et al. Sensitivity and specificity of multimodal and ultrasound screening for ovarian cancer, and stage distribution of detected cancers: results of the prevalence screen of the UK Collaborative Trial of Ovarian Cancer Screening (UKCTOCS). Lancet Oncol. 2009;10(4):327–40.
106. Partridge E, Kreimer AR, Greenlee RT, Williams C, Xu JL, Church TR, The PLCO Project Team, et al. Results from four rounds of ovarian cancer screening in a randomized trial. Obstet Gynecol. 2009;113(4):775–82.
107. Tinelli A, Pellegrino M, Malvasi A, Lorusso V. Laparoscopical management ovarian early sex cord-stromal tumors in postmenopausal women: a proposal method. Arch Gynecol Obstet. 2011;283 Suppl 1:87–91.
108. Nezhat FR, DeNoble SM, Liu CS, Cho JE, Brown DN, Chuang L, et al. The safety and efficacy of laparoscopic surgical staging and debulking of apparent advanced stage ovarian, fallopian tube, and primary peritoneal cancers. JSLS. 2010;14(2):155–68.

Ovarian Cancer in the Pediatric Population

8

Anne C. Fischer

Introduction

Pediatric ovarian tumors are an uncommon type of childhood cancer. On the one hand, they are the most frequent neoplasms of the female genital tract in childhood and yet account for only 1 % of all malignancies in children (<17 years). An ovarian mass can be due to both neoplastic and nonneoplastic processes. Nonneoplastic conditions include follicular cysts, corpus luteal cysts, and endometriomas, whereas neoplastic processes include both benign tumors, such as mature cystic teratomas, as well as malignant tumors that range from being highly malignant to having only a low malignant potential.

Generally these tumors are classified into three main pathologic categories, including epithelial, stromal, and germ cell tumors: The predominance of pediatric ovarian tumors are germ cell tumors as opposed to the majority of epithelial tumors in adults. This difference highlights the importance of considering patient age when evaluating an ovarian mass. Germ cell tumors include teratomas and gonadoblastomas as well as endodermal sinus tumors, also called yolk sac tumors, embryonal carcinomas, polyembryomas, and choriocarcinomas. Less frequent, non-germ cell tumors include sex cord–stromal tumors and epithelial tumors. Sex cord–stromal tumors include thecoma–fibroma, Sertoli–Leydig cell tumors, and juvenile granulosa cell tumors.

Though uncommon in children, the clinical spectrum of ovarian tumors ranges from largely benign mature teratomas to life-threatening, widely metastatic cancers. Pain was the most common symptom, although presence of an abdominal mass was frequent and other nonspecific symptoms. Precocious puberty and/or increasing abdominal girth may present concurrently, so abdominal and endocrine symptoms should raise the index of suspicion. Torsion is infrequently associated with underlying malignancies; although historically torsion was presumed to be secondary to an underlying mass.

Studies have reported wide variability in malignancy rates, from 16 to 55 %, depending on the inclusion criteria of the study, the type of referral center, and the number of surgical resections for benign ovarian masses, such as for functional cysts, torsions, and dermoids. Therefore the risk of malignancy in these different populations is highly variable depending on the same aforementioned factors impacting the malignancy rate. In a Surveillance, Epidemiology, and End Results (SEER) database study, we determined that the age-adjusted incidence of malignant pediatric ovarian tumors approximated 0.102 per 100,000 per year in children younger than 9 years of age, ten times higher in those aged

A.C. Fischer, MD, PhD
Department of Pediatric Surgery,
William Beaumont Hospital,
Medical Office Building, 3535 West 13 Mile Road,
Suite 748, Royal Oak, MI 48073, USA

Department of Surgery, Oakland University
William Beaumont Medical School,
Royal Oak, MI 48073, USA
e-mail: anne.fischer@beaumont.edu

S.A. Farghaly (ed.), *Advances in Diagnosis and Management of Ovarian Cancer*,
DOI 10.1007/978-1-4614-8271-0_8, © Springer Science+Business Media New York 2014

10–19 years of age, compared to 100 times higher at 11.446 per 100,000 for adult women older than 20 years of age.

Ultrasound is 100 % accurate in localizing any process to the ovaries; however, ultrasound has not been conclusively shown to distinguish benign from malignant neoplasms. Almost all neoplasms present as unilateral masses and rarely are metastatic at diagnosis. Fortunately, ovarian malignancies in children are frequently found at an early stage and most respond favorably to chemotherapy. Most children with ovarian malignancies clinically do well with few recurrences tumors given the profound impact that platinum-based therapies have had on this field.

The option of conservative surgical therapy depends on the stage of disease at the time of diagnosis and only recently have efforts been more concerted to balance the need for effective treatment with conservation of ovarian function and fertility, despite ovarian preservation being the putative dogma.

Incidence

Ovarian neoplasms are uncommon in children and account for 1 % of all malignancies in pediatric patients less than 17 years of age, although they are the most common pediatric gynecologic tumor [1, 2]. The literature available is replete with mainly case reports and series, given the limited number of cases seen at a center annually. The overall incidence of an ovarian mass in childhood approximates 2.6 cases/100,000 cases per year, whereas the incidence of those that are tumors may vary from 16 up to 55 % of these case series in Finland [3]. Thus, the true incidence of malignant ovarian tumors was not known in the pediatric population given the wide range of reported malignancy rates in different case series of ovarian masses.

Our analysis of the Surveillance, Epidemiology, and End Results (SEER) 2008 database, the largest cancer database in the USA, identified 1,037 pediatric ovarian tumors diagnosed over three decades from 1973 to 2005 [4]. The SEER program of the National Cancer Institute (NCI) is compiled from 17 population-based cancer registries, encompassing 26 % of the US population. The analysis of all malignant pediatric ovarian tumors in the SEER database demonstrated an age-adjusted tenfold increase in incidence with each decade of life. The age-adjusted incidence of malignant pediatric ovarian tumors was 0.102 per 100,000 per year in children younger than 9 years of age, 1.072 per 100,000 in children aged 10–19 years of age, and 11.446 per 100,000 in adult women older than 20 years of age.

Epidemiological Aspects

The low percentage of malignancies among overall ovarian masses, which encompass functional cysts, benign masses, and neoplasms, is demonstrated in several large case series. Approximately 14- to 15-year reviews of ovarian lesions at three centers, Dallas Children's Medical Center, Children's Hospital of Philadelphia, and Texas Children's Hospital, reviewed a total of 424, 251, 102 ovarian lesions, respectively; each series reported approximately a 10 % malignancy rate among all ovarian lesions [5–7]. The variation in the incidence of neoplasms reported from different series is likely impacted by age cutoffs and referral patterns for those institutions for an ovarian mass. Typically the mean age of patients with a malignancy was similar to those with a nonneoplastic lesion [5–7] but can nonetheless be impacted by the age range referred to a given institution.

Most people in the SEER database analysis of ovarian malignancies were Caucasian (76.6 %), non-Hispanic (77.0 %), presented with local disease (57.4 %) and treated with surgery (79.3 %). The percentage of ovarian malignancies in each age range was distributed as follows: 10 % of all malignancies occurred in patients ≤9 years of age, 28.2 % in those between 10 and 14, and up to 61.7 % in patients 15–19 years of age [4]. On the other hand, case series best demonstrate how frequently an ovarian mass is malignant out of *all ovarian lesions* presenting at different ages. This last metric is more clinically applicable in the evaluation of a patient presenting with an ovarian mass. The percentage of malignancies among all ovarian lesions varies by age; the subset aged 1–8 years had the highest percentage (22 %) of malignant neoplasms among ovarian lesions in comparison to 10 % seen in older girls [5]. This finding was further substantiated by a threefold greater odds ratio for malignancy in the 1–8 year group compared to the 15–19 year olds [5].

Anatomic Aspects of Ovarian Masses

Ovarian masses include neoplastic and nonneoplastic lesions. Neoplastic lesions include benign or malignant neoplasms. Ovarian germ cell tumors are the most common malignancy in children, and epithelial cell tumors are the least common, in contrast to the predominance of epithelial tumors in adult women. The significance of this difference anatomically is the fact that most pediatric tumors present at a low stage, and even those at more advanced stages present with localized spread as opposed to gross metastases. A majority of adult ovarian cancers are epithelial neoplasms, derived from the coelomic epithelium covering the surface of the ovary so the tumor can spread widely throughout all surface peritoneum in the peritoneal cavity; they are not locally contained, requiring extensive staging and debulking procedures.

There are some assumptions made about the malignant potential in nonneoplastic conditions associated with the presentation of an ovarian mass which are detailed below. Nonneoplastic conditions include functional cysts, corpus luteal cysts, and endometriomas, and even the ovarian enlargement resulting from the venous engorgement secondary to torsion is often assumed to be hiding a malignant component. Historically, it was presumed that all ovaries containing any lesion discovered in children should be removed surgically for concern of malignancy; however, given better imaging and identification of serum tumor markers, a conservative fertility-sparing approach to the management of ovarian masses has been developed.

Ovarian Masses Associated with Torsion

Ovarian masses presenting as torsion were historically presumed to have an underlying pathology; however, torsion is most commonly associated with normal ovaries [8]. Ovarian enlargement or a discrepancy in ovarian volume is the most characteristic ultrasound (US) finding in torsion and is merely the end result of progressive edema and venous congestion. Previous reports have shown no underlying ovarian pathology was found in over half the cases [9–13]. Given the abdominal location and fair mobility of the ovary in a child and the long utero-ovarian ligament, the normal adnexa are at risk of torsion. Torsion of the ovary usually occurs with the twisting of the associated fallopian tube (adnexal torsion) around the broad ligament; although, in very rare cases the ovary rotates just around the mesovarium, or the fallopian tube rotates around the mesosalpinx in an isolated fashion. If this diagnosis is not detected in a timely fashion, then the twisting results in a compromised blood supply to the vascular pedicle and subsequent infarction in adnexal structures leading to necrosis and peritonitis. A dual blood supply was presumed to be the reason why Doppler ultrasonography is not definitive in the diagnosis of torsion. However, a dual blood supply exists in only 56 % cases; 40 % of ovaries are supplied by the ovarian artery alone and 4 % by the uterine artery [14].

Torsed ovaries are associated with a markedly lower overall malignancy rate of 0.5–1.9 % compared with the typical 10 % malignancy rate reported for all ovarian masses, in the Healthcare Cost and Utilization Project Kids' Inpatient Database (KID) and in the largest reported case series (682 patients) [8, 9]. The anatomic distortion from the edema of venous congestion can confound decision making intraoperatively, resulting in an inappropriately more aggressive use of oophorectomy in the acute setting. Torsed ovaries should be "detorsed" laparoscopically with conservation of the ovary despite an ischemic or necrotic appearance and follow-up US surveillance to assess for a persistent mass [12, 13, 15]. The historical theories regarding blood clots and emboli from detorsion have proven to be unfounded: there was no diagnosis of pulmonary thromboembolism in any ovarian-related hospitalization in the KID database [8].

Ovarian Cysts in A Changing Hormonal Milieu

Functional cysts are normal physiologically and most resolve spontaneously in 1–2 months. They include follicular, corpus luteum, and theca-lutein types, all of which are benign and self-limited. Simple cysts result from the persistence of a maturing follicle that does not ovulate or involute. Most ovarian cysts <3 cm are normal follicles and require no further evaluation. They can vary with the development and hormonal milieu of the patient.

Ovarian cysts are the rule in 98 % of newborn girls and over 20 % are larger than 9 mm [16]: nearly all simple cysts resolve. Although a neonatal simple cyst >2.5 cm is considered pathologic, surveillance is done to ensure regression since most simple cysts >4–5 cm will resolve spontaneously with the maturation of the hypothalamic-pituitary-ovarian axis. Most resolve by 10–12 months of age due to withdrawal of maternal hormonal stimulation [17]. Follicle-stimulating hormone (FSH) and luteinizing hormone (LH) levels peak in the newborn at 3–4 months of age and then reach prepubertal levels at 2–3 years of age [18]. Even large cysts, up to 8.7 cm, can spontaneously resolve: resolution of a large cyst typically can take time, up to 10 months, which can be concerning for the risk of torsion [19, 20].

The management of large simple cysts (>4–5 cm) and complex cysts is controversial in comparing the risks of expectant management versus surgery. The decision for expectant management is substantiated by the high likelihood of oophorectomy as the outcome of surgical intervention as opposed to preservation of ovarian function if surgical intervention is avoided [21, 22]. Expectant management can be considered in those cysts that are (1) ovarian in origin, (2) with no associated mass besides debris and septa, (3) have normal tumor markers (alpha-fetoprotein [AFP]and β-human chorionic gonadotropin [β-HCG]), and (4) are asymptomatic [22]. Although the risk of malignancy is essentially nonexistent, most surgeons advocate the removal of complex cysts to prevent complications of bleeding and rupture. Ovarian salvage with perinatal torsions is unexpected, given that the majority of torsions of antenatally diagnosed ovarian cysts occur before the first postnatal US [21]. However, viable ovarian tissue has been shown to recover in perinatal torsion over time, supporting nonoperative intervention [22]. Simple cysts are best treated with fenestration as opposed to aspiration which is fraught with recurrences; complex cysts should be treated with cystectomy with the goal to maximize preservation of ovarian tissue. A neonatal cyst can be managed by laparoscopy but may require a minilaparotomy.

Ovarian cysts are least common in prepubertal girls due to a low hormonal milieu and cysts <1 cm are considered normal requiring no further evaluation. Larger cysts require further evaluation given any association with sexual precocity. The persistence of any ovarian cyst or a complex cyst in the prepubertal child warrants surgical resection. Nonfunctional ovarian cysts will present as nonresolving cystic masses, and although rare, benign cystic epithelial tumors, such as serous and mucinous cystadenomas, do occur, can be asymptomatic, and require excision [23].

Most common in adolescence ovarian cysts typically present up to 3 cm in diameter and resolve in the second half of the menstrual cycle. Dysfunctional ovulation causes a persistence of the functional cyst which then can continue to enlarge: those cysts that measure 6–8 cm can take up to 3 months to resolve [24]. Complex cysts typically result from hemorrhage into the functional cyst but should raise a concern for a dermoid or other neoplasms, so tumor markers, serum AFP, and β-HCG should be measured. Those cysts that persist over 3–6 months, increase in size, exceed 6 cm, or are symptomatic require intervention. A laparoscopic cyst aspiration (with cytologic analysis of the aspirated fluid) or cystectomy (with pathologic sampling of the cyst wall) should be performed. A laparoscopic cystectomy with preservation of the remaining

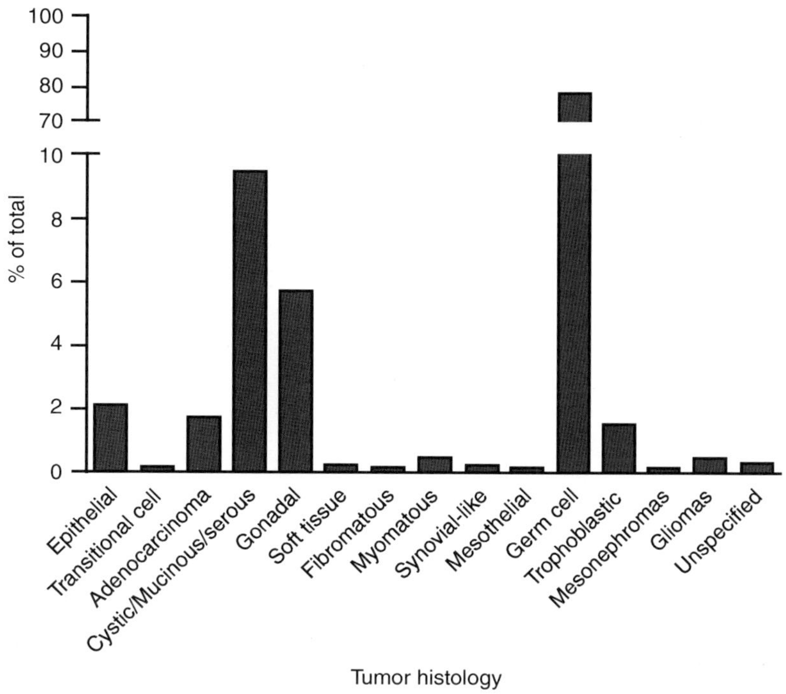

Fig. 8.1 Distribution of tumor histopathology shown as a percentage of total ovarian tumors in SEER database study (From Brookfield et al. [4]; with permission)

ovary is preferred over an aspiration, due to a high rate of recurrence following aspirations [25].

Histopathologic Types of Tumors

The clinical spectrum of ovarian tumors is varied. Malignancies are classified into three main histopathologic categories, reflecting the three cell types with neoplastic potential in gonadal tissue, which includes the primordial germ, stromal, and epithelial cells. Primordial germ cells give rise to germ cell tumors. The cells of the sex cords develop rarely into stromal tumors, such as ovarian granulosa cell tumors or Sertoli–Leydig cell tumors, or mixtures of these components. Then coelomic epithelium covering the ovary may evolve into epithelial neoplasms, which are the most common cell type in ovarian cancer in adults.

The SEER database analysis best demonstrates the distribution of tumor histology as is shown in Figure 8.1. Table 8.1 shows a corresponding list of the histopathologic classification of pediatric ovarian tumors. Germ cell neoplasms were the most common tumor identified across all ages, constituting nearly 80 % of all ovarian tumors in every age group of the pediatric population (Figure 8.2). The distribution of tumor histopathology included germ cell tumors (77.4 %)

Table 8.1 Histologic classification of ovarian tumors

Germ cell tumors
Undifferentiated
Dysgerminoma
Embryonic
Teratoma
Embryonal carcinoma
Extraembryonic
Endodermal sinus tumor
Choriocarcinoma
Sex cord–stromal tumors
Granulosa-theca cell
Sertoli-Leydig cell tumor
Epithelial tumors
Serous cystadenoma/cystadenocarcinoma
Mucinous cystadenoma/cystadenocarcinoma
Miscellaneous
Lymphoma
Leukemia
Polyembryoma
Ovarian myxoma
Mesothelioma
Gonadoblastoma

and serous or mucinous cystic neoplasms (9.6 %) which accounted for the majority of pathologic types of malignancies [4]. Sex cord–stromal neoplasms were the next frequent, accounting for 5.7 % which in other reports constituted up to 12.3 % of all tumors [1].

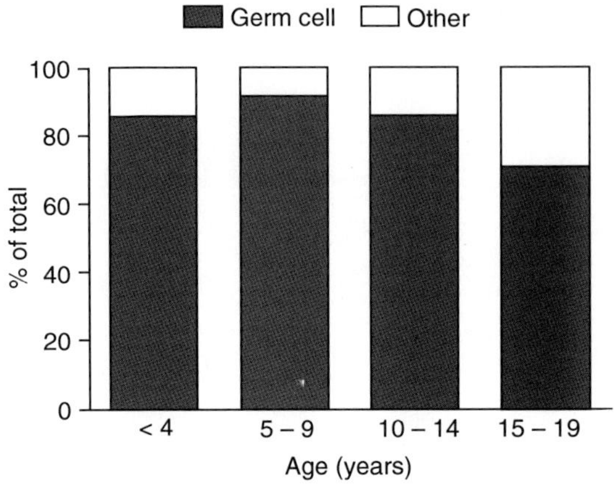

Fig. 8.2 Germ cell tumor shown as a percent of total ovarian tumors by age group (From Brookfield et al. [4]; with permission)

Malignant Germ Cell Tumors

Germ cell tumors (GCTs) arise from the fetal yolk sac: Their heterogeneity stems from the variations in the developmental age, histopathology, and malignant potential of the primordial germ cell. GCTs account for typically 75–80 % of all neoplastic pediatric ovarian masses in most series [3, 4]. All GCTs arise from the primordial germ cell but can express different tumor markers and have different malignant potentials, resulting from the differences in the stage of germ cell development at tumorigenesis and the tumor microenvironment secondary to the location of the clone. The most undifferentiated GCTs are dysgerminomas. Germ cells that undergo some degree of differentiation before becoming neoplastic either differentiate into *embryonic* tumors (embryonal carcinoma or teratoma) or *extraembryonic* tumors (endodermal sinus tumors or choriocarcinoma) as is shown in Figure 8.3 [26].

Teratomas

Teratomas are the most common ovarian tumors and are either mature (benign), immature (contain

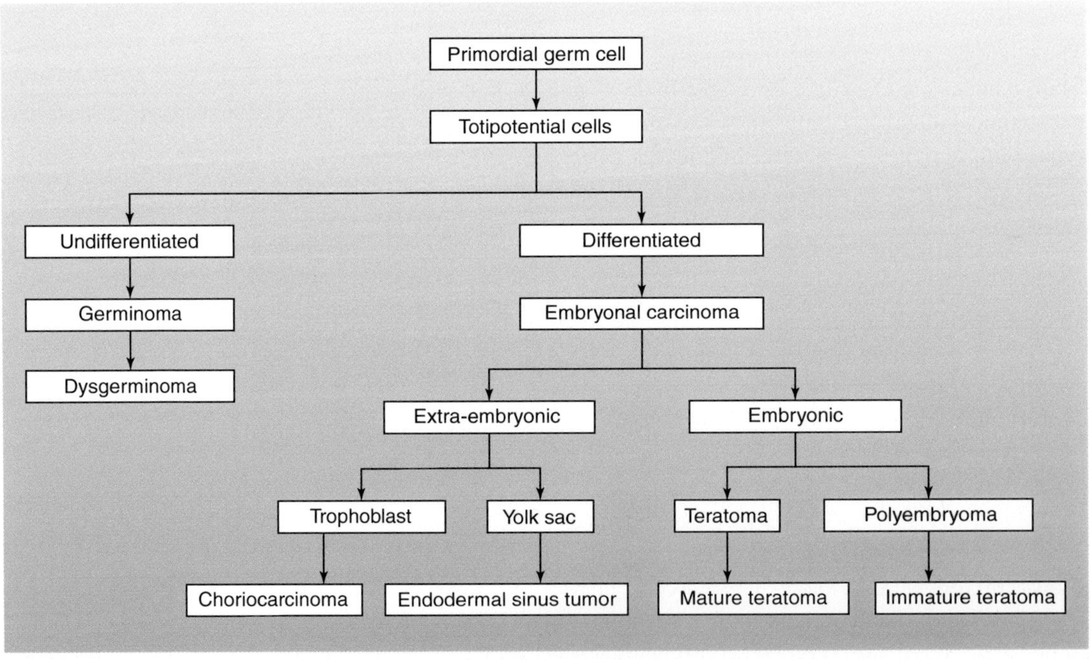

Fig. 8.3 Histologic derivation of ovarian germ cell tumors

Table 8.2 Grading of immature ovarian teratomas

Grade 0	All tissues mature; no mitotic activity
Grade 1	Some immaturity but with neuroepithelium absent or limited to one low-magnification field; no more than one focus in a slide
Grade 2	Immaturity present; neuroepithelium common but no more than three low-power microscopic fields in one slide
Grade 3	Immaturity and neuroectoderm prominent; no more than four low-power fields per section

Table 8.3 Ovarian tumor markers

Pathology	Tumor markers	Incidence of bilaterality
Teratoma	±AFP	10 %
Dysgerminoma	LDH-1	15 %
Endodermal Sinus Tumor	AFP	Low
Choriocarcinoma	β-HCG	Low
Epithelial tumors	CA-125	15 %

malignant potential), or malignant. The mature teratoma is composed of mature representative tissue from all three germ layers: ectoderm, mesoderm, and endoderm. Immature teratomas have a gross similar appearance to that of a mature teratoma but uniquely have various foci of immature tissues present, usually neuroepithelium. Immature teratomas in children behave in a malignant fashion only if they are clinically advanced (advanced stage) or contain foci of malignant germ cell elements (yolk sac tumor). Clusters of yolk sac tumor may be very small and associated intimately with immature neural tissue and thus do not stain avidly for AFP and are overlooked. These foci of immature elements are assumed to be responsible for the metastatic potential of an immature teratoma.

All grading systems quantify the degree of immaturity in the lesion. Immature tumors are graded from I to III based on the amount of neuroepithelium or the degree of immature elements present in the mass (see Table 8.2). Grade I is the most differentiated with the least risk of malignancy, and grade III is the least differentiated with the greatest risk of malignancy. The histologic level of differentiation is determined by the presence of immature elements: the more immature neural elements result in a higher histologic grade which correlates with a more aggressive biology of the tumor in adults [27]. This grading of the extent of immature lesions has shown potential prognostic significance only in adults, and chemotherapy is required to reduce recurrences in adults with this aggressive phenotype. In contrast, an intergroup study of Children's Oncology Group and the Pediatric Oncology Group examined the need for adjuvant therapy in children and concluded that surgery alone is an adequate treatment for an immature teratoma, even in the presence of an elevated AFP suggestive of a component of *YOLK Sac* tumor [28]. Table 8.3 correlates serum tumor markers with underlying histopathology. Five-year survival for pure immature teratomas by histologic grade was 81, 60, and 30 % for grade I to III, respectively [29]. Survival among pure immature teratomas has shown 74 % 5-year survival for all grades of stage I and 38 % survival for stages II and III [27]. Many teratomas are associated with the presence of peritoneal implants of mature glial tissue, *gliomatosis peritonei*, which is a distinct entity and does not change tumor stage or alter prognosis.

Germinomas

Malignant dysgerminomas arise from the primordial undifferentiated germ cells and are the most common pure germ cell malignancy in the ovary, accounting for 50 % of malignant ovarian GCTs [30]. They can occur in dysgenetic gonads, those abnormal gonads containing gonadoblastoma [31], or phenotypic females with karyotypic abnormalities. The majority of pure dysgerminomas present as stage I disease and are highly responsive to chemotherapy and radiation and are histologically identical to a seminoma in males. Bilateral disease occurs in 10–15 % of cases [32]. The 10-year survival rates for a dysgerminoma confined to one ovary and treated with surgery is 92 %; however, there is a noted 17 % recurrence rate and 6 % mortality rate [32].

Yolk Sac Tumor (*Endodermal Sinus Tumor*)

Endodermal sinus tumor, also called a yolk sac tumor, is of extraembryonic germ cell origin and is the second most common pure GCT [33]. It is typically associated with elevations of AFP [33] (see Table 8.3) and has an aggressive biology with peritoneal spread and metastases to the liver, lung, and brain [34, 35]. There are four general histopathologic patterns but these patterns are not clinically relevant. The "pseudopapillary or festoon" pattern and "microcystic or reticular" pattern are the most common. The "solid" pattern is usually found only focally and can resemble embryonal carcinoma; the "hepatoid" pattern closely resembles fetal liver and is a variant of the "solid" pattern. The fourth pattern is the "polyvesicular vitelline" pattern.

Endodermal sinus tumors can be associated with gonadoblastomas in some cases. Gonadoblastomas are benign tumors typically and occur exclusively in phenotypic females with at least a portion of the Y chromosome; thus they present clinically as male pseudohermaphrodites and have dysgenetic gonads. Germinomas frequently develop with gonadoblastomas [36].

Mixed Cell Tumors: Embryonal Carcinoma and Choriocarcinoma

Mixed GCTs contain multiple malignant cell types and carries the phenotypic biology and diagnosis of the "worst" acting cellular element. They constitute up to 30 % of malignant GCTs [37]. Both embryonal carcinoma and choriocarcinoma are rare in isolation but are more commonly seen in mixed tumors: both produce β-HCG, and embryonal carcinoma can produce precocious puberty. The two histopathologic forms of embryonal carcinoma—the pseudotubular and papillary patterns—can be confused with yolk sac tumors, but the cells are AFP negative and lack the eosinophilic hyaline globules characteristic of yolk sac tumors. Embryonal carcinoma stains positive for CD30 by immunohistochemical staining.

Choriocarcinoma also rarely occurs as a pure lesion, and when it appears in infants, it represents metastases from maternal or placental gestational trophoblastic primary tumor [38, 39]. These tumors are very friable and hemorrhagic and require the presence of two cell types—cytotrophoblasts and the syncytiotrophoblasts—which stain for β-HCG for diagnostic confirmation.

Polyembryoma is a very rare malignant lesion with a poor prognosis, occurring as a component of a mixed lesion. Both AFP and β-HCG can be elevated and also this tumor presents often with symptoms of precocious puberty [40].

Non-Germ Cell Tumors

Non-germ cell tumors include both sex cord–stromal tumors (stromal histology) and the epithelial tumors (epithelial histology). Tumors of epithelial or stromal cells of origin each accounts for the remaining 15–20 % of ovarian malignancies that are not germ cells.

Sex Cord–Stromal Tumors

Sex cord–stromal tumors include Sertoli–Leydig cell tumors and juvenile granulosa cell tumors, arising from the stromal components of the ovary and are hormonally active. Juvenile granulosa cell tumors, constituting 10–20 % of pediatric ovarian tumors, have a malignant potential although they follow a benign clinical course in children unlike adults. The pure granulosa tumor is highly malignant, mixed tumors are less malignant, and the pure thecoma is benign. The majority (>95 %) develop in postpubertal girls with estrogen excess and can be associated with pseudo-precocious puberty in 80 % of girls with breast enlargement, vaginal bleeding, and galactorrhea [41, 42]. Menstrual irregularities and swelling are the presenting symptoms. Most cases are limited to the ovary at presentation with <5 % being bilateral so that a unilateral salpingo-oophorectomy and appropriate staging is usually adequate therapy. Serum inhibin levels are associated with determining recurrence. Prognosis is excellent with 84–92 % survival.

Sertoli–Leydig cell tumors, arrhenoblastomas, are rare and account for <0.5 % of all malignant ovarian neoplasms [43]. The less well-differentiated and retiform histologies are most commonly found in children, most often localized to the ovary, and represent a low-grade malignancy. Clinically they present with androgen excess, precocious puberty in young children, and hirsutism or virilization in adolescents. An elevated AFP is associated with this tumor [44]. Prognosis depends on the stage and degree of differentiation of the tumor; usually it is a low-grade malignancy, so a unilateral salpingo-oophorectomy with staging is sufficient. Multiagent chemotherapy is utilized for advanced, metastatic, or recurrent disease [45].

In stromal cell tumors, mitotic activity in conjunction with tumor stage correlates with patient outcome. Tumors with >20 mitoses per high-power field (HPF) had an event-free survival (EFS) that was half of those with <20 mitoses per HPF [46]. Those tumors with high proliferative activity are the high risk category and difficult to treat.

Epithelial Tumors

In adults, epithelial tumors represent the majority of ovarian tumors, but in contrast less than 20 % of those in childhood are derived from the surface epithelium of the ovary and are rare to present before menarche [47]. The histologic subtypes in children are limited to serous or mucinous tumors which can be characterized as benign, borderline (of low malignant potential), or malignant. Approximately 84 % of epithelial lesions in two case series were benign or of low malignant potential [6, 48].

Borderline epithelial tumors are defined as neoplasms with varying nuclear atypia that lacks stromal invasion of the ovary and occur three times more frequently in children than adults [39]. Cystadenomas are usually benign with 7 % being borderline and 4 % being malignant [49–52]. Borderline tumors are indolent and can be bilateral. They can present locally extensive and proper workup would require applying the proper operative staging of epithelial tumors using adult guidelines since they are an epithelial histology, as opposed to the pediatric guidelines designed for germ cell tumors.

Adenocarcinoma of the ovary is very rare, presenting as two cases in a 40-year center review, and has very poor outcomes [37, 53, 54].

Metastatic Disease to the Ovary

Lymphoma can be a primary ovarian tumor [55] or metastatic to the ovary. Leukemia can cause ovarian enlargement masquerading as an ovarian tumor [56]. Gastric carcinoma can also be metastatic to the ovary [57].

Molecular Pathology of Ovarian Tumors

Mature Teratomas

Ovarian mature GTCs are thought to arise primarily from benign germ cells in meiosis and not from a malignant transformation of the germ cell. The entry into meiosis of primordial germ cells is a gradual process that continues until birth. Over 95 % of mature ovarian teratomas are karyotypically normal with only 5 % showing gains of a single whole chromosome [58, 59]. Analysis of molecular loci has shown that the majority has entered but not completed meiosis and thus is diploid [58].

Immature Teratomas

Immature and mature teratomas appear to have a different mechanism of origin and thus represent different biologic entities rather than occurring along the same spectrum of maturation. The origins of immature teratomas appear to come from meiotic stem cells and others from mitotic cells, implying a failure of early meiotic arrest [60], whereas mature teratomas originate from germ cells entering but not completing meiosis, a normal process of maturation. The frequency of chromosomal abnormalities is higher in immature teratomas than mature teratomas. Chromosomal analysis suggests that immature ovarian teratomas of premeiotic origin show a greater malignant potential and deviations in karyotype suggest a worse prognosis [61, 62]. The majority of patients with cytogenetically abnormal immature teratomas have recurrent disease. In contrast those with karyotypically normal immature teratomas have remained disease-free [60–62].

Malignant Ovarian Germ Cell Tumors

Immature teratomas may develop genetic changes found in malignant teratomas which correlate with the histologic malignant transformation of malignant GCTs. Malignant ovarian teratomas are presumed to originate from the malignant transformation of a germ cell. The genetics of malignant ovarian teratomas are similar to those of testicular tumors with similar ploidy and genetic features. Malignant teratomas often are aneuploid and 75 % may contain the isochromosome 12p, i(12p), common in malignant testicular teratomas [63]. Other genetic features include 42 and 32 % have gains of chromosomes 21 and 1q, respectively, whereas 25 and 42 % have loss of chromosomes 13 and 8, respectively [64–66].

The association between sex chromosomal abnormalities and the development of GCT is well established. Individuals with 46XY and 45X/46XY gonadal dysgenesis have a 10–50 % risk of developing a gonadal germ cell tumor [67].

Dysgerminomas, in particular, are associated with abnormal karyotypes in phenotypic females: 46XY as in gonadal dysgenesis or complete androgen insensitivity, or 45X/46XY as in mixed gonadal dysgenesis.

Table 8.4 Criteria for suspicious malignant ovarian masses

Adnexal masses with extra-ovarian spread
Ultrasonically suspicious masses >8 cm
Thick cyst wall by ultrasound
Lengthened utero-ovarian ligament
Numerous vessels starting from the mesovarium with a comb-like pattern
Peritoneal metastasis
External ovarian vegetations
Intracystic vegetations

Adapted from Canis et al. [80]

Clinical Presentation

Although rare in presentation, ovarian tumors must be included in the differential diagnosis of abdominal pain or an abdominal mass in female children. Pain is the most common symptom, although the presence of an abdominal mass was frequent and other symptoms are often nonspecific. Precocious puberty and increasing abdominal girth are also suspicious for an underlying ovarian malignancy. The symptoms of abdominal pain and increased girth, with nausea and vomiting, also typify appendicitis, which is the primary diagnosis that causes the majority of these operations being performed on an emergency basis without a complete workup or tumor markers. Exquisite tenderness may suggest peritoneal irritation from rupture or torsion of the mass.

The largest case series of ovarian masses analyzed differences in presentation between those that are benign or malignant masses [5]. Perimenarchal patients tend to have a greater number of benign lesions such as cysts and neoplasms, while those younger patients that are hormonally quiescent are less likely to present with an ovarian mass at all. The greatest percentage of malignancies in all ovarian lesions was in those patients aged 1–8 years, with malignancy being present in up to a quarter of the time. As a result, a higher index of suspicion for malignancy is needed in the patient aged 1–8 years, as indicated by a threefold increase in the odds ratio. Conversely, it is exceedingly rare for a child less than 1 year to have a malignant neoplasm [5, 68, 69].

The presenting symptoms of patients with malignancies can significantly overlap with those with benign conditions. Complaints of an abdominal mass or precocious puberty are statistically more often associated with an underlying malignancy [6, 68, 69]. Precocious puberty in the setting of a mass can be associated with sex cord–stromal tumors, including Sertoli–Leydig cell tumors, and GCTs, such as embryonal carcinoma and polyembryoma. Evidence of unusual hormonal activity is more often associated with either estrogen production from a juvenile granulosa cell tumor or androgen production with resultant virilization from a Sertoli–Leydig cell tumor [70, 71]. Not infrequently, a similar level of hormone production can be seen with autonomously functioning benign follicular cysts [22]. In contrast over 50 % of epithelial tumors in children present as asymptomatic masses incidentally detected [6].

A recent largest single institution review analyzed the features of benign ovarian masses compared to malignancies to best unravel the diagnostic dilemma of an ovarian mass on presentation. The findings and odds ratios suggestive of a potential malignancy included masses in those aged 1–8 years of age, a chief complaint of a mass or precocious puberty, imaging findings of a mass greater than 8 cm, or a mass that is solid in character (shown in Table 8.4) [5]. Laboratory investigations showing elevated β-HCG, AFP, or cancer antigen 125 (CA-125) were worrisome for malignant neoplasm but are not definitive if normal.

Management Strategy

Evaluation

The work-up involves comprehensive exam, preoperative imaging, and testing for serum tumor markers, and if they are abnormal, then consult with a pediatric oncologist. Preoperative imaging will often reveal a pelvic mass, easily detected by US, computed tomography (CT) scan, or magnetic resonance imaging (MRI), depending on the initial complaints prompting the radiologic evaluation. Malignant masses were generally thought to be greater than 5 cm [48, 68], whereas others advocate the use of >8 cm to be the size cutoff for concern of malignancy [72]. In a case series, all malignancies exceeded 6 cm, whereas ≥8 cm allowed for a statistically significant odds ratio with the greatest accuracy (Table 8.4). The caveat is that using the 8-cm cutoff, two of 46 malignancies (4.3 %) would have been missed by size alone [5].

Radiologic studies are not always able to distinguish benign lesions from malignancies. Classically, solid masses are thought to have a higher risk of malignancy, although heterogeneous and cystic masses can also harbor underlying malignant neoplasm [7]. Solid masses, either by ultrasound or by CT scan had the highest frequency (33–60 %) of malignancy; solid features were only evident in 14–15 % of all malignancies [5]. Conversely, the majority of radiologic reads identified either a heterogeneous or cystic mass, which were associated with malignancy in only 15–20 % and 4–5 % of the time, respectively, which is consistent with previous reports [73]. While findings of a cystic lesion may be relatively reassuring, heterogeneous masses should still be approached with a heightened suspicion for malignancy, especially if additional concerning factors are present.

If an ovarian mass >8 cm is seen on preoperative imaging, serum levels of AFP, β-HCG, and CA-125 should be evaluated before surgery, and a chest CT scan should be obtained to rule out metastatic disease. If signs of precocious puberty are apparent, then FSH, LH, estradiol, and lactate dehydrogenase (LDH) serum levels should be obtained.

Tumor Markers

β-HCG, AFP, and CA-125 are all potential serum tumor markers for ovarian malignancies. GCTs will often produce AFP and/or β-HCG, depending on their subgrouping (see Table 8.3) [74]. Dysgerminomas can result in elevations of serum lactic dehydrogenase (LDH), β-HCG, or CA-125 [74]. Yolk sac and Sertoli–Leydig cell tumors are both associated with AFP elevations. CA-125 is most commonly associated with epithelial type tumors [6]. However, the caveat is that tumor markers do not exclude the possibility of malignancy when they are not elevated.

Thus, tumor markers are not definitive measurements preoperatively but are of greatest value, if elevated, in the ability to monitor postoperatively for complete resection of disease, as well as to detect relapse [75, 76]. Tumor markers should be drawn preoperatively whenever possible, but elevations can still be detected immediately postop due to the relatively long half-lives of both AFP and β-HCG [75].

Operative Management

Operative Staging

Proper staging at the time of surgery is critical in determining the need for postoperative chemotherapy; cisplatin-based adjuvant chemotherapy has markedly improved the long-term survival in GCTs. Over 80 % of ovarian neoplasms in any age group are GCTs [4], and thus they result from the undifferentiated primordial germ cell. In contrast, adult ovarian malignancies are primarily epithelial. This difference explains the two different staging systems since epithelial spread requires sampling of many peritoneal surfaces

Table 8.5 Modified FIGO staging classification for GCTs

Stage	Extent of disease
I	Limited to ovary, peritoneal washings negative for malignant cells; no clinical, radiographic, or histologic evidence of disease beyond the ovaries. The presence of gliomatosis peritonei does not result in changing stage I disease to a higher stage. Tumor markers normal after half-life decline
II	Microscopic residual or positive lymph nodes <2 cm; peritoneal washings negative for malignant cells. The presence of gliomatosis peritonei does not result in changing stage II disease to a higher stage; tumor markers positive or negative
III	Lymph node involvement (metastatic nodule) >2 cm; gross residual or biopsy only; contiguous visceral involvement (omentum, intestine, bladder); peritoneal washings positive for malignant cells; tumor markers positive or negative
IV	Distant metastases, including liver

and more extirpative surgery for clearance or debulking, whereas most germ cell tumors present at a low stage and have evidence of local spread, so the staging system for GCTs is focused on sampling what is visibly abnormal. Thus the modified International Federation of Gynecology and Obstetrics (FIGO) staging is best utilized for GCTs, and the American Joint Committee on Cancer (AJCC) and FIGO staging for primary ovarian carcinoma is utilized for epithelial-based tumors in children as in adults (see Table 8.5) [77, 78].

The surgical incision is based on the size of the mass to remove it without rupture and the best means to accomplish an appropriate staging procedure. Often this entails a transverse Pfannenstiel incision with vertical fascial incision depending on the size of the tumor and likelihood of malignancy. Intraoperative staging entails (1) sampling ascites for cytology, (2) lymph node sampling, (3) omentectomy, and (4) peritoneal biopsies with (5) assessment of the contralateral ovary. The steps of lymph node dissections, biopsies of peritoneal surfaces, and an omentectomy, which are standard in the staging in adults, are usually omitted in pediatric germ cell cases unless gross visible involvement is noted. There is no adverse impact on survival given this modification of staging for pediatric GCTs, and thus the new guidelines omit the need for these steps 2–4, listed above, without evidence of gross disease [68]. These new guidelines apply presumed GCTs.

Epithelial tumors should be staged according to the adult staging guidelines since lymph nodes are positive in up to 38 % of FIGO stage I epithelial tumors [79]. Bilateral biopsies are important since lymph node metastases are not clinically evident or visibly obvious.

Surgical Management

Ovarian lesions can be approached from a midline incision or a Pfannenstiel approach depending on the size of the tumor and likelihood of malignancy. It is often impossible to know at the time of surgery if the lesion is malignant or neoplastic at all.

Laparoscopy is controversial and discouraged by the Children's Oncology Group, since it is essential to remove the tumor intact to avoid the upstaging associated with rupturing the tumor or violating the capsule intraoperatively [74]. A careful intraoperative inspection is also critical.

When a mixed cystic and solid mass is encountered at laparoscopy or laparotomy, careful inspection is critical to best differentiate if the mass is benign or malignant. Adnexal masses with extraovarian spread, ovarian masses >8 cm in diameter, with peritoneal metastases, and external ovarian or intracystic vegetations can predict malignancy with 100 % sensitivity (see Table 8.4) [80].

Tumor markers can guide surgical decision making. If tumor markers are elevated, after incidental detection of an >8-cm solid or mixed mass, then a staging laparotomy should proceed and unilateral oophorectomy or salpingo-oophorectomy. Oophorectomy should be done if signs of precocious puberty exist. If tumor markers are normal and there are no clinical signs of precocious puberty, then excision of the mass >8 cm with an attempt at ovarian salvage to spare the ovary is warranted.

Recommended surgical therapy for specific pathologies is discussed below.

Most immature teratomas with a reassuring grade and cell type are typically treated with a unilateral salpingo-oophorectomy and a staging procedure. If the tumor is a distinct encapsulated teratoma, then the ipsilateral fallopian tube can be preserved. Surgery alone is curative even in the presence of elevated levels of AFP or microscopic foci of yolk sac tumors since chemotherapy is used for postoperative cases of relapse [28, 81]. For metastatic or recurrent disease, multiagent chemotherapy is utilized: the response to chemotherapy is excellent in the settings of a recurrence [28, 81, 82]. Extensive GCTs usually require multiple biopsies to confirm extent of disease without resecting vital structures since multiagent chemotherapy is very effective in reducing the extent of disease at the second-look procedure if planned after four rounds of chemotherapy to achieve a complete response.

Since most dysgerminomas have stage I disease, surgery alone is advised. Approximately 8–15 % of dysgerminomas are bilateral, and thus suspicious areas on the contralateral ovary are biopsied. Lymphatic spread typically involves pelvic and para-aortic lymph nodes, so ipsilateral nodes should be sampled to stage the patient. If the dysgerminoma is greater than stage I disease, then cytoreductive surgery to remove all operable tumor is advised, followed by multiagent chemotherapy [30, 83].

Therapy for endodermal sinus tumor involves a staging laparotomy and unilateral salpingo-oophorectomy, unless intraperitoneal and hematogenous spread have resulted in presentation at a higher stage.

Embryonal carcinoma, mixed GCTs, and choriocarcinoma all typically require a staging laparotomy with unilateral salpingo-oophorectomy and postoperative multiagent chemotherapy to reduce recurrence.

Borderline and malignant epithelial tumors typically are managed with conservative therapy since they present early. Thus they are managed with (1) a unilateral salpingo-oophorectomy for stage IA borderline tumors involving one ovary, (2) staging, and (3) biopsy of the contralateral ovary with a serous cystadenoma or if suspicious as in cases of a mucinous cystadenoma. Conservative management of stage II or III borderline tumors can also allow for preservation of fertility. However, in the rare case of an invasive tumor with peritoneal spread, patients presenting with more advanced stages should be managed as adults with staging laparotomy, cytoreductive surgery, and multiagent chemotherapy [84]. They may require total abdominal hysterectomy with bilateral salpingo-oophorectomy.

Fertility-Sparing Approaches

Malignant ovarian neoplasms in children arise predominately from the germ cell element of the ovary. Although the characteristics of each tumor type (germ cell, stromal, epithelial) differ, the majority of malignant ovarian tumors present at a low stage and can be treated with fertility-sparing surgery.

Given that most lesions present as an ovarian mass without clear evidence of being a malignancy, most advise ovarian-sparing operations for all benign-appearing lesions with normal tumor markers [7]. If the mass is secondary to torsion, then laparoscopic detorsion is first done, even if the ovary is ischemic or necrotic in appearance, and then surveillance by US is done to ensure the mass does not persist and that there is return of ovarian function [11, 12]. If the tumor is a bilateral teratoma, then an attempt to enucleate a lesion on one ovary is attempted to preserve fertility. Typically in a mature teratoma, if a fallopian tube is not involved and the tumor is clearly encapsulated, then the fallopian tube is preserved. Although oophorectomy has been the traditional treatment for teratomas, many authors report no adverse sequelae from resection of the mass alone in mature teratomas [7, 84]. The resection can be done laparoscopically, and the incidence of recurrent mature cystic teratomas in adults following cystectomy alone is 3–4 % [85]. In patients <40 years who had multiple or bilateral mature cystic teratomas resected, such as dermoids, there is a 2–3 % incidence of developing subsequent germ cell tumors [86].

Chemotherapy

Cisplatin-based adjuvant chemotherapy has vastly improved survival of GCTs of the ovary even in advanced cases with a dramatic improvement over the last few decades. Chemotherapy is required to manage those tumors that present spreading beyond the confines of the ovary. The current management with bleomycin, etoposide, and cisplatin has improved event-free survival (EFS) and overall survival (OS) for stage I GCTs to 95.1 %. Patients with stage II disease have EFS and OS of 87.5 and 93.8 % with four cycles of standard cisplatin, etoposide, and low-dose bleomycin [87]. High-dose cisplatin does not improve survival but is associated with more toxicity, so carboplatin is being tested to replace cisplatin.

Stromal cell tumors with high mitotic activity remain a challenge to treat. Those with mitoses >20 HPF have an EFS of 48 % compared to those <20 mitoses HPF with an EFS of 100 % [46]. The majority present at a low tumor stage, and prognosis is excellent, but for those with a higher proliferative activity, taxanes are being combined with cisplatin-based therapy to better improve outcomes.

Although the specific histopathologies of each tumor type in pediatric ovarian malignancies differ, the majority of malignant ovarian tumors present at a low stage and can be treated with fertility-sparing surgery. Platinum-based chemotherapy regimens have improved the outcome for that small subset that present with advanced stages of disease. Proper staging is critical to identify that small subset for best targeted chemotherapy.

References

1. Hassan E, Creatsas G, Deligeorolgu E, Michalas S. Ovarian tumors during childhood and adolescence. A clinicopathological study. Eur J Gynaecol Oncol. 1999;20:124.
2. Piver MS, Patton T. Ovarian cancer in children. Semin Surg Oncol. 1986;2:163.
3. Lindfors O. Primary ovarian neoplasms in infants and children: a study of 81 cases diagnosed in Finland and Sweden. Ann Chir Gynaecol Fenn Suppl. 1971; 177:1–6.
4. Brookfield KF, Cheung MC, Koniaris L, Sola J, Fischer AC. A population-based analysis of 1,037 malignant ovarian tumors in the pediatric population. J Surg Res. 2009;156(1):45–9.
5. Oltmann S, Garcia N, Huang R, Hicks B, Fischer AC. Can We preoperatively risk stratify ovarian masses for malignancy? J Pediatr Surg. 2010; 45(1):130–4.
6. Morowitz M, Huff D, von Allmen D. Epithelial ovarian tumors in children: a retrospective analysis. J Pediatr Surg. 2003;38:331–5; discussion 331–5.
7. Cass DL, Hawkins E, Brandt ML, Chintagumpala M, Bloss RS, Milewicz AL, Minifee PK, Wesson DE, Nuchtern JG, et al. Surgery for ovarian masses in infants, children, adolescents: 102 consecutive patients treated in a 15 year period. J Pediatr Surg. 2001;36:693.
8. Gutherie BD, Adler MD, Powell EC. Incidence and trends of pediatric ovarian torsion hospitalizations in the United States, 2000–2006. Pediatrics. 2010;125: 532–8.
9. Oltmann SC, Fischer AC, Barber R, Fischer A, Barber R, Huang R, et al. Pediatric ovarian malignancy presenting as ovarian torsion: incidence and relevance. J Pediatr Surg. 2010;45:135–9.
10. Cass DL. Ovarian torsion. Semin Pediatr Surg. 2005;14:86–92.
11. Kokoska ER, Keller MS, Weber TR. Acute ovarian torsion in children. Am J Surg. 2000;180:462–5.
12. Celik A, Ergun O, Aldemir H, Aldemir H, Ozcan C, Ozok G, et al. Long-term results of conservative management of adnexal torsion in children. J Pediatr Surg. 2005;40(4):704–8.
13. Aziz D, Davis V, Allen L, Langer J. Ovarian torsion in children: is oophorectomy necessary? J Pediatr Surg. 2004;39(5):750–3.
14. Fischer AC. Ovarian masses and torsion. In: Ledbetter DJ, Johnson PRV, editors. Endocrine surgery in children. New York: Springer; 2011.
15. Chang YJ, Yan DC, Kong MS, Wu CT, Chao HC, Luo CC, Hsia SH. Adnexal torsion in children. Pediatr Emerg Care. 2008;24(8):534–7.
16. Vogtlander MF, Rijntjes-Jacobs EG, van den Hoonaard TL, Versteegh FG. Neonatal ovarian cysts. Acta Paediatr. 2003;92:498–501.
17. Luzzatto C, Midrio P, Toffolutti T, Suma V. Neonatal ovarian cysts: management and follow up. Pediatr Surg Int. 2000;16:56–9.
18. Dolgin SE. Ovarian masses in the newborn. Semin Pediatr Surg. 2000;9:121–7.
19. Campbell BA, Garg RS, Garg K, Garg V, Othersen Jr HB, Smith CD. Perinatal cysts: a nonsurgical approach. J Pediatr Surg. 1992;27:1618–9.
20. Chiaramonte C, Piscopo A, Cataliotti F. Ovarian cysts in newborns. Pediatr Surg Int. 2001;17:171–4.
21. Brandt ML, Luks FI, Filiatrault D, Garel L, Desjardins JG, Youssef S. Surgical indications in antenatally

diagnosed ovarian cysts. J Pediatr Surg. 1991;26: 276–81.
22. Brandt ML, Helmrath MA. Ovarian cysts in infants and children. Semin Pediatr Surg. 2005;14:78–85.
23. Barton S, Laufer MR. Recurrent bilateral serous cystadenomas in a premenarchal girl: a case report and literature review. J Pediatr Adolesc Gynecol. 2010; 23(1):e27–9.
24. Magrina JF, Cornella JL. Office management of ovarian cysts. Mayo Clin Proc. 1997;72:653–6.
25. Lipitz S, Seidman DS, Menczer J, Bider D, Oelsner G, Moran O, Shaley J. Recurrence rate after fluid aspiration from sonographically benign-appearing ovarian cysts. J Reprod Med. 1992;37(10):845–8.
26. Teilum G. Classification of endodermal sinus tumour (mesoblastoma vitellinum) and so-called "embryonal carcinoma" of the ovary. Acta Pathol Microbiol Scand. 1965;64(4):407–29.
27. Norris HJ, Zirkin HJ, Benson WL. Immature (malignant) teratoma of the ovary: a clinical and pathologic study of 58 cases. Cancer. 1976;37:2359–72.
28. Cushing B, Giller R, Ablin A, Cohen L, Cullen J, Hawkins E. Surgical resection alone is effective treatment for ovarian immature teratoma in children and adolescents: a report of the pediatric oncology group and the children's cancer group. Am J Obstet Gynecol. 1999;181:353–8.
29. O'Connor DM, Norris HJ. The influence of grade on the outcome of stage I ovarian immature (malignant) teratomas and the reproducibility of grading. Int J Gynecol Pathol. 1994;13:283–9.
30. Pawinski A, Favalli G, Ploch E, Sahmoud T, van Oosterom AT, Pecorelli S. PVB chemotherapy in patients with recurrent or advanced dysgerminoma: a phase II study of the EORTC Gynaecological Cancer Cooperative Group. Clin Oncol. 1998;10(5): 301–5.
31. Ayhan A, Tuncer ZS, Yanik F, Bükülmez O, Yanik A, Küçükali T. Malignant germ cell tumors of the ovary: Hacettepe hospital experience. Acta Obstet Gynecol Scand. 1995;74(5):384–90.
32. Gordon A, Lipton D, Woodruff D. Dysgerminoma: a review of 158 cases from the Emil Novak ovarian tumor registry. Obstet Gynecol. 1981;58: 497–504.
33. Laufer MR. Adnexal Masses. In: Goldstein's pediatric & adolescent gynecology. Emans SJH, Laufer MR, 6th Edition. Lippincott Williams Wilkins, Philadelphia; 2012. p. 397–404.
34. Kurman RJ, Norris HJ. Endodermal sinus tumor of the ovary: a clinical and pathologic analysis of 71 cases. Cancer. 1976;38:2404–19.
35. Gershenson DM, Del Junco G, Herson J, Rutledge FN. Endodermal sinus tumor of the ovary: the MD Anderson experience. Obstet Gynecol. 1983;61: 194–202.
36. Scully RE. Gonadoblastoma: a review of 74 cases. Cancer. 1970;25:1340–56.
37. Gribbon M, Ein SH, Mancer K. Pediatric malignant ovarian tumors: a 43-year review. J Pediatr Surg. 1992;27:480–4.
38. Belchis D, Mowry J, Davis J. Infantile choriocarcinoma. Re-examination of a potentially curable entity. Cancer. 1993;72:2028–32.
39. Flam F, Lundstrom V, Silfversward C. Choriocarcinoma in mother and child: case report. Br J Obstet Bynaecol. 1989;96:241–4.
40. Takeda A, Ishizuka T, Goto T, Goto S, Ohta M, Tomoda Y, Hoshino M. Polyembryoma of ovary producing alpha-fetoprotein and HCG: immunoperoxidase and electron microscopic study. Cancer. 1982;49(9):1878–89.
41. Koksal Y, Reisli I, Gunel E, Caliskan U, Bulun A, Kale G. Galactorrhea-associated granulosa cell tumor in a child. Pediatr Hematol Oncol. 2004;21:101–6.
42. Chan LF, Storr HL, Scheimberg I, Perry LA, Banerjee K, Miraki-Moud F. Pseudo-precocious puberty caused by a juvenile granulosa cell tumour secreting androstenedione, inhibin and insulin-like growth factor-I. J Pediatr Endocrinol Metab. 2004;17:679–84.
43. Lazar EL, Stolar CJ. Evaluation and management of pediatric solid ovarian tumors. Semin Pediatr Surg. 1998;7:29–34.
44. Tetu B, Ordonez NG, Silva EG. Sertoli-Leydig cell tumor of the ovary with alpha-fetoprotein production. Arch Pathol Lab Med. 1986;110:65–8.
45. Gershenson DM, Copeland LI, Kavanagh JJ, Stringer CA, Saul PB, Wharton JT. Treatment of metastatic stromal tumors of the ovary with cisplatin, doxorubicin, and cyclophosphamide. Obstet Gynecol. 1987;70:765–9.
46. Schneider DT, Janig U, Calaminus G, Göbel U, Harms D. Ovarian sex cord-stromal tumors: a clinicopathological study of 72 cases from the Kiel Pediatric Tumor Registry. Virchows Arch. 2003;443: 549–60.
47. Breen JL, Maxon WS. Ovarian tumors in children and adolescents. Clin Obstet Gynecol. 1977;20:607–23.
48. Tsai JY, Saigo PE, Brown C, La Quaglia MP. Diagnosis, pathology, staging, treatment, and outcome of epithelial ovarian neoplasia in patients age <21 years. Cancer. 2001;91:2065–70.
49. Deprest J, Moerman P, Corneillie P, Ide P. Ovarian borderline mucinous tumor in a premenarchal girl: review on ovarian epithelial cancer in young girls. Gynecol Oncol. 1992;45(2):219–24.
50. Leake JF, Currie JL, Rosenshein NB, Woodruff JD. Long-term follow-up of serous ovarian tumors of low malignant potential. Gynecol Oncol. 1992;47(2): 150–8.
51. Elchalal U, Dgani R, Piura B, Anteby SO, Anteby SO, Zalel Y, Czernobilsky B, Schenker JG. Current concepts in management of epithelial ovarian tumors of low malignant potential. Obstet Gynecol Surv. 1995;50(1):62–70.
52. Barakat RR. Borderline tumors of the ovary. Obstet Gynecol Clin North Am. 1994;21(1):93–105.

53. Skinner MA, Schlatter M, Heifetz S, Skinner MA. Ovarian neoplasms in children. Arch Surg. 1993;128: 849–54.
54. Kr S, Wakhlu A, Kokai GK, McDowell H, Jones MO. Ovarian adenocarcinoma in premenarchal girls. J Pediatr Surg. 2001;36:511–5.
55. Chakrabarti B, Bhaduri B, Barik S, Gupta D, Chakravorty S. Primary ovarian lymphoma in a child. J Indian Med Assoc. 2011;109(9):679–80.
56. Heaton DC, Duff GB. Ovarian relapse in a young woman with acute lymphoblastic leukaemia. Am J Hematol. 1989;30(1):42–3.
57. Cacciaguerra S, Miano AE, Di Benedetto A, Vasquez E, Magro G, Fraggetta F. Gastric carcinoma with ovarian metastases in an adolescent. Pediatr Surg Int. 1998;14(1–2):98–9.
58. Surti U, Hoffner L, Chakravarti A, Ferrell RE. Genetics and biology of human ovarian teratomas: I. Cytogenetic analysis and mechanism of origin. Am J Hum Genet. 1990;47:635–43.
59. Parrington JM, West LE, Povey S. The origin of ovarian teratomas. J Med Genet. 1984;21:4–12.
60. Ohama K, Nomura K, Okamato E, Fukuda Y, Ihara T, Fujiwara A. Origin of immature teratoma of the ovary. Am J Obstet Gynecol. 1985;152:896–900.
61. King ME, DiGiovanni LM, Yung JF, Clarke-Pearson DL. Immature teratoma of the ovary grade 3, with karyotype analysis. Int J Gynecol Pathol. 1990;9(2): 178–84.
62. Ihara T, Ohama K, Satoh H, Fujii T, Nomura K, Fujiwara A. Histologic grade and karyotype of immature teratoma of the ovary. Cancer. 1984;54(12): 2988–94.
63. Ulbright TM. Gonadal teratomas: a review and speculation. Adv Anat Pathol. 2004;11:10–23.
64. Hoffner L, Deka R, Chakravarti A. Cytogenetics and origins of pediatric germ cell tumors. Cancer Genet Cytogenet. 1994;74:54–8.
65. Hoffner L, Shen-Schwarz S, Deka R, Chakravarti A, Surti U. Genetics and biology of human ovarian teratomas: III. Cytogenetics and origins of malignant ovarian germ cell tumors. Cancer Genet Cytogenet. 1992;62:58–65.
66. Thompson FH, Emerson J, Alberts D, Liu Y, Guan XY, Burgess A, et al. Clonal chromosome abnormalities in 54 cases of ovarian carcinoma. Cancer Genet Cytogenet. 1994;73:33–45.
67. Rutgers JL, Scully RE. Pathology of the testis in intersex syndromes. Semin Diagn Pathol. 1987;4:275–91.
68. Billmire D, Vinocur C, Rescorla F, Cushing B, London W, Schlatter M, et al. Outcome and staging evaluation in malignant germ cell tumors of the ovary in children and adolescents: an intergroup study. J Pediatr Surg. 2004;39:424–9.
69. Templeman C, Fallat ME, Blinchevsky A, Hertweck SP. Noninflammatory ovarian masses in girls and young women. Obstet Gynecol. 2000;96:229–33.
70. Niedziela M. Virilizing ovarian tumor in a 14-year-Old female with prior familial multinodular goiter. Pediatr Blood Cancer. 2008;51:543–5.
71. Calaminus G, Wessalowski R, Harms D, Göbel U. Juvenile granulosa cell tumors of the ovary in children and adolescents: results from 33 patients registered in a prospective cooperative study. Gynecol Oncol. 1997;65:447–52.
72. Hayes-Jordan A. Surgical management of the incidentally identified ovarian mass. Semin Pediatr Surg. 2005;14:106–10.
73. Brown MF, Hebra A, McGeehin K, Ross III AJ. Ovarian masses in children: a review of 91 cases of malignant and benign masses. J Pediatr Surg. 1993;28:930–2.
74. Von Allmen D. Malignant lesions of the ovary in childhood. Semin Pediatr Surg. 2005;14:100–5.
75. Childrens Oncology Group. Treatment of children with germ cell tumors handbook. 2004. www.childrensoncologygroup.org.
76. Pectasides D, Pestasides E, Kassanos D. Germ cell tumors of the ovary. Cancer Treat Rev. 2008;34: 427–41.
77. Thalberg SA. New gynecologic cancer staging. Obstet Gynecol. 1990;76(1):158.
78. Benedet JL, Bender H, Jones 3rd H, Ngan HY, Pecorelli S. FIGOstaging classifications and clinical practice guidelines in the management of gynecologic cancers. FIGO Committee on Gynecologic Oncology. Int J Gynaecol Obstet. 2000;70(2):209–62.
79. Morice P, Joulie F, Camatte S, Atallah D, Rouzier R, Pautier P, et al. Lymph node involvement in epithelial ovarian cancer: analysis of 276 pelvic and paraaortic lymphadenectomies and surgical implications. J Am Coll Surg. 2003;197:198–205.
80. Canis M, Bassil S, Wattiez A, Pouly JL, Manhes H, Mage G, Bruhat MA, et al. Fertility following laparoscopic management of benign adnexal cysts. Hum Reprod. 1992;7:529–31.
81. Terenziani M, D'Angelo P, Bisogno G, Boldrini R, Cecchetto G, Collini P, et al. Teratoma with a malignant somatic component in pediatric patients: the Associazione Italiana Ematologia Oncologia Pediatrica (AIEOP) experience. Pediatr Blood Cancer. 2010;54(4):532–7.
82. Topuz S, Iyibozkurt AC, Akhan SE, Keskin N, Yavuz E, Salihoglu Y, et al. Malignant germ cell tumors of the ovary: a review of 41 cases and risk factors for recurrence. Eur J Gynaecol Oncol. 2008;29(6): 635–7.
83. Thomas GM, Dembo AJ, Hacker NF, DePetrillo AD. Current therapy for dysgerminoma of the ovary. Obstet Gynecol. 1987;70(2):268–75.
84. Templeman CL, Hertweck SP, Scheetz JP, Perlman SE, Fallat ME. The management of mature cystic teratoma in children and adolescents: a retrospective analysis. Hum Reprod. 2000;15:2669–72.

85. Azizkhan RG, Caty MG. Teratomas in childhood. Curr Opin Pediatr. 1996;8:287–92.
86. Yanai-Inbar I, Scully RE. Relations of ovarian dermoid cysts and immature teratomas: an analysis of 350 cases of immature teratoma and 10 cases of dermoid cyst with microscopic foci of immature tissue. Int J Gynecol Pathol. 1987;6:203–12.
87. Rogers PC, Olson TA, Cullen JW, Billmire DF, Marina N, Rescorla F, et al. Treatment of children and adolescents with stage II testicular and stages I and II ovarian malignant germ cell tumors: a pediatric intergroup study- POG 9048 and COG 8891. J Clin Oncol. 2004;22:3563–9.

Management of Patients with Early-Stage Ovarian Cancer

9

Samir A. Farghaly

Introduction

Worldwide, the annual number of new patients who have ovarian cancer are about 225,500 and about 140,200 die of this disease. The American Cancer Society estimates that in 2013, about 22,240 new cases of ovarian cancer will be diagnosed and 15,500 women will die of ovarian cancer in the USA. The mortality rates for ovarian cancer have not improved in 40 years. The other cancers have shown a marked reduction in mortality, due to the availability of early detection tests and improved treatments. Early-stage ovarian cancer (International Federation of Gynecology and Obstetrics [FIGO] stages I to IIA) is approximately 30 % of patients with ovarian cancer; the disease is restricted to the true pelvis when it is diagnosed. In these early stages, there is a reasonable chance of cure. The standard primary therapy for epithelial ovarian cancer (EOC) involves staged procedures with pelvic and para-aortic lymphadenectomy, followed by adjuvant chemotherapy consisting of carboplatin and paclitaxel. In the literature, lymph node metastasis has been detected in 6–18 % and 23–31 % of patients with pT1 and pT2, respectively. Systematic resection and pathological examination of retroperitoneal lymph nodes have clinical significance for accurate assessment of staging and prognosis. Systematic lymphadenectomy is not always performed on patients during initial surgery for early-stage disease. This procedure may involve para-aortic lesions, and therefore it may increase surgical morbidity, such as increased operation time, increased blood loss, lymph cyst formation, and edema in the leg. Moreover, the therapeutic value of systematic lymphadenectomy remains controversial, especially in early disease. Following surgery, patients with early ovarian cancer—FIGO stages I to IIA, except stage IA, grade 1—benefit from 3 to 6 cycles of platinum-based chemotherapy, in terms of both overall survival (increase in 5-year survival rate from 74 to 82 %; $P<0.008$) and disease-free survival (increase from 65 to 76 %; $P<0.001$). The protocols of most of the available studies established six cycles of platinum-based chemotherapy. It is also unclear whether combined chemotherapy with carboplatin and paclitaxel is superior to monotherapy with carboplatin (area under the curve [AUC] 5) in early stages. Fertility-sparing surgery (FSS) for women of childbearing age with early-stage ovarian cancer had been discussed over the past 20 years. Preservation of the reproductive tract organs in young women who want to conceive is an understood need. Hysterectomy and bilateral salpingo-oophorectomy have been considered part of the initial surgical approach to ovarian cancer, regardless of the stage of the disease. Preservation of the adnexa and uterus is recommended in patients

S.A. Farghaly, MD, PhD
Department of Obstetrics and Gynecology,
The Weill Cornell Medical College/Weill Cornell Graduate School of Medical Sciences,
and The New York Presbyterian Hospital- Weill Cornell Medical Center, Cornell University,
New York, NY, USA
e-mail: samirfarghaly@yahoo.com

S.A. Farghaly (ed.), *Advances in Diagnosis and Management of Ovarian Cancer*,
DOI 10.1007/978-1-4614-8271-0_9, © Springer Science+Business Media New York 2014

with non-epithelial tumors and epithelial borderline ovarian cancer, in those patients.

Screening for Ovarian Cancer

Routine EOC screening of the general population has not been recommended by any professional society (Table 9.1) [1]. Women who are high risk for EOC on the basis of *BRCA* mutations or who have a family history of breast or ovarian cancer require a different "screening" approach. There is no evidence that measurement of cancer antigen 125 (CA-125) and transvaginal ultrasonography every 6 months provides a survival benefit, but the National Comprehensive Cancer Network does recommend this strategy for high-risk patients.

Table 9.1 Recommendations for ovarian cancer screening

Professional group	Recommendation
US Preventive Services Task Force	Does not recommend routine screening, concluding that "the potential harms outweigh the potential benefits"
American Cancer Society	Does not recommend routine screening; possible screening for women with a family history of ovarian cancer, although "it is not known how helpful" the tests will be in improving survival
American College Of Obstetricians and Gynecologists	Does not recommend routine screening; suggests evaluation of signs and symptoms of ovarian cancer (e.g., pelvic mass, pelvic or abdominal pain, urinary frequency or urgency, increased abdominal size or bloating, or difficulty eating or feeling of fullness)
National Comprehensive Cancer Network	Does not recommend routine screening; recommends screening of high-risk women (i.e., those with either a family history of ovarian or breast cancer or a documented BRCA mutation) with transvaginal ultrasonography and CA-125 measurements every 6 month, starting at the age of 35 years or 5–10 years before the earliest age at diagnosis of ovarian cancer in relatives; recommends strong consideration of risk-reducing prophylactic salpingo-oophorectomy at the completion of childbearing in women with a BRCA mutation

Early Detection of Ovarian Cancer

Early detection is very important to the successful treatment of ovarian cancer. It is estimated that 15 % of ovarian cancer is localized to the ovary, 17 % is regional, and 62 % occurs as distant disease. With tumor spread into the pelvis and upper abdomen, patients often complain of pelvic or abdominal pain or pressure, abdominal swelling, dyspepsia, and early satiety. As the disease progresses, patients note weight loss and increasing pain, and they can develop bowel or urinary tract disorders. Many patients will note a several-month history of vague abdominal discomfort which does not represent marked underlying pathology. A study from the University of Washington [2] noted that ovarian cancer patients' symptoms occurred 20–30 times per month as compared with two to three times for the clinic population. The severity of symptoms was also significantly higher in cancer patients and of more recent onset. The authors also noted that 44 % of women with ovarian cancer had a triad of bloating, increased abdominal size, and urinary urgency, as compared with only 8 % of clinic controls. They also observed that the important distinction between cases and controls seems to be in the frequency, severity, and duration of the symptoms. Several researchers in the USA and in other countries have found similar results. The same group [2] established a positive symptom index (any of those six symptoms that occurred more than 12 times per month in less than 1 year) and had a sensitivity of 56.7 % for early-stage disease and 79.5 % for advanced disease. More specificity was 90 % for patients older than 50 years and 86.7 % for patients younger than 50 years. Ovarian cancer should be included in the differential diagnosis and testing for the disease should be included in the work-up, if these symptoms are present.

Diagnosis and Staging

Palpation of an adnexal mass during a pelvic examination is considered a diagnostic evaluation for ovarian cancer. Ultrasound examination is a useful noninvasive diagnostic test. Between 13 and 21 % of women undergoing surgery for an adnexal mass will have an ovarian malignancy. Surgical option for management depends on several factors: age, menopausal status, family history, size and complexity of the mass, associated symptoms, CA-125, unilaterality versus bilaterality, and characteristics on ultrasound. Management may include observation with repeat examination, radiographic imaging, and laparoscopy or laparotomy. The preoperative evaluation of a woman with suspected ovarian cancer includes measurement of CA-125, which is elevated in greater than 80 % of patients with advanced EOC. Sensitivity is lower for stage I disease (50 %). CA-125 is highest in serous and lowest in mucinous EOC. In addition, CA-125 is not specific for EOC and found to be elevated in endometriosis, pelvic inflammatory disease, endometrial, and pancreatic cancers. Surgery is necessary for the diagnosis, staging, and treatment of EOC. The bulk of the ovarian tumor could be found on peritoneal surfaces. This peritoneal disease results from shedding of ovarian tumor cells into the peritoneal cavity, circulation of these cells throughout the abdomen and pelvis, and l implantation onto peritoneal surfaces. This is dependent upon the development of sufficient neovasculature to support cell survival and tumor growth. Optimal surgical cytoreduction before the administration of chemotherapy is a common practice in management of ovarian cancer. Optimal cytoreduction could be achieved by reducing the largest residual tumor nodule that remains after debulking surgery to 0.5 cm or less and greater than 1 cm for suboptimal debulking. The goals of initial surgery in ovarian cancer are to diagnose and stage disease and to provide therapeutic benefit with cytoreduction. Accurate histologic diagnosis and staging are required before systemic treatment is established.

Ovarian malignancies are surgically staged according to the FIGO staging system (Table 9.2).

Table 9.2 FIGO staging and prognosis of ovarian cancer

FIGO stage	Characteristics	Stage distribution (%)	10-year survival rate (%)
I	Disease confined to the ovaries		
IA	One ovary, capsule intact, no ascites		
IB	Both ovaries, capsule intact, no ascites	20	73
IC	Stage IA or IB plus ascites or washings, capsule ruptures, tumor on ovarian surface		
II	Disease confined to the pelvis	5	45
III	Disease confined to the abdominal cavity, including surface of the liver; pelvic, inguinal, or para-aortic lymph nodes; omentum or bowel	58	21
IIIA	Negative lymph nodes, plus microscopic seeding of peritoneal surface		
IIIB	Negative lymph nodes, peritoneal implants <2		
IIIC	Positive lymph nodes and/or abdominal implants >2 cm		
IV	Spread to the liver parenchyma, lung, pleura, or other extra-abdominal sites	17	<5

Staging laparotomy includes inspection of the peritoneal cavity, including the parabolic gutters, pelvis, and domes of the diaphragm; total abdominal hysterectomy (TAH) and bilateral salpingo-oophorectomy (BSO); liver palpation and biopsy (if indicated); lymph node sampling; omentectomy; and peritoneal washings. The extent of surgical cytoreduction should be fully documented.

Treatment Options for Early-Stage Ovarian Cancer

Treatment of early-stage ovarian cancer is dependent on the stage of the disease and extent of surgical cytoreduction. Approximately 25 % of women with ovarian cancer have disease confined to one or both ovaries (FIGO stage I) or to the pelvis (FIGO stage II). Treatment options for stage 1 and stage 2 ovarian epithelial cancers may include:

(A) Surgery: Total hysterectomy, bilateral salpingo-oophorectomy, partial omentectomy, and surgical staging of the lymph nodes and other tissues in the pelvis and abdomen. Selected premenopausal women in stage I with the lowest-grade tumors in one ovary may be treated salpingo-oophorectomy to preserve fertility.

(B) Chemotherapy: Patients with stage IA or B disease, grade 1 (or sometimes grade 2) do not need further therapy after surgery. The higher-risk patients (stage IC, stage I/grade 3) are treated with platinum-based chemotherapy to reduce their risk of recurrence.

(C) Clinical trials with chemotherapy, radiation therapy, or targeted molecular therapy.

Data from the International Collaborative Ovarian Neoplasm trial 1 (ICON1) and Adjuvant Chemotherapy in Ovarian Neoplasm (ACTION) have compared a platinum-containing adjuvant chemotherapy regimen with observation after surgery. They reported over 900 patients with over 4 years of median follow-up; the hazard ratio for recurrence-free survival is 0.64 (95 % confidence interval [95 % CI], 0.50–0.82; $P = .001$) in favor of adjuvant chemotherapy, and the hazard ratio for overall survival (OS) is 0.67 (95 % CI, 0.50–0.90; $P = .008$) in favor of adjuvant chemotherapy. A subgroup analysis suggested that the benefits of chemotherapy were in non-optimally staged patients, establishing the clinical importance of surgical staging in early-stage ovarian cancer [3].

The Gynecologic Oncology Group (GOG) studies have shown that patients with stage IA or IB disease (limited to one or both ovaries with no ascites and negative peritoneal washings) and with well- or moderately differentiated histology have a 5-year disease-free survival (DFS) rate of 91 % and a 5-year OS rate of 94 % with surgery alone. This subset of patients is generally not treated with adjuvant therapy. However, it is critical that these patients are fully staged. It has been shown that one-third of apparent early-stage patients will have more advanced stage disease when full staging is done. Also, it was observed that chemotherapy improves progression-free survival (PFS) for patients with stage IA or IB poorly differentiated disease, stage IC, or stage II disease, and these patients should receive adjuvant chemotherapy [4].

GOG in phase 3 study of patients with early-stage ovarian cancer (GOG protocol 157) compared 3 versus 6 cycles of paclitaxel and carboplatin. The 5-year probability of recurrence was 20.1 % for six cycles versus 25.4 % for three cycles, a 24 % reduction in recurrence risk. But the OS was similar for both regimens and the decrease in recurrence was not statistically significant. In addition, analysis of patients from this trial showed that those with high-grade serous histology had a significantly lower risk of recurrence with six compared with three cycles. Based on these findings, it is recommended that a minimum of three cycles of paclitaxel and carboplatin for patients with early-stage disease who are treated with adjuvant chemotherapy and six cycles for those with high-grade serous cancers.

Borderline Ovarian Tumors

Borderline tumors of the ovary are characterized by serous, mucinous or endometrioid histology type, and lack of stromal invasion. The median age at diagnosis is 45, with greater than 34 % of patients being less than 40 years of age. These tumors are managed with TAH and BSO. Twenty-five percent borderline tumors are reclassified as invasive on final review of the histopathology. The surgical management could be limited to unilateral salpingo-oophorectomy with complete surgical staging if patients desire fertility preservation. If the patient has bilateral ovarian tumor, and complete resection can be achieved, ovarian cystectomy is reasonable treatment option.

Complete surgical staging, including exploration of the entire abdominal cavity, peritoneal washings, infrasonic omentectomy, and multiple

Table 9.3 Oncologic and obstetric outcomes in patients with borderline ovarian tumors undergoing fertility-preserving surgery

Author	Patients	Pregnancies	Live births	Recurrences	Deaths
Zanetta et al. [5]	189	44	N/A	35	0
Lim-Tan et al. [6]	35	8	6	6	0
Morice et al. [7]	44	17	10	9	0
Boran et al. [8]	62	13	10	4	0
Fauvet et al. [9]	162	30	18	27	0
Donnez et al. [10]	16	12	12	3	0
Seracchiolo et al. [11]	19	6	6	1	0
Camatte et al. [12]	17	8	8	9	0
Morris et al. [13]	43	25	16	14	1
Gotlieb et al. [14]	39	22	21	3	0
Total	626	185 (50 %)	107 (58 %)	111(18 %)	1 (0.2 %)

Table 9.4 The obstetric outcomes in patients with malignant germ cell tumors treated conservatively

Author	Patients	Pregnancies	Live births	Recurrences	Deaths
Kanazawa et al. [15]	21	11	9	1	1
Gershenson et al. [16]	71	37	30	10	4
Zanetta et al. [17]	138	41	28	16	3
Perrin et al. [18]	45	8	7	4	2
Tangir et al. [19]	64	47	38	5	3

peritoneal biopsies, is important, as 20 % of patients may have noninvasive as well as invasive metastatic implants (Table 9.3).

Malignant germ cell tumors account for 5 % of ovarian malignancies, and the median age of affected patients is 19 years. Generally, most of those patients have stage I disease. The management of those patients includes (1) examination and palpation of the ileac and aortocaval nodes with biopsy of abnormal areas intact removal of the tumor, (2) examination and palpation of the omentum with removal of suspicious areas sparing of the fallopian tube if not adherent to the tumor, (3) collection of cytologic washings or harvesting of ascites fluid, and (4) removal of the tumor, (5) sparing the tube and the ovary. It was shown that 90–95 % of malignant germ cell tumors of the ovary are curable with the use of postoperative systemic chemotherapy [20] (Table 9.4).

Biopsy of a normal-appearing contralateral ovary is not recommended as this can result in tissue pelvic adhesion and possible mechanical infertility.

Platinum-Based Chemotherapy for Early-Stage Ovarian Cancer

Adjuvant platinum-based chemotherapy has been established as the optimal of care for women with high-risk early-stage EOC [21]. Gynecologic Cancer Intergroup (GCIG) consensus statement [22] and a Cochrane meta-analysis [23] advocated the use of platinum-based chemotherapy. National Comprehensive Cancer Network (NCCN) [24] guidelines recommend three to six cycles of a carboplatin/taxane combination. The GOG-157 trial [25] and other case series [26, 27] show that carboplatin-paclitaxel (CP) is frequently used as the standard of care for early epithelial ovarian cancer. This is due to concerns about suboptimal surgical staging. The GOG definition of comprehensive surgical staging includes total hysterectomy, bilateral salpingo-oophorectomy, resection of all gross disease, aspiration of free peritoneal fluid, peritoneal washings for cytology, infracolic omentectomy, selective bilateral pelvic and aortic node dissections, peritoneal biopsies from four pelvic locations and bilateral paracolic areas, and right diaphragm cytology or biopsy. The ACTION trial [28] found that only 151 (34 %) women were optimally staged. In a study of series of 100 women with apparent early-stage EOC, they underwent a second, comprehensive surgical staging procedure at which 23 were found to have stage III disease [20]. It has been shown that comprehensive surgical staging is critical in all women with early-stage ovarian cancer [29]. It may avoid the need for chemotherapy for some, as subset analysis of the 151 (34 %) optimally staged women in the ACTION trial [28] showed no benefit of adjuvant chemotherapy. The majority of women labeled as having early-stage EOC will have undergone less than comprehensive surgery. Some of these will have occult stage III disease.

It is known that the risk of paclitaxel-related neuropathy increases with cumulative dose [30], and if paclitaxel is used in the initial regimen, the ability to administer sufficient doses to women who relapse will be reduced. This additional toxicity could be justified if there was an overall survival benefit. The ICON three trial [31] compared carboplatin with carboplatin plus paclitaxel. In this trial, 20 % of the population had stage I or II disease. There was no benefit in survival either in the trial as a whole or in the 413 women with early-stage disease.

Published studies (Table 9.5) showed 5-year relapse-free survival (RFS) and 5-year overall survival (OS) in patients with early-stage ovarian cancer treated with systemic chemotherapy following comprehensive surgical staging.

The role of chemotherapy in early-stage epithelial ovarian cancer and the completeness of surgical staging are interlinked. The improved survival of women with suboptimally staged, early-stage ovarian cancer noted in ACTION 2003 is likely to be due to chemotherapy-related treatment of occult disease. The National Institute for Health and Care Excellence (NICE) guidelines (NCCC OC 2011) do not recommend systematic lymphadenectomy but advocate lymph node assessment by palpation and sampling of any suspiciously enlarged nodes. It argues that the morbidity of a comprehensive para-aortic lymphadenectomy cannot be justified. In addition, it has been shown that platinum-taxane combination chemotherapy and platinum-based chemotherapy without taxane were effective in prolonging survival with a significant dose–response relationship among patients with late-stage ovarian cancer. Among those with early-stage tumors, platinum-taxane combination appeared more effective than other chemotherapy regimens [29].

Minimally Invasive Surgery for Patients with Early-Stage Ovarian Cancer

The major deterrents to the general acceptance of laparoscopic staging of EOC have been:

1. Ovarian cancer represents a major surgical challenge, as it entails more extensive surgery than other gynecological cancers.
2. Comprehensive surgical staging is of undoubtful importance, as subsequent treatment plans and prognosis will be determined by the stage of disease.
3. The common and earliest mode of dissemination of ovarian cancer is by exfoliation of cells into the peritoneal cavity.
4. Last, ovarian neoplasms are often cystic masses and thus are prone to intraoperative rupture.

The real possibility of inadequate staging, port-site recurrence, and intraperitoneal spillage has been counted against the use of minimally invasive surgery for surgical treatment of ovarian cancer.

Laparoscopic Surgery for Ovarian Cancer

Results of published studies addressing laparoscopic staging of EOC are listed in Table 9.6.

The search for clear evidence-based data supportive of treatment decisions in EOC remains unclear. Previous trials, involving open surgery for the staging process of EOC, have shown inconsistencies in surgical staging, with a low rate of completely staged patients.

Childers et al. noted a mean operating time of 149 min in patients who did not undergo a

Table 9.5 Published studies of adjuvant chemotherapy on early-stage ovarian cancer

Study	Study type	Stage	Systemic therapy	Women	5-year RFS	5-year OS
Young et al. [32]	Prospective/randomized	Stage IG3/stage II	Melphalan/32P	68/73	80 %/80 %	81 %/78 %
Bolis et al. [33]	Prospective/randomized	Stage IC	Cisplatin/32P	82/79	85 %/65 %	81 %/79 %
Trope et al. [34]	Prospective/randomized	Stage I	Carboplatin/observation	81/81	70 %/71 %	86 %/85 %
Trimbos et al. [28]	Prospective/randomized	IA–IIA except IA/B G1	Platinum/observation	224/224	76 %**/68 %	85 %/78 %
ICON 1 [3]	Prospective/randomized	Uncertain benefit immediate chemotherapy	Platinum/observation	241/236	73***/62 %	79 %*/70 %
Bell [35]	Prospective/randomized	I and II except IA/B G1/2	CP × 6/CP × 3	225/232	80 %/75 %	83 %/81 %
Bamias et al. [26]	Retrospective/ nonrandomized	I–IIB except IA/b G1	CP × 4	69	79 %	87 %
Shimada et al. [27]	Retrospective/ nonrandomized	I–II	CAP × 3 or CP × 3	69/31		92 % (total group)
Platinum-based adjuvant therapy for early-stage EOC; single or combination chemotherapy (Adams [20])	Retrospective/ nonrandomized	IA–IIC	CP × 6/C × 6	60/35	57 %/54 %	73 %/62 %
Adams [20] (Subgroup PS0/1 stage 1)	Retrospective/ nonrandomized	IA–IC	CP × 6/C × 6	33/20	60 %/80 %	60 %/80 %

CAP cisplatin 50 mg/m^2, docorubicin 40 mg/m^2, and cyclophosphamide 400 mg/m^2
*$P = 0.03$, **$P = 0.02$, ***$P = 0.01$

Table 9.6 Studies on laparoscopic surgical staging of early-stage ovarian cancer

Study, *n*	Time in OR, min	EBL, mL	Complications	Conversion	Hospital stay, day	PLN, *n*	PALN, *n*	Upstaging, %	Follow-up, month	DFS, %	Overall survival, %
Querleu and Leblanc [36], 9	227	<30	0	0	2.8	–	8.6	11.1	NA	NA	NA
Pomel et al. [37], 10	313	NA	1 hemoperitoneum, 1 pulmonary embolus	0	4.7	7.5	8.5	10	NA	100	100
Childers et al. [38], 18	149/196	NA	0	0	1.6	–	–	35.7	NA	NA	NA
Tozzi et al. [39], 24	176	NA	1 chylous ascites, 1 hematoma, 2 lymphocysts	0	7	19.4	19.6	20.8	46.4 (2–72)	91.6	100
Leblanc et al. [40], 42	238	NA	1 hematoma, 2 lymphocysts	0	3.1	14	20	19	54 (8–116)	90.5	97.6
Chi et al. [41], 20	321	235	0	0	3.1	12.3	6.7	10	NA	NA	NA
Ghezzi et al. [42], 15	377		1 hematoma, 1 lymphedema	0	3	25.2	6.5	27.6	16 (4–33)	100	100
Park et al. [43], 17	321	231	1 ureter injury, 1 vein injury	0	9.4	13.7	8.9	5.9	17 (5–61)	88.2	94.1
Park et al. [44], 19	220	240	1 great vessel injury	5.3 %	8.9	27.2	6.6	21.1	17 (2–40)	100	100
Colomer et al. [45], 200	223	NA	1 vein injury (conversion)	5 %	3	18	11.3	20	24.7 (1–61)	95	100
Nezhat et al. [46], 36	229	195	2 lymphocyst	0	2.4	14.8	12.2	19.4	55.9	83.3	100
Lee et al. [47], 26	228	230	2 umbilical hernia	3.7 %	6.4	23.5	9.9	3.8 %	12 (1–42)	100	100
Schreuder et al. [48], 25	235	100	2 hemorrhage, 2 port-site hematomas	0	4	8	6	32	43 ± 31.5	92	92

hysterectomy during their laparoscopic staging and a mean operating time of 196 min in patients who did undergo a hysterectomy [38]. It has been shown that total hysterectomy in a laparoscopic staging procedure is not justifiable [49, 50]. In women who wish to preserve fertility, it has been reported that leaving the uterus and the remaining ovary seems to be safe [51]. Eltabbakh et al., in a study, performed laparoscopic-assisted vaginal hysterectomy with bilateral salpingo-oophorectomy and pelvic lymph node sampling in patients staged for endometrial cancer. They reported reduction in operating time and a significant increase in the amount of pelvic lymph nodes harvested [52].

Many gynecologic oncologists are reluctant to adopt laparoscopic staging of ovarian cancer. This is based on doubts about, the number of lymph nodes obtained, possible risk of port-site metastases, lack of tactile sensation, and risk of intraoperative mass rupture [39, 41–44, 53, 54].

Nagarsheth et al. demonstrated that the risk of port-site metastases (ranging from 0 to 2.3 %) is comparable to the incidence of implantation metastases observed after conventional laparotomy [55, 56]. The risk seems to be higher in patients with recurrent ovarian cancer or primary peritoneal malignancies in the presence of ascites [54, 57].

Intraoperative mass rupture laparoscopic staging procedure of early-stage ovarian cancer is thought to be a risk [58]. Upstaging of the tumor (having a higher stage after secondary staging procedure then presumed after the initial operation) may create the need for adjuvant chemotherapy in patients with early-stage disease [43].

A multivariate analysis reported that accidental capsular rupture did not affect the prognosis in stage I and II ovarian cancer [56].

Vergote et al. reported that tumor rupture during surgery has a negative effect on prognosis [59]. It has been shown that the incidence of iatrogenic rupture of ovarian cancer cysts is similar in the laparoscopy and laparotomy groups [37, 44].

The rate of upstaging reported ranged between 0 [36] and 41.7 % [53]. The upstaging rates in laparotomic staging were reported to be ranging from 21.2 [43] to 47 % [39].

The complication rate for the laparoscopic staging procedure in early-stage ovarian cancer ranged from 4.2 [53] to 37.5 % [60], and the complication rate in laparoscopy is similar to with laparotomy [41, 42]. It has been noted that laparoscopic-assisted ovarian tumorectomy is a feasible surgical procedure in patients with early-stage ovarian cancer [61, 62].

Postoperative hospital stay for laparoscopic staging ranges from 2 to 10.6 days [53, 60]. Jung et al. found a mean postoperative stay of 10.6 days. The postoperative stay in the laparotomy control groups ranges from 5.8 to 14.5 days [41, 44].

Port-site metastasis following laparoscopic surgery is well documented. It is noteworthy that if the following protective measures are applied, it will decrease undoubtedly the risk of the development of port-site metastases: trocar fixation, prevention of insufflation gas leaks, rinsing of instruments with 1 % povidone-iodine solution, minilaparotomy protection, rinsing off trocars before removal, closure of all abdominal layers including peritoneum, and rinsing of all wounds with 1 % povidone-iodine solution. The issue of insufflation gas, which is used during laparoscopic surgery, is an important one. It has been shown that the use of helium as a laparoscopic insufflation agent for cancer surgery results in less tumor implantation and growth at port-sites. Helium significantly slows down cell growth and has a minimal effect on the reduction of pH. These two factors are important in the development of port-site malignancy recurrence [63].

Robotic Surgery for Ovarian Cancer

There are several limitations to laparoscopic-assisted surgery. First, the learning curve is long; second, the hand movements are counterintuitive; third, the long instruments working through a fixed entry point cause small movements.

The da Vinci robotic platform (Fig. 9.1) is employed in robot-assisted laparoscopic surgery. It consists of three components: the surgeon's console, which directs the movements of the robotic arms, the vision system, and the patient-side cart, which in the latest system has four arms. After placement of port sites and docking

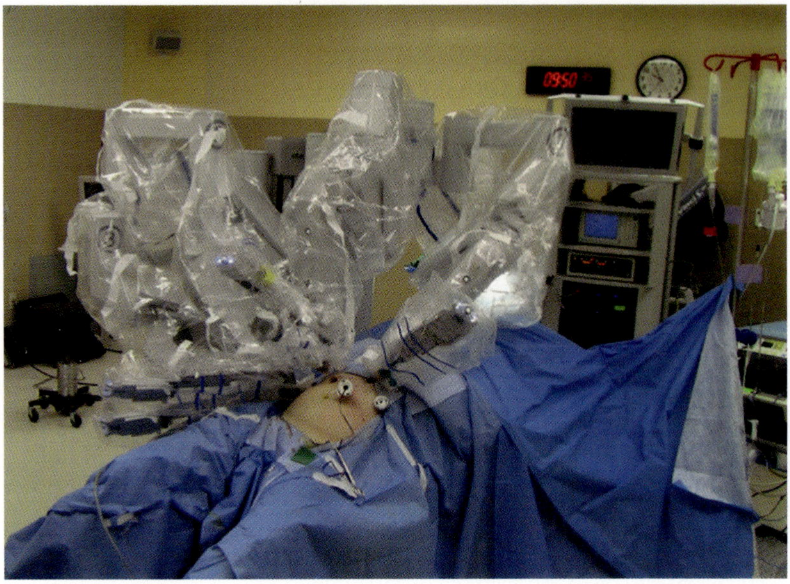

Fig. 9.1 Robotic platform docked off patient's right shoulder in 10° reverse Trendelenburg position, 10° rotation to left

the patient-side cart, the surgeon sits at the console and is able to view the pelvis through a three-dimensional vision system in high definition.

Furthermore, the camera system is stabilized by the robotic platform and easily controlled by the surgeon through foot pedals and arm movements. At the console, the surgeon controls the robotic arms and the EndoWrist instruments with natural hand and wrist motions that mimic movements performed in open surgery.

There are only a few publications that relate to robotic surgery for ovarian cancer patients. In a case analysis of robotic approach for epithelial ovarian cancer [64], twenty-five patients that underwent robotic surgical treatment were compared with those treated by laparoscopy and laparotomy. Complete debulking was achieved in 84 % of patients in the robotic group, 93 % in the laparoscopy group, and 56 % in the laparotomy group ($P<0.001$). The authors noted that optimal debulking is more important than the type of surgical method, as there was no difference in the overall and progression-free survival for robotic and laparotomy patients. To, thoroughly, explore all four quadrants of the abdomen, Magrina et al. [64] have suggested the rotation of operative table and redocking the robot at the patient's head. Also, the authors noted that it was easier to resect para-aortic lymph nodes to higher levels and upper abdominal metastases. Also, the reverse-docking position was useful when the transverse colon needed mobilization for bowel resection.

Fertility-Sparing Surgery in Young Women with Early-Stage Ovarian Cancer

Fertility-sparing surgery for ovarian neoplasms has been used in borderline tumors of the ovary, early-stage malignant ovarian germ cell tumors, granulosa cell tumors, Sertoli-Leydig cell tumors, and ovarian dysgerminomas, with satisfactory fertility and oncological outcomes. The acceptable standard is to implement adequate operative staging to reveal occult advanced disease with acceptable therapeutic results and satisfactory prognosis [65].

The guidelines of the American College of Obstetrics and Gynecology (ACOG) in 2007, fertility-sparing surgery for reproductive-age patients with invasive EOC is recommended for highly or moderately differentiated stage IA disease with non-clear cell histology.

The European Society for Medical Oncology (ESMO) in 2008 indicated that fertility-sparing techniques in EOC is recommended in patients with unilateral stage I tumor without dense adhesions with moderate or highly differentiated, non-clear cell histology. The number of published studies related to FSS in young patients with EOC is limited, and the patient's samples are small to allow a consensus regarding the selection criteria of the optimal candidate for FSS.

Borderline Ovarian Tumors

Patients with borderline ovarian tumors (BOTs) are good candidates for FSS, which has shown increased safety and efficacy in those patients.

The standard surgical procedures include total hysterectomy, BSO, peritoneal washings, multiple peritoneal biopsies, resection of implants, omentectomy, and appendectomy (in patients with mucinous BOTs) [64, 66].

Lymphadenectomy is usually not indicated due to the rarity of lymph node metastasis [67–70].

Type of Surgery

Salpingo-oophorectomy in patients with BOTs has been reported to be associated with better oncologic outcome as less-extensive surgery has been associated with higher recurrence rates. However, cystectomy as FSS could be the only option, in some patients, due to previous history of unilateral oophorectomy or salpingo-oophorectomy or bilateral involvement of BOTs.

Several studies have suggested that bilateral adnexectomy in patients with bilateral BOTs was associated with an insignificant increase in recurrence rate. This indicates that cystectomy should be limited to patients with a previous history of unilateral adnexectomy or bilateral BOTs.

The rates of bilateral involvement of BOTs have been reported to be 25–50 % for serous-type tumors and 5–10 % for mucinous-type tumors [71, 72]. The need for histopathologic evaluation of the contralateral ovary during fertility-sparing surgery is paramount, and wedge biopsy of the remaining ovary may cause mechanical infertility or ovarian failure [73–75].

A study of 14 patients who underwent wedge biopsy of the contralateral ovary found that none was positive, and one patient with normal results had recurrent disease in the remaining ovary [73]. This would indicate that histopathologic evaluation of the normal appearing contralateral ovary is not helpful in reducing the risk of recurrence in the remaining ovary.

In another study, all patients who underwent wedge biopsy of the normal-appearing contralateral ovary, none was positive for BOTs, whereas 11 of the 22 patients who underwent cystectomy to remove benign-appearing cysts of the contralateral ovary had BOTs on the contralateral ovary [76]. This illustrate that thorough inspection of the surface of the contralateral ovary and biopsies of suspicious lesions are adequate for screening.

FSS laparoscopic surgery has several advantages over laparotomy. Farghaly [43] described a technique for video laparoscopic fertility-sparing surgery in patients with low malignant potential (LMP) ovarian tumors. This technique was shown to be feasible, accurate, and safe.

Also, two studies [43, 44] have suggested the feasibility, safety, and accuracy of laparoscopic surgery for patients with early-stage epithelial ovarian cancer.

Recurrence rates were found to be similar in patients undergoing laparoscopy or laparotomy and FSS for early ovarian cancer [10, 72, 77–79].

Border line ovarian tumors with a micropapillary histologic pattern [80, 81] have been associated with more common bilateral ovarian involvement, extraovarian implants, and invasive implants [82, 83]. In a study of 15 patients with that pattern, the rates of bilateral ovarian involvement, extraovarian implants, and recurrence were high [84].

It has been shown, in a study of ten patients with microinvasion, that five of these patients had recurrent disease, all lesions developed on the remaining ovary, and all patients with recurrence were successfully treated [84].

Other Potential Options to Preserve Fertility

Where FSS is not indicated, because the normal ovarian tissue cannot be preserved due to massive bilateral ovarian involvement and only the uterus can be preserved, have several options for fertility preservation. These include embryo freezing, oocyte freezing, and ovarian tissue freezing. Embryo freezing has been shown to offer reasonable success rate of 20–30 % [85]. This option could be considered for patients with BOTs, before definitive surgery [86]. In this treatment, a life partner or sperm donor is required, and patients must delay cancer treatment for 2–6 weeks. Oocyte freezing is also a viable option for fertility preservation in patients with BOTs. More than 230 pregnancies from frozen oocytes have been reported worldwide, with live-birth rates per oocyte thawed of 1.9–4.6 % [87]. Oocyte freezing does not require a life partner or sperm donor, and it requires a 2–6-week delay in cancer treatment. Ovarian tissue freezing is another option and three pregnancies have been reported [87–89]. A delay in cancer treatment and a life partner or sperm donor is not required. A restoration of endocrine function and embryo development from this technique has been reported, but cancer cells may be transmitted [90]. As of now, the cryopreserved fragments have not been reimplanted [91]. Donor oocytes could be an alternative option for fertility preservation [92, 93].

Oncologic Outcomes After FSS

FSS is a safe treatment option for early-stage ovarian cancer patients with acceptable oncologic safety profile [94]. Satoh et al., in a study of stage I EOC patients who underwent fertility-sparing surgery [50], reported that 8.5 % relapsed with 27 % of the relapsed patients presenting recurrence in the remaining ovary. In patients with stage IA disease with clear cell histology or stage IC with unilateral ovarian involvement and favorable histology, authors emphasized the need of a complete surgical staging and an adjuvant platinum-based chemotherapy. In other studies, the mean relapse rates were estimated to be around 10 % [94–99].

Kajiyama et al. [99] concluded that patients with stage IC (surface involvement/positive cytology) their outcome was significantly poorer than those of patients with stage IA after FSS.

Zanetta et al. reported that none of the women undergoing bilateral oophorectomy had microscopic foci of cancer in the normal-looking contralateral ovary [94].

It has been shown that the negative impact of unfavorable histology on survival has mainly been related to advanced-stage disease III and IV [100, 101]. The reason for that was increased chemotherapy resistance to carboplatin and paclitaxel regimens, and in stage IA, no adjuvant treatment was necessary.

Reproductive Outcomes After Fertility-Sparing Surgery

Impaired fertility in young women with early-stage ovarian cancer represents a therapeutic challenge. Chemotherapy and surgical treatments often compromise the ovarian function, resulting in infertility and premature menopause [102–104]. The rate of women with successful conception after FSS is approximately 30 % of all patients; however, it is higher in women in the child-bearing age, ranges from 66 to 100 %. It has been shown that only a small percentage of patients required assisted reproductive techniques for a successful conception and pregnancy [50, 94, 105, 106]. The incidence of spontaneous abortions reported to be between 11 and 33 %. In a study by Satoh et al. [50], 5.0 % of the patients who received platinum-based chemotherapy presented a persistent secondary amenorrhea up to 224 months after completion of four to six cycles of systemic chemotherapy. 9.1 % of the patients who successfully conceived have been stated to receive an infertility treatment before pregnancy. In addition, it has been reported that none of the patients who successfully conceived and gave birth presented any cancer-related problems during the perinatal period, and rates of congenital malformations and abnormal fetal outcomes have been the same as in the general population [50, 107].

Chemotherapy-Induced Gonadotoxicity Following FSS

To decrease chemotherapy-induced gonadotoxicity after FSS, hormonal protection has been utilized to affect the ovarian tissue by pituitary downregulation to enter into a state of inactivity and so to make it less susceptible to cytotoxic agents. Several agents have been used, such as GnRH agonists, oral contraceptives, and tamoxifen. Tan et al. applied different doses of triptorelin in combination with busulfan in sexually mature, virgin, female mice. Results have demonstrated a dose-dependent protective effect against gonadotoxic chemotherapy of a gonadotropin-releasing hormone (GnRH) analogue on ovarian reserve [107].

All clinical studies assessing the protective effect of GnRH agents have been conducted in patients with hematologic malignancies, breast cancer, and lupus erythematodes chemotherapy and have shown a reduction of premature ovarian failure in patients receiving GnRH analogue or OC during systemic chemotherapy [108].

References

1. American Cancer Society. Cancer facts and figures 2013. Atlanta, GA: American Cancer Society. 2013. Available at http://www.cancer.org/cancer/ovarian cancer/Detailed Guide/Ovarian-Cancer-Key-Statistics. Accessed 23 May 2013.
2. Goff BA. Ovarian cancer: screening and early detection. Obstet Gynecol Clin North Am. 2012;39(2):183–94.
3. Colombo N, Pecorelli S. What have we learned from ICON1 and ACTION? Int J Gynecol Cancer. 2003;13 Suppl 2:140–3.
4. Chan JK, Tian C, Teoh D, Monk BJ, Herzog T, Kapp DS, Bell J. Survival after recurrence in early-stage high-risk epithelial ovarian cancer: a Gynecologic Oncology Group study. Gynecol Oncol. 2010;116(3):307–11.
5. Zanetta G, Meni A, Brancatelli G, Chiari S, Lissoni AA, Ratti M, Buda A. Comparison of methods for monitoring young women with stage I borderline ovarian tumor after conservative surgery. Minerva Ginecol. 2001;53(1 Suppl 1):10–1.
6. Lim-Tan SK, Cajigas HE, Scully RE. Ovarian cystectomy for serous borderline tumors: a follow-up study of 35 cases. Obstet Gynecol. 1988;72(5):775–81.
7. Morice P, Camatte S, Wicart-Poque F, Atallah D, Rouzier R, Pautier P, Pomel C, Lhommé C, Duvillard P, Castaigne D. Results of conservative management of epithelial malignant and borderline ovarian tumors. Hum Reprod Update. 2003;9(2):185–92. Review.
8. Boran N, Cil AP, Tulunay G, Ozturkoglu E, Koc S, Bulbul D, Kose MF. Fertility and recurrence results of conservative surgery for borderline ovarian tumors. Gynecol Oncol. 2005;97(3):845–51.
9. Fauvet R, Poncelet C, Boccara J, Descamps P, Fondrinier E, Daraï E. Fertility after conservative treatment for borderline ovarian tumors: a French multicenter study. Fertil Steril. 2005;83(2):284–90.
10. Donnez J, Munschke A, Berliere M, Pirard C, Jadoul P, Smets M, Squifflet J. Safety of conservative management and fertility outcome in women with borderline tumors of the ovary. Fertil Steril. 2003;79(5):1216–21.
11. Seracchioli R, Venturoli S, Colombo FM, Govoni F, Missiroli S, Bagnoli A. Fertility and tumor recurrence rate after conservative laparoscopic management of young women with early-stage borderline ovarian tumors. Fertil Steril. 2001;76(5):999–1004.
12. Camatte S, Deffieux X, Castaigne D, Thoury A, Fourchotte V, Pautier P, Lhommé C, Duvillard P, Morice P. Laparoscopic treatment of borderline ovarian tumor: analysis of 54 patients and clinical outcomes. Gynecol Obstet Fertil. 2005;33(6):395–402.
13. Morris RT, Gershenson DM, Silva EG, Follen M, Morris M, Wharton JT. Outcome and reproductive function after conservative surgery for borderline ovarian tumors. Obstet Gynecol. 2000;95(4):541–7.
14. Gotlieb WH, Flikker S, Davidson B, Korach Y, Kopolovic J, Ben-Baruch G. Borderline tumors of the ovary: fertility treatment, conservative management, and pregnancy outcome. Cancer. 1998;82(1):141–6.
15. Kanazawa K, Suzuki T, Sakumoto K. Treatment of malignant ovarian germ cell tumors with preservation of fertility: reproductive performance after persistent remission. Am J Clin Oncol. 2000;23(3):244–8.
16. Gershenson DM, Miller AM, Champion VL, Monahan PO, Zhao Q, Cella D, Williams SD, Gynecologic Oncology Group. Reproductive and sexual function after platinum-based chemotherapy in long-term ovarian germ cell tumor survivors: a Gynecologic Oncology Group Study. J Clin Oncol. 2007;25(19):2792–7.
17. Zanetta G, Bonazzi C, Cantù M, Binidagger S, Locatelli A, Bratina G, Mangioni C. Survival and reproductive function after treatment of malignant germ cell ovarian tumors. J Clin Oncol. 2001;19(4):1015–20.
18. Perrin LC, Low J, Nicklin JL, Ward BG, Crandon AJ. Fertility and ovarian function after conservative surgery for germ cell tumors of the ovary. Aust N Z J Obstet Gynaecol. 1999;39(2):243–5.
19. Tangir J, Zelterman D, Ma W, Schwartz PE. Reproductive function after conservative surgery and chemotherapy for malignant germ cell tumors of the ovary. Obstet Gynecol. 2003;101(2):251–7.

20. Adams G, Zekri J, Wong H, Walking J, Green JA. Platinum-based adjuvant chemotherapy for early-stage epithelial ovarian cancer: single or combination chemotherapy? BJOG. 2010;117(12):1459–67.
21. Winter-Roach BA, Kitchener HC, Dickinson HO. Adjuvant (post-surgery) chemotherapy for early stage epithelial ovarian cancer. Cochrane Database Syst Rev. 2009;(3):CD004706.
22. Stuart GC, Kitchener H, Bacon M, Dubois A, Friedlander M, Ledermann J, Marth C, Thigpen T, Trimble E, participants of 4th Ovarian Cancer Consensus Conference (OCCC), Gynecologic Cancer Intergroup. 2010 Gynecologic Cancer InterGroup (GCIG) consensus statement on clinical trials in ovarian cancer: report from the Fourth Ovarian Cancer Consensus Conference. Int J Gynecol Cancer. 2011;21(4):750–5.
23. Winter-Roach BA, Kitchener HC, Dickinson HO. Adjuvant (post-surgery) chemotherapy for early stage epithelial ovarian cancer. Cochrane Database Syst Rev. 2009;3, CD004706. doi:10.1002/14651858.CD004706.pub3. Review.
24. Trimbos JB, Vergote I, Bolis G, Vermorken JB, Mangioni C, Madronal C, Franchi M, Tateo S, Zanetta G, Scarfone G, Giurgea L, Timmers P, Coens C, Pecorelli S, EORTC-ACTION collaborators, European Organisation for Research and Treatment of Cancer-Adjuvant ChemoTherapy in Ovarian Neoplasm. Impact of adjuvant chemotherapy and surgical staging in early-stage ovarian carcinoma: European Organisation for Research and Treatment of Cancer-Adjuvant ChemoTherapy in Ovarian Neoplasm trial. J Natl Cancer Inst. 2003; 95(2):113–25.
25. Darcy KM, Brady WE, McBroom JW, Bell JG, Young RC, McGuire WP, Linnoila RI, Hendricks D, Bonome T, Farley JH, Gynecologic Oncology Group. Associations between p53 overexpression and multiple measures of clinical outcome in high-risk, early stage or suboptimally-resected, advanced stage epithelial ovarian cancers A Gynecologic Oncology Group study. Gynecol Oncol. 2008; 111(3):487–95.
26. Bamias A, Papadimitriou C, Efstathiou E, Rodolakis A, Vlahos G, Voulgaris Z, Bozas G, Fountzilas G, Aravantinos G, Razis E, Gika D, Dimopoulos MA. Four cycles of paclitaxel and carboplatin as adjuvant treatment in early-stage ovarian cancer: a six-year experience of the Hellenic Cooperative Oncology Group. BMC Cancer. 2006;6:228.
27. Shimada M, Kigawa J, Kanamori Y, Itamochi H, Oishi T, Minagawa Y, Ishihara K, Takeuchi Y, Okada M, Terakawa N. Outcome of patients with early ovarian cancer undergoing three courses of adjuvant chemotherapy following complete surgical staging. Int J Gynecol Cancer. 2005;15(4):601–5.
28. Trimbos JB, Parmar M, Vergote I, Guthrie D, Bolis G, Colombo N, Vermorken JB, Torri V, Mangioni C, Pecorelli S, Lissoni A, Swart AM, International Collaborative Ovarian Neoplasm 1, European Organisation for Research and Treatment of Cancer Collaborators-Adjuvant ChemoTherapy un Ovarian Neoplasm. International Collaborative Ovarian Neoplasm trial 1 and Adjuvant ChemoTherapy In Ovarian Neoplasm trial: two parallel randomized phase III trials of adjuvant chemotherapy in patients with early-stage ovarian carcinoma. J Natl Cancer Inst. 2003;95(2):105–12.
29. Du XL, Parikh RC, Lairson DR, Giordano SH, Cen P. Comparative effectiveness of platinum-based chemotherapy versus taxane and other regimens for ovarian cancer. Med Oncol. 2013;30(1):440. doi:10.1007/s12032-012-0440-4.
30. Seliger G, Mueller LP, Kegel T, Kantelhardt EJ, Grothey A, Groe R, Strauss HG, Koelbl H, Thomssen C, Schmoll HJ. Phase 2 trial of docetaxel, gemcitabine, and oxaliplatin combination chemotherapy in platinum- and paclitaxel-pretreated epithelial ovarian cancer. Int J Gynecol Cancer. 2009;19(8):1446–53.
31. Ozols RF, Markman M, Thigpen JT. ICON3 and chemotherapy for ovarian cancer. Lancet. 2002; 360(9350):2086–7; author reply 2088.
32. Young RC, Brady MF, Nieberg RK, Long HJ, Mayer AR, Lentz SS, Hurteau J, Alberts DS. Adjuvant treatment for early ovarian cancer: a randomized phase III trial of intraperitoneal 32P or intravenous cyclophosphamide and cisplatin–a gynecologic oncology group study. J Clin Oncol. 2003;21(23):4350–5.
33. Bolis G, Scarfone G, Polverino G, Raspagliesi F, Tateo S, Richiardi G, Melpignano M, Franchi M, Mangili G, Presti M, Villa A, Conta E, Guarnerio P, Cipriani S, Parazzini F. Paclitaxel 175 or 225 mg per meters squared with carboplatin in advanced ovarian cancer: a randomized trial. J Clin Oncol. 2004;22(4):686–90.
34. Tropé CG, Kisic J, Vergote I. Prognostic factors in platinum-resistant ovarian carcinoma treated with ifosfamide-etoposide. Eur J Gynaecol Oncol. 2000; 21(3):255–9.
35. Bell J, Brady MF, Young RC, Lage J, Walker JL, Look KY, Rose GS, Spirtos NM. Randomized phase III trial of three versus six cycles of adjuvant carboplatin and paclitaxel in early stage epithelial ovarian carcinoma: a Gynecologic Oncology Group study. Gynecol Oncol. 2006;102(3):432–9.
36. Querleu D, Leblanc E. Laparoscopic infrarenal para-aortic lymph node dissection for restaging of carcinoma of the ovary or fallopian tube. Cancer. 1994; 73:1467–71.
37. Pomel C, Provencher D, Dauplat J, et al. Laparoscopic staging of early ovarian cancer. Gynecol Oncol. 1995;58:301–6.
38. Childers JM, Lang J, Surwit EA, Hatch KM. Laparoscopic surgical staging of ovarian cancer. Gynecol Oncol. 1995;59:25–33.
39. Tozzi R, Köhler C, Ferrara A, Schneider A. Laparoscopic treatment of early ovarian cancer: surgical and survival outcomes. Gynecol Oncol. 2004;93: 199–203.
40. Leblanc E, Querleu D, Narducci F, Occelli B, Papageorgiou T, Sonoda Y. Laparoscopic staging of

early stage invasive adnexal tumors: a 10-year experience. Gynecol Oncol. 2004;94:624–9.
41. Chi DS, Abu-Rustum NR, Sonoda Y, et al. The safety and efficacy of laparoscopic surgical staging of apparent stage I ovarian and fallopian tube cancers. Am J Obstet Gynecol. 2005;192:1614–9.
42. Ghezzi F, Cromi A, Uccella S, et al. Laparoscopy versus laparotomy for the surgical management of apparent early stage ovarian cancer. Gynecol Oncol. 2007;105:409–13.
43. Park JY, Bae J, Lim MC, et al. Laparoscopic and laparotomic staging in stage I epithelial ovarian cancer: a comparison of feasibility and safety. Int J Gynecol Cancer. 2008;18:1202–9.
44. Park JY, Kim DY, Suh DS, et al. Comparison of laparoscopy and laparotomy in surgical staging of early-stage ovarian and fallopian tubal cancer. Ann Surg Oncol. 2008;15:2012–9.
45. Colomer AT, Jiménez AM, Bover Barceló MI. Laparoscopic treatment and staging of early ovarian cancer. J Minim Invasive Gynecol. 2008;15:414–9.
46. Nezhat FR, Ezzati M, Chuang L, Shamshirsaz AA, Rahaman J, Gretz H. Laparoscopic management of early ovarian and fallopian tube cancers: surgical and survival outcome. Am J Obstet Gynecol. 2009;200:83.e1–6.
47. Lee M, Kim SW, Paek J, et al. Comparisons of surgical outcomes, complications, and costs between laparotomy and laparoscopy in early-stage ovarian cancer. Int J Gynecol Cancer. 2011;21:251–6.
48. Schreuder HW, Pattij TO, Zweemer RP, van Baal MW, Verheijen RH. Increasing experience in laparoscopic staging of early ovarian cancer. Gynecol Surg. 2012;9(1):89–96. doi:10.1007/s10397-011-0692-6.
49. Schlaerth AC, Chi DS, Poynor EA, Barakat RR, Brown CL. Long-term survival after fertility-sparing surgery for epithelial ovarian cancer. Int J Gynecol Cancer. 2009;19(7):1199–204.
50. Zanetta G, Chiari S, Rota S, Bratina G, Maneo A, Torri V, Mangioni C. Conservative surgery for stage I ovarian carcinoma in women of childbearing age. Br J Obstet Gynaecol. 1997;104(9):1030–5.
51. Muzii L, Palaia I, Sansone M, Calcagno M, Plotti F, Angioli R, Panici PB. Laparoscopic fertility-sparing staging in unexpected early stage ovarian malignancies. Fertil Steril. 2009;91(6):2632–7.
52. Eltabbakh GH. Effect of surgeon's experience on the surgical outcome of laparoscopic surgery for women with endometrial cancer. Gynecol Oncol. 2000;78(1):58–61.
53. Jung US, Lee JH, Kyung MS, Choi JS. Feasibility and efficacy of laparoscopic management of ovarian cancer. J Obstet Gynaecol Res. 2009;35(1):113–8.
54. Nezhat FR, Ezzati M, Chuang L, Shamshirsaz AA, Rahaman J, Gretz H. Laparoscopic management of early ovarian and fallopian tube cancers: surgical and survival outcome. Am J Obstet Gynecol. 2009;200(1):83–6.
55. Spirtos NM, Eisekop SM, Boike G, Schlaerth JB, Cappellari JO. Laparoscopic staging in patients with incompletely staged cancers of the uterus, ovary, fallopian tube, and primary peritoneum: a Gynecologic Oncology Group (GOG) study. Am J Obstet Gynecol. 2005;193(5):1645–9.
56. Kodama S, Tanaka K, Tokunaga A, Sudo N, Takahashi T, Matsui K. Multivariate analysis of prognostic factors in patients with ovarian cancer stage I and II. Int J Gynaecol Obstet. 1997;56(2):147–15367.
57. Nagarsheth NP, Rahaman J, Cohen CJ, Gretz H, Nezhat F. The incidence of port-site metastases in gynecologic cancers. JSLS. 2004;8(2):133–9.
58. Tozzi R, Schneider A. Laparoscopic treatment of early ovarian cancer. Curr Opin Obstet Gynecol. 2005;17(4):354–8.
59. Vergote I, De BJ, Fyles A, Bertelsen K, Einhorn N, Sevelda P, Gore ME, Kaern J, Verrelst H, Sjovall K, Timmerman D, Vandewalle J, Van GM, Trope CG. Prognostic importance of degree of differentiation and cyst rupture in stage I invasive epithelial ovarian carcinoma. Lancet. 2001;357(9251):176–82.
60. Krivak TC, Elkas JC, Rose GS, Sundborg M, Winter WE, Carlson J, MacKoul PJ. The utility of hand-assisted laparoscopy in ovarian cancer. Gynecol Oncol. 2005;96(1):72–6.
61. Amara DP, Nezhat C, Teng NN, Nezhat F, Nezhat C, Rosati M. Operative laparoscopy in the management of ovarian cancer. Surg Laparosc Endosc. 1996;6(1):38–45.
62. Farghaly SA. Laparoscopic – assisted ovarian tumorectomy for patients with early- stage ovarian cancer: Farghaly's procedure. JAAGL. 2001;8(3):S17. supplement.
63. Farghaly SA. Observations on port-site metastases following laparoscopic surgery for ovarian cancer. Am J Obstet Gynecol. 2004;190(5):1490.
64. Magrina JF, Zanagnolo V, Noble BN, et al. Robotic approach for ovarian cancer: perioperative and survival results and comparison with laparoscopy and laparotomy. Gynecol Oncol. 2011;121:100–5.
65. Eskander RN, et al. Fertility preservation in patients with gynecologic malignancies. Am J Obstet Gynecol. 2011;205(2):103–10.
66. Laurent I, Uzan C, Gouy S, et al. Results after conservative treatment of serous borderline tumors of the ovary with a micropapillary pattern. Ann Surg Oncol. 2008;15:3561–6.
67. Seidman JD, Kurman RJ. Ovarian serous borderline tumors: a critical review of the literature with emphasis on prognostic indicators. Hum Pathol. 2000;31:539–57.
68. Camatte S, Morice P, Thoury A, et al. Impact of surgical staging in patients with macroscopic 'stage I' ovarian borderline tumours: analysis of a continuous series of 101 cases. Eur J Cancer. 2004;40:1842–9.
69. Desfeux P, Camatte S, Chatellier G, et al. Impact of surgical approach on the management of macroscopic early ovarian borderline tumors. Gynecol Oncol. 2005;98:390–5.
70. Cho YH, Kim DY, Kim JH, et al. Is complete surgical staging necessary in patients with stage I mucinous

epithelial ovarian tumors? Gynecol Oncol. 2006; 103:878–82.
71. Acs G. Serous and mucinous borderline (low malignant potential) tumors of the ovary. Am J Clin Pathol. 2005;123(Suppl):S13–57.
72. Tinelli R, Tinelli A, Tinelli FG, et al. Conservative surgery for borderline ovarian tumors: a review. Gynecol Oncol. 2006;100:185–91.
73. Morice P, Camatte S, El Hassan J, et al. Clinical outcomes and fertility after conservative treatment of ovarian borderline tumors. Fertil Steril. 2001; 75:92–6.
74. Weinstein D, Polishuk WZ. The role of wedge resection of the ovary as a cause for mechanical sterility. Surg Gynecol Obstet. 1975;141:417–8.
75. Park JY, Kim DY, Kim JH, et al. Surgical management of borderline ovarian tumors: the role of fertility-sparing surgery. Gynecol Oncol. 2009;113:75–82.
76. Farghaly SA. Video laparoscopic fertility- sparing surgery in patients with low malignant potential (LMP) ovarian tumors: Farghaly's technique. Min Inv Gynecol. 2008;15(6):84S.
77. Romagnolo C, Gadducci A, Sartori E, et al. Management of borderline ovarian tumors: results of an Italian multicenter study. Gynecol Oncol. 2006; 101:255–60.
78. Maneo A, Vignali M, Chiari S, et al. Are borderline tumors of the ovary safely treated by laparoscopy? Gynecol Oncol. 2004;94:387–92.
79. Tinelli R, Malzoni M, Cosentino F, et al. Feasibility, safety, and efficacy of conservative laparoscopic treatment of borderline ovarian tumors. Fertil Steril. 2009;92:736–41.
80. Burks RT, Sherman ME, Kurman RJ. Micropapillary serous carcinoma of the ovary. A distinctive low-grade carcinoma related to serous borderline tumors. Am J Surg Pathol. 1996;20:1319–30.
81. Seidman JD, Kurman RJ. Subclassification of serous borderline tumors of the ovary into benign and malignant types. A clinicopathologic study of 65 advanced stage cases. Am J Surg Pathol. 1996;20:1331–45.
82. Prat J, De Nictolis M. Serous borderline tumors of the ovary: a long-term follow-up study of 137 cases, including 18 with a micropapillary pattern and 20 with microinvasion. Am J Surg Pathol. 2002;26:1111–28.
83. Deavers MT, Gershenson DM, Tortolero-Luna G, et al. Micropapillary and cribriform patterns in ovarian serous tumors of low malignant potential: a study of 99 advanced stage cases. Am J Surg Pathol. 2002;26:1129–41.
84. Laurent I, Uzan C, Gouy S, et al. Results after conservative treatment of serous borderline tumours of the ovary with stromal microinvasion but without micropapillary pattern. BJOG. 2009;116:860–2.
85. Abusief ME, Hornstein MD, Jain T. Assessment of United States fertility clinic websites according to the American Society for Reproductive Medicine (ASRM)/Society for Assisted Reproductive Technology (SART) guidelines. Fertil Steril. 2007;87:88–92.
86. Gallot D, Pouly JL, Janny L, et al. Successful transfer of frozen-thawed embryos obtained immediately before radical surgery for stage IIIa serous borderline ovarian tumour: case report. Hum Reprod. 2000;15:2347–50.
87. Donnez J, Dolmans MM, Demylle D, et al. Livebirth after orthotopic transplantation of cryopreserved ovarian tissue. Lancet. 2004;364:1405–10.
88. Oktay K, Cil AP, Bang H. Efficiency of oocyte cryopreservation: a meta-analysis. Fertil Steril. 2006;86: 70–80.
89. Meirow D, Levron J, Eldar-Geva T, Hardan I, Fridman E, Zalel Y, et al. Pregnancy after transplantation of cryopreserved ovarian tissue in a patient with ovarian failure after chemotherapy. N Engl J Med. 2005;353:318–21.
90. Demeestere I, Simon P, Buxant F, Robin V, Fernandez SA, Centner J, et al. Ovarian function and spontaneous pregnancy after combined heterotopic and orthotopic cryopreserved ovarian tissue transplantation in a patient previously treated with bone marrow transplantation: case report. Hum Reprod. 2006;21:2010–4.
91. Kim SS, Radford J, Harris M, Varley J, Rutherford AJ, Lieberman B, et al. Ovarian tissue harvested from lymphoma patients to preserve fertility may be safe for autotransplantation. Hum Reprod. 2001;16:2056–60.
92. Fain-Kahn V, Poirot C, Uzan C, Prades M, Gouy S, Genestie C, et al. Feasibility of ovarian cryopreservation in borderline ovarian tumours. Hum Reprod. 2009;24:850–5.
93. Navot D, Fox JH, Williams M, Brodman M, Friedman Jr F, Cohen CJ. The concept of uterine preservation with ovarian malignancies. Obstet Gynecol. 1991;78:566–8.
94. Lawal AH, B-Lynch C. Borderline ovarian cancer, bilateral surgical castration, chemotherapy and a normal delivery after ovum donation and in vitro fertilisation-embryo transfer. Br J Obstet Gynaecol. 1996;103:931–2.
95. Kwon YS, Hahn HS, Kim TJ, Lee IH, Lim KT, Lee KH, et al. Fertility preservation in patients with early epithelial ovarian cancer. J Gynecol Oncol. 2009; 20(1):44–7.
96. Borgfeldt C, Iosif C, Måsbäck A. Fertility-sparing surgery and outcome in fertile women with ovarian borderline tumors and epithelial invasive ovarian cancer. Eur J Obstet Gynecol Reprod Biol. 2007;134(1):110–4.
97. Kajiyama H, Shibata K, Mizuno M, et al. Long-term survival of young women receiving fertility-sparing surgery for ovarian cancer in comparison with those undergoing radical surgery. Br J Cancer. 2011; 105(9):1288–94.
98. Kajiyama H, Shibata K, Mizuno M, et al. Fertility-sparing surgery in patients with clear-cell carcinoma of the ovary: is it possible? Hum Reprod. 2011; 26(12):3297–302.

99. Kajiyama H, Shibata K, Suzuki S, et al. Fertility-sparing surgery in young women with invasive epithelial ovarian cancer. Eur J Surg Oncol. 2010;36(4):404–8.
100. Braicu E-I, Sehouli J, Richter R, Pietzner K, Denkert C, Fotopoulou C. Role of histological type on surgical outcome and survival following radical primary tumour debulking of epithelial ovarian, fallopian tube and peritoneal cancers. Br J Cancer. 2011;105(12):1818–24.
101. Bamias A, Psaltopoulou T, Sotiropoulou M, Haidopoulos D, Lianos E, Bournakis E, et al. Mucinous but not clear cell histology is associated with inferior survival in patients with advanced stage ovarian carcinoma treated with platinum-paclitaxel chemotherapy. Cancer. 2010;116(6):1462–8.
102. Partridge AH, Ruddy KJ, Gelber S, Schapira L, Abusief M, Meyer M, Ginsburg E. Ovarian reserve in women who remain premenopausal after chemotherapy for early stage breast cancer. Fertil Steril. 2010;94(2):638–44.
103. Lutchman Singh K, Muttukrishna S, Stein RC, McGarrigle HH, Patel A, Parikh B, et al. Predictors of ovarian reserve in young women with breast cancer. Br J Cancer. 2007;96(12):1808–16.
104. Hancke K, Isachenko V, Isachenko E, Weiss JM. Prevention of ovarian damage and infertility in young female cancer patients awaiting chemotherapy-clinical approach and unsolved issues. Support Care Cancer. 2011;19(12):1909–19.
105. Morice P, Leblanc E, Rey A, Querleu D, Blanchot J, Duvillard P, et al. Conservative treatment in epithelial ovarian cancer: results of a multicentre study of the GCCLCC (Groupe des Chirurgiens de Centre de Lutte Contre le Cancer) and SFOG (Société Française d'Oncologie Gynécologique). Hum Reprod. 2005;20(5):1379–85.
106. Oven Ustaalioglu BB, Bilici A, Kefeli U, Seker M, Salepci T, Unal O, Gumus M. A retrospective analysis of women's chances to become pregnant after completion of chemotherapy: a single center experience. J BUON. 2011;16(2):349–52.
107. Tan SJ, Yeh YC, Shang WJ, Wu GJ, Liu JY, Chen CH. Protective effect of a gonadotropin-releasing hormone analogue on chemotherapeutic agent-induced ovarian gonadotoxicity: a mouse model. Eur J Obstet Gynecol Reprod Biol. 2010;149(2):182–5.
108. Blumenfeld Z, von Wolff M. GnRH-analogues and oral contraceptives for Efertility preservation in women during chemotherapy. Hum Reprod Update. 2008;14(6):543–52.

Treatment of Advanced Stage Ovarian Cancer

10

John Butler and Alexandra Lawrence

Introduction

Two thirds of women with epithelial ovarian cancer are diagnosed with advanced stage disease (FIGO stage III/IV), and the management of these patients usually involves a combination of surgery, chemotherapy and palliative treatments. Despite advances in both chemotherapy and surgery, the majority of these patients will have disease recurrence and ultimately die from their disease. Unlike most other tumour sites, there appears to be a significant survival benefit from surgical debulking of advanced stage disease. Recent major studies have been conducted to address the timing of surgery with relation to chemotherapy, radicality of surgery, intraperitoneal chemotherapy and use of targeted chemotherapy agents in addition to standard chemotherapy (Table 10.1).

Table 10.1 Ovarian cancer staging by International Federation of Gynecology and Obstetrics Critera (FIGO, 2002)

Stage I: Growth limited to the ovaries
IA: Tumour limited to one ovary; capsule intact, no tumour on ovarian surface; no malignant cells in ascites or peritoneal washings
IIB: Tumour limited to both ovaries; capsules intact, no tumour on ovarian surface; no malignant cells in ascites or peritoneal washings
IC: Tumour limited to one or both ovaries with capsule rupture or tumour on ovarian surface; malignant cells in ascites or peritoneal washings
Stage II: Tumour involves one or both ovaries with pelvic extensions
IIA: Extension or implants on uterus or tube(s), or both; no malignant cells in ascites or peritoneal washings
IIB: Extension to other pelvic tissues; no malignant cells in ascites or peritoneal washings
IIC: Pelvic extension with malignant cells in ascites or peritoneal washings
Stage III: Tumour involves one or both ovaries with peritoneal metastasis outside the pelvis or retroperitoneal or inguinal node metastasis
IIIA: Microscopic peritoneal metastasis beyond pelvis
IIIB: Macroscopic peritoneal metastasis beyond pelvis 2 cm or less in greatest dimension
IIIC: Peritoneal metastasis beyond pelvis more than 2 cm in greatest dimension or regional lymph node metastasis, or both
Stage IV: Distant metastasis (excludes peritoneal metastasis) to liver parenchyma or other visceral organs or a malignant pleural effusion

J. Butler, MD
Department of Gynaecological Oncology, St. Bartholomew's Hospital, West Smithfield, London, UK
e-mail: john.butler@bartshealth.nhs.uk

A. Lawrence, MD, MRCOG (✉)
Department of Gynaecological Oncology, St. Bartholomew's Hospital, West Smithfield, London EC1A 7BE, UK

Queen's Hospital, Rom Valley Way, Romford, UK
e-mail: alexandra.lawrence@bartshealth.nhs.uk

S.A. Farghaly (ed.), *Advances in Diagnosis and Management of Ovarian Cancer*,
DOI 10.1007/978-1-4614-8271-0_10,

Diagnosis

Patients with advanced stage ovarian cancer may present with a variety of symptoms such as bloating, pelvic or abdominal pain, early satiety and urinary symptoms. There may be abnormal findings at pelvic or abdominal examination, or abnormalities found in imaging studies or surgery for other conditions. Ovarian cancer diagnosis may be made after a staging laparotomy for suspected ovarian cancer, image-guided needle biopsy, laparoscopic assessment and biopsy or biopsy during other operations. Cytology of ascites or pleural fluid is not recommended to make the diagnosis as they may not provide sufficient diagnostic accuracy to both confirm and classify ovarian cancer. Cases of suspected and confirmed advanced stage ovarian cancer should be discussed by multidisciplinary teams including a gynaecological oncology surgeon, medical or clinical oncologist, radiologist, pathologist, clinical nurse specialist and palliative care team with at least one member having assessed the patient. This multi-professional discussion will ensure that holistic management of patients can be planned and pathways of care organised which often involve a combination of surgery and chemotherapy alongside other hospital and community services.

Surgery in Ovarian Cancer

Surgery has been conducted for patients with ovarian cancer since the 1930s and in 1975 Griffiths et al. published a landmark paper demonstrating an inverse relationship between residual tumour diameter after surgery and survival [1, 2]. After the benefits of platinum-based chemotherapy (cisplatin and carboplatin) were established in the 1980s, there have been no randomised controlled studies to compare the outcomes of patients receiving and not receiving surgery in addition to chemotherapy and surgery continues to be performed. The timing of initial surgery may be before chemotherapy (primary surgery) or after chemotherapy (delayed primary surgery). Secondary surgery (a subsequent laparotomy) may be performed during chemotherapy (interval debulking surgery – IDS) or after completion of chemotherapy (second-look laparotomy). The roles of surgery include diagnosis, staging, palliation and cytoreduction.

Table 10.2 Definitions of cytoreduction

Complete cytoreduction	No visible residual disease
Optimal	All residual deposits <1 cm maximal dimension
Suboptimal	Residual deposits 1 cm or greater

In the platinum era the benefit of surgical debulking persisted. In Bristow's meta-analysis of 53 studies including 6,885 patients with stage III or IV disease, for every 10 % in cytoreduction median survival improved by 5.5 % [3]. There is uncertainty whether this represents inherent tumour biology – or benefit gained from surgical aggression and radicality.

Cytoreduction is usually classified as complete when there is no visible residual disease at the end of surgery, optimal if there are only small tumour deposits at the end of surgery (usually <1 cm maximum diameter) and suboptimal if there is greater than 1 cm of disease after surgery (Table 10.2). As the definition of optimal debulking has changed over time and between studies, more recent studies have classified optimal as complete cytoreduction, suboptimal as <1 cm deposits [4]. The benefits of surgery may include (1) resection of areas of tumour that are poorly vascularised and in which chemotherapy may be less effective, (2) higher growth fraction in well-perfused small residual tumour masses that may be more chemosensitive, (3) treating a smaller volume of disease may need less chemotherapy and reduce the opportunity for resistant tumour clones to develop, (4) resection of drug-resistant tumour cells and (5) host immunocompetence improved with removal of tumour bulk [5]. Complete and optimal debulking rates are higher when patients are operated on by gynaecological oncologists in specialised hospitals, compared to general gynaecologists or general surgeons [3, 6, 7]. It remains unclear whether these improved outcomes in optimally debulked patients are due to the surgery or patient and disease factors [8].

Table 10.3 Routine preoperative tests for patients with advanced ovarian cancer

Type of test	Test
Routine blood tests	Full blood count, renal function, liver function, (including albumin), clotting profile, blood grouping
Tumour markers	CA-125 (±CEA, CA19-9, HE-4, beta HCG, LDH, alpha fetoprotein, inhibin)
Imaging	CT thorax, abdomen and pelvis *or* CT thorax and abdomen and MRI pelvis
Cardiorespiratory	Electrocardiogram, ± echocardiogram, ± lung function, ± sleep studies, ± CPEX testing
Other ±	Colonoscopy, gastroscopy, stoma counselling

Cytoreductive Surgery

The aims of cytoreductive surgery is to (1) remove all sites of macroscopic disease, (2) assess areas for microscopic disease spread to allow accurate staging to guide treatment and inform prognosis and (3) minimise morbidity.

Evaluation of Patients for Surgery

The patient should, if possible, be reviewed by a surgical and medical oncologist and then discussed at a multidisciplinary meeting with relevant imaging and blood tests (Table 10.3).

Initial management options include:

1. Primary cytoreductive surgery
2. Laparoscopy ± proceed to primary cytoreductive surgery
3. Image-guided biopsy to establish ovarian cancer diagnosis and proceed to primary cytoreductive surgery
4. Image-guided biopsy to establish ovarian cancer diagnosis and proceed to primary chemotherapy
5. Palliative surgery
6. Supportive care ± palliative chemotherapy

The use of image-guided biopsy prior to surgery (option 3 above) is reserved for cases in which the primary cancer is in doubt. Gastric cancer with omental disease, ascites and Krukenberg tumours may masquerade as an ovarian cancer and should be excluded if there is any doubt preoperatively [9].

Selection of Patients for Primary Cytoreductive Surgery

Survival benefit from primary cytoreductive surgery in advanced ovarian cancer is gained for patients where complete or optimal cytoreduction can be achieved rather than different prognoses according to specific sites of disease [10]. Furthermore, women with tumours that cannot be reduced to less than 2 cm will suffer surgical morbidity but probably derive no survival benefit from surgery [11]. A variety of predictive factors have been assessed. Bristow et al. identified a Gynecologic Oncology Group (GOG) performance status of ≥2, CT features of peritoneal thickening, peritoneal implants (≥2 cm), bowel mesentery involvement (≥2 cm), suprarenal para-aortic lymph nodes (≥1 cm), omental extension (spleen, stomach or lesser sac) and pelvic sidewall involvement and/or hydroureter to be most strongly associated with surgical outcome [12]. Using the scoring system (Table 10.4) in all patients with a score of less than four optimal or complete debulking was achieved, whereas in those with a score of 4 or greater, 87.5 % of patients were suboptimally debulked (Fig. 10.1) [12].

Ferrandina et al. validated this approach in a European centre and identified five independent variables: ECOG performance status ≥2, CT findings of peritoneal thickening, peritoneal implants ≥2 cm, bowel mesentery involvement, suprarenal aortic lymph nodes ≥1 cm and diaphragmatic disease (widespread infiltrating carcinomatosis or confluent nodules) [13]. With each of these allocated a score of 1, a predictive index value can be calculated (PIV) with corresponding rates of unnecessary surgery and also inappropriate unexploration.

Vergote and colleagues report the Leuven criteria to determine patients where primary cytoreductive surgery should not be performed [4].

Table 10.4 Final model of predictive index parameters, including 13 radiographic features and GOG performance status >2

Predictive index parameter	Point value	Sensitivity	Specificity	PPV	NPV	Accuracy
Peritoneal Thickening	2	71.4 % (15/21)	90.0 % (18/20)	88.2 % (15/17)	75.0 % (18/24)	80.5 % (33/41)
Peritoneal Implants ≥2 cm	2	57.1 % (12/21)	95.0 % (19/20)	92.3 % (12/13)	67.9 % (19/28)	75.6 % (31/41)
Small bowel mesentery disease ≥2 cm	2	33.3 % (7/21)	100 % (20/20)	100 % (7/7)	58.8 % (20/34)	65.9 % (27/41)
Large bowel mesentery disease ≥2 cm	2	38.1 % (8/21)	90.0 % (18/20)	80.0 % (8/10)	58.1 % (18/31)	63.4 % (26/41)
Omentum extension to stomach, spleen, or lesser sac	2	42.9 % (9/21)	85.0 % (17/20)	75.0 % (9/12)	58.6 % (17/29)	63.4 % (26/41)
Extension to pelvic sidewall, parametria, or hydroureter	2	42.9 % (9/21)	85.0 % (17/20)	75.0 % (9/12)	58.6 % (17/29)	63.4 % (26/41)
Ascites-large volume (seen on all cuts)	2	38.1 % (8/21)	90.0 % (18/20)	80.0 % (8/10)	58.1 % (18/31)	63.4 % (26/41)
Performance Status ≥2	2	33.0 % (7/21)	95.0 % (19/20)	87.5 % (7/8)	57.6 % (19/33)	63.4 % (26/41)
Suprarenal paraaortic lymph nodes ≥1 cm	2	23.8 % (5/21)	100 % (20/20)	100 % (5/5)	55.6 % (20/36)	61.0 % (25/41)
Diaphragm or lung base disease ≥2 cm, or confluent plaque	1	42.9 % (9/21)	75.0 % (15/20)	64.3 % (9/14)	55.6 % (15/27)	58.5 % (24/41)
Inguinal canal disease or lymph nodes ≥2 cm	1	19.0 % (4/21)	100 % (20/20)	100 % (4/4)	54.1 % (20/37)	58.5 % (24/41)
Liver lesion ≥2 cm on surface, or parenchymal lesion any size	1	14.3 % (3/21)	90.0 % (18/20)	80.0 % (8/10)	58.1 % (18/31)	56.1 % (23/41)
Porta hepatis or gallbladder fossa disease ≥1 cm	1	14.3 % (3/21)	100 % (20/20)	100 % (3/3)	52.6% (20/38)	56.1 % (23/41)
Infrarenal paraaortic lymph nodes ≥2 cm	1	14.3 % (3/21)	100 % (20/20)	100 % (3/3)	52.6 % (20/38)	56.1 % (23/41)

There is currently no perfect model that can completely predict patients where optimal debulking may be achieved so that patients do not receive unnecessary surgery. Variation between surgeons and centres makes any predictive model difficult to apply universally and the lack of reproducibility of CT interpretation highlights the caution that should be observed with any model [14]. In particular radical upper abdominal procedures have been introduced to many gynaecological oncology centres with associated improvements in optimal debulking and survival and will alter rates of optimal and complete debulking [15]. Chi et al. reported a significant increase in both cytoreduction, survival and progression-free survival when extensive upper abdominal procedures were performed on patients with advanced ovarian cancer [15] (Fig. 10.2).

This often requires close working with hepatobiliary and colorectal surgeons both for preoperative evaluation and intraoperative support. These procedures are associated with significant surgical morbidity and it is essential to audit quality of life alongside disease specific

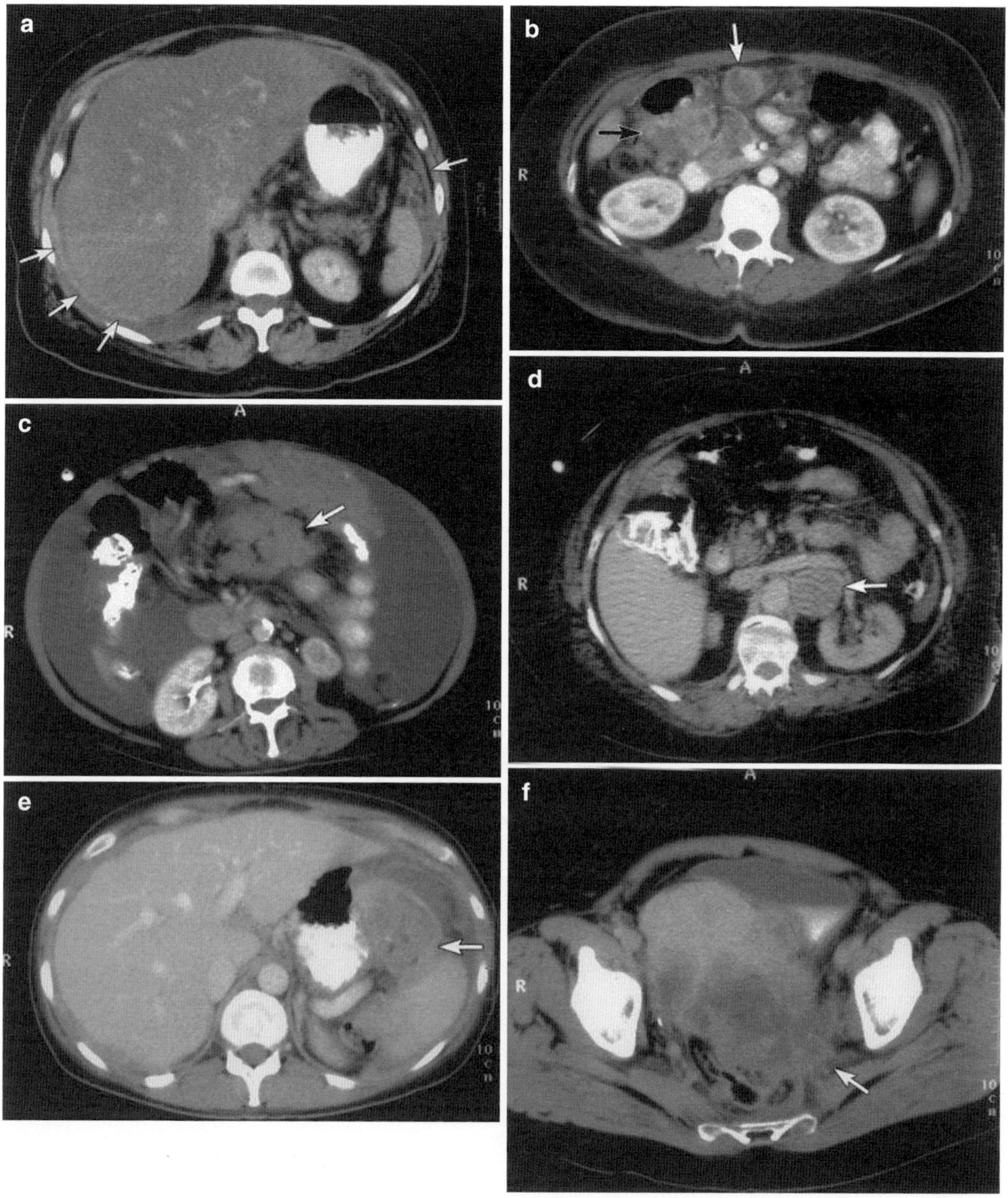

Fig. 10.1 shows representative CT findings: (**a**) peritoneal thickening, (**b**) peritoneal implant ≥2 cm and large bowel mesentery disease ≥2 cm, (**c**) small bowel mesentery disease ≥2 cm, (**d**) suprarenal para-aortic lymph node ≥1 cm (the left renal vein can be seen running ventral to the tumour mass), (**e**) omental tumour extension to spleen and (**f**) tumour infiltration of parametrial soft tissue and extension to pelvic sidewall Bristow et al. [12]

measures as this approach becomes more widespread.

For many patients although there may be no survival benefit from primary surgery if optimal debulking is not achieved, surgery may improve symptoms such as those from large ovarian cysts or obstructed bowel and establish diagnosis.

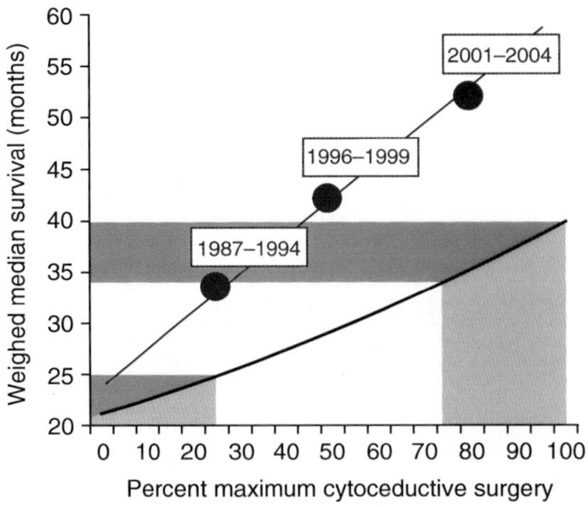

Fig. 10.2 Median overall survival as a function of percent maximum or optimal cytoreductive surgery. Memorial Sloan Kettering Cancer Center survival 1987–2004 superimposed on model by Bristow et al. (Modified with permission Bristow et al. [3])

Operative and Perioperative Management

Preoperative evaluation will help determine the likely extent of surgery in particular the likelihood of bowel resection, stoma formation and upper abdominal procedures. It is important that any relevant multi-professional support is available if procedures outside the repertoire of the lead surgeon may be performed. For patients where a stoma is likely, preoperative stoma siting and counselling are useful not only to ensure a good anatomical location of any stoma but also help with psychological aspects of bowel diversion. Patients should also be counselled about the potential benefits and risks of intraperitoneal chemotherapy if optimal or complete debulking is achieved and consent taken for intraperitoneal catheter placement.

Bowel Preparation

In elective colorectal surgery there is no evidence of any improved outcomes with preoperative mechanical bowel preparation although rates of anastomotic leakage are non-significantly lower in patients receiving bowel preparation [16]. For patients with presumed advanced stage ovarian cancer, we recommend that mechanical bowel preparation is used with concurrent intravenous hydration to avoid intravascular volume depletion and electrolyte imbalance particularly in the elderly [17, 18]. An enema before surgery is also often used to ensure the lower bowel is completely empty. Bowel preparation should not be used in patients with bowel obstruction.

Fast-Track Surgery/Enhanced Recovery After Surgery (ERAS)

Across all surgical specialties, fast-track surgery and ERAS protocols have been introduced to improve recovery after surgery. Techniques include preoperative nutrition, epidural or local anaesthesia, optimal pain control, early feeding and aggressive postoperative rehabilitation [19]. Although there has been no robust evidence of benefits of this approach in ovarian cancer patients, it is associated with earlier return of bowel function, shorter hospital stay and reduced hospital costs [20–22].

Surgery

The goals of the initial surgical procedure are to (1) make a pathological diagnosis of ovarian malignancy, (2) quantify the extent of initial disease, (3) achieve complete cytoreduction and (4) quantify the extent of residual disease. After administration of general anaesthesia, ± epidural anaesthetic and a dose of prophylactic intravenous antibiotics (e.g. 1.2 g co-amoxiclav), the patient is placed in a modified Lloyd Davies position, cleaned, draped and catheterised to facilitate operative exposure from rectum to xiphisternum. A midline incision is then performed from the symphysis pubis that may be infraumbilical initially; however, to fully assess the upper abdomen, supraumbilical extension is usually necessary. Upon entering the peritoneal cavity, any ascites present should be aspirated. If no ascites is present a peritoneal lavage is performed and specimen sent for cytological examination and then all peritoneal surfaces should then methodically be inspected. In advanced ovarian cancer this assessment is essential to determine whether optimal or complete cytoreduction is possible. If optimal cytoreduction is not possible, representative biopsies should be taken which may include unilateral or bilateral oophorectomy, hysterectomy and omentectomy and the abdomen closed so that operative morbidity is minimised (Fig. 10.3).

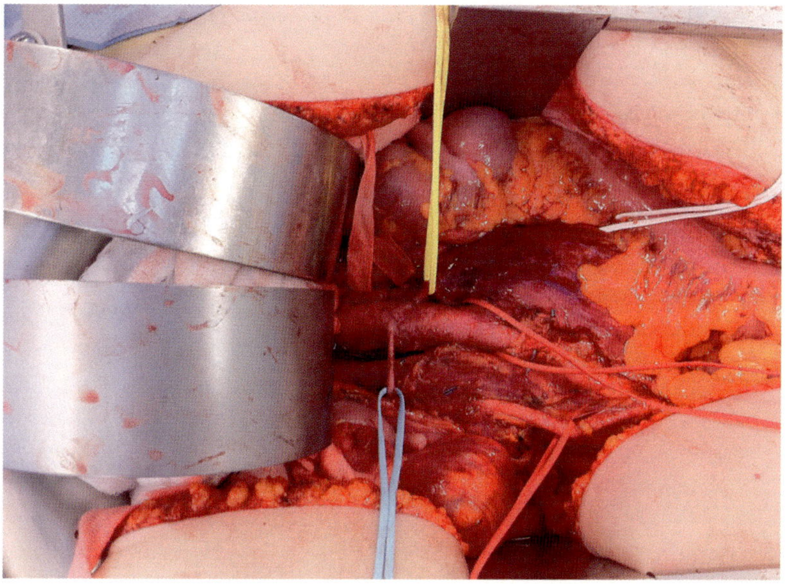

Fig. 10.3 shows a para-aortic node dissection. *White vessel loop* marks to left ureter, *red loops* to right ureter and aortic bifurcation, *yellow loop* to inferior mesenteric artery and *blue loop* to anomalous accessory right renal artery supplying lower renal pole

Relative contraindications to an attempt at primary debulking include extensive upper abdominal disease or carcinomatosis, large tumour burden in bowel mesentery or porta hepatis, bulky omental disease with splenic extension, suprarenal lymphadenopathy, patient co-morbidity and patient wishes (e.g. stoma formation). If ovarian cancer is confirmed, these patients should receive adjuvant chemotherapy and be considered for interval debulking surgery. For patients where optimal or complete debulking is deemed possible, standard and extended procedures should be performed to achieve cytoreduction and the disease status at the end of surgery clearly documented (Table 10.5). Appendicectomy should be performed unless it is known that the tumour is not mucinous and there is no evidence of metastatic disease to the appendix. If optimal or complete cytoreduction is achieved, consideration should be given to placing an intraperitoneal port for the administration of adjuvant chemotherapy.

Postoperative care is usually on the high dependency or intensive care unit. Fluid balance in particular needs active monitoring and treatment as there are often marked third space fluid losses and depleted intravascular fluid volumes. This is exacerbated with low serum albumin levels. Unless there is a coagulopathy, prophylactic low molecular weight heparin should be given. Early mobilisation and physiotherapy reduce the incidence of chest sepsis and thrombosis.

Pathological Review

Following surgery all specimens should undergo pathological evaluation and a final stage and histology recorded alongside sites of residual disease.

Chemotherapy

If a diagnosis of ovarian cancer is confirmed, patients with advanced stage disease should be considered for adjuvant chemotherapy. The options include intravenous chemotherapy, combination intraperitoneal and intravenous chemotherapy or a clinical trial. A variety of regimens are used with a platinum agent (carboplatin or cisplatin) and taxane (paclitaxel or docetaxel).

GOG 172 reported an improved medial overall survival of 67 months with intraperitoneal cisplatin and paclitaxel compared to 49 months with IV treatment [23]. These improvements in survival are associated with greater rates of toxicity and adverse events with less than half of patients tolerating six cycles of IP chemotherapy [24]. A further trial is underway to examine if there is a survival benefit with IP carboplatin and paclitaxel (PETROC/OV21).

Table 10.5 Procedures in the management of primary advanced stage ovarian cancer

Standard procedures	
	Bilateral salpingo-oophorectomy
	Total hysterectomy
	Omentectomy
	Simple peritonectomy (pelvic, paracolic gutters or anterolateral diaphragmatic area)
	Pelvic lymphadenectomy
	Infrarenal para-aortic lymphadenectomy
	Intraperitoneal port placement
Extended procedures	
	Radical pelvic dissection
	Bowel resection
	Bowel anastomosis
	Ileostomy/colostomy
	Suprarenal para-aortic lymphadenectomy
	Diaphragm or other complex peritoneal stripping
	Full-thickness resection of diaphragm
	Splenectomy
	Partial hepatectomy
	Partial gastrectomy
	Partial cystectomy
	Ureteric reimplantation/anastomosis
	Distal pancreatectomy
Palliative procedures	
	Paracentesis
	Thoracentesis
	Pleurodesis
	Anterograde or retrograde ureteric stents
	Bowel diversion
	Gastrostomy tube
	Venous access systems (implanted port or peripherally inserted central catheter line)
	Intestinal stents
	Inferior vena cava filter

Targeted Agents

Two recent trials have reported on the role of bevacizumab in ovarian cancer (ICON-7, GOG 128) [25, 26]. These trials demonstrate a small improvement in progression-free survival in patients who have not been optimally debulked but no improvement in overall survival. It is likely that the major benefit of drugs from these agents will be gained if suboptimally debulked patients remain on maintenance bevacizumab until progression. The high costs of these drugs may preclude their widespread introduction.

Neoadjuvant Chemotherapy and Delayed Primary Surgery

In many patients with advanced ovarian cancer, optimal or complete cytoreduction cannot be achieved due to patient co-morbidity, pattern of disease, surgical expertise or unwillingness of patient to undergo extensive surgery (e.g. stoma). Furthermore, in patients who respond to chemotherapy, if primary surgery is performed after chemotherapy surgical radicality, complications and side effects may be reduced. Vergote et al. reported outcomes of 632 patients with advanced stage disease (IIC–IV) randomised to primary debulking surgery followed by platinum-based chemotherapy or to neoadjuvant platinum-based chemotherapy (NACT) followed by debulking surgery (delayed primary debulking surgery) after three cycles of chemotherapy. There appeared to be no difference in overall survival between the two groups, and less morbidity in NACT patients [4].

NACT therefore appears a reasonable approach in patients where optimal debulking is unlikely to be achieved with primary debulking surgery, or there is coexistent co-morbidity that may be improved with chemotherapy such as ascites, pleural effusions and hypoalbuminaemia. The study had low rates of complete (19.2 %) and optimal debulking (41 %) and this may reflect surgical expertise or case selection that limits the universal application of the findings.

Delayed Primary Surgery

The goals of delayed primary surgery after NACT are identical to that of primary debulking surgery (PDS) – complete cytoreduction. Vergote et al. reported worse outcomes for patients with optimal primary debulking surgery than after NACT. Although there was no overall significant difference in survival rates, survival for patients with complete and optimal debulking was lower in patients after PDS than NACT [4]. A question remains around the management of patients who have after three cycles of NACT by CT assessment have progressive disease, partial response or mixed response and only suboptimal debulking is felt possible. We recommend that laparoscopy or mini-laparotomy be performed to assess resectability although there is no robust evidence base for this.

Interval Debulking Surgery

For patients where maximal surgical effort has been performed by an ovarian cancer surgeon, there is no benefit from an interval debulking procedure [27]. In patients where maximal surgical effort has not been undertaken either due to surgical expertise or patient factors, consideration should be given to interval debulking with a similar approach to patients managed by neoadjuvant chemotherapy.

Laparoscopic and Robotically Assisted Surgery

The advantages of laparoscopic surgery have been well established in gynaecological surgery, in particular reduced surgical morbidity, length of stay, adhesion formation, blood loss and post-operative pain. This has been advanced further with the introduction of robotically assisted surgery that offers the potential of more complex procedures to be performed. In order to allow a full oncological assessment, all peritoneal surfaces should be inspected and retroperitoneal structures palpated if not visualised. Concerns with laparoscopic surgery include the lack of visualisation of all peritoneal structures and the lack of haptic feedback particularly with robotic surgery. Laparoscopy has a role in the assessment of patients suitable for optimal cytoreduction and a scoring system has been developed [28]. Vergote et al. reported successful optimal cytoreduction in 61 of 77 (79 %) patients with preoperative imaging suggestive of unresectable advanced ovarian carcinoma [29]. This approach both increases the rate of optimal debulking surgery and reduces rates of primary cytoreductive surgery [30]. Hand-assisted laparoscopic surgery (HALS) has been developed that allows the tactile benefits of laparotomy to be applied to laparoscopy, this will expand the role of laparoscopy in ovarian cancer to enable palpation of areas that cannot be fully assessed laparoscopically [31]. Robotically assisted laparoscopic surgery allows more complex dissections to be performed than 'straight stick' laparoscopy due to articulated instruments. Complex urological, gynaecological and exenterative procedures may be performed robotically and these have been applied to ovarian cancer in selected patients [32]. It is essential that any novel techniques applied to the management of patients with ovarian cancer have multidisciplinary review to ensure that the patient is fully counselled regarding both the risks and benefits of more novel surgical approaches.

Palliative Surgery

Unfortunately, most patients diagnosed with advanced stage ovarian cancer will die from recurrent or progressive disease. Bowel obstruction is the most frequent cause of admission for ovarian cancer patients in their last year of life [33]. Many patients can be managed initially with nasogastric suction tube, bowel rest and intravenous hydration.

Surgery can have an important role in palliation of symptoms usually in order to relieve bowel obstruction. The management of bowel obstruction will depend on the disease status of the patient, life expectancy with and without surgery, nutritional and medical status and site/s of obstruction. The goal of any intervention is to improve symptoms and quality of life; it is rarely appropriate to perform secondary debulking for patients with recurrent ovarian cancer causing bowel obstruction.

Patients with recurrent ovarian cancer and bowel obstruction have high rates of perioperative mortality and morbidity, but successful palliation can be achieved. Kolomainen et al. reported successful palliation (oral intake at least 60 days postoperatively) in 59 of 90 patients (66 %) undergoing surgery with only the absence of ascites, a predictor for successful palliation [34].

For distal large bowel obstruction (sigmoid and descending colon), colorectal stents may be considered. This may require balloon dilatation and for a selected group of patients surgery and stoma formation may be avoided [35].

Recurrent or advanced ovarian cancer may cause ureteric obstruction and ureteric stents or a nephrostomy may be considered to relieve obstruction to preserve or improve renal function. For many patients with terminal disease, insertion of a stent or nephrostomy may be inappropriate due to the poor prognosis.

Recurrence

Most patients with advanced ovarian cancer experience disease recurrence. For patients with advanced ovarian cancer who progress despite primary treatment (cytoreductive surgery and platinum-based chemotherapy), the prognosis is poor and there is no role for further surgery outside a palliative setting. On the other hand, patients who have had a complete response to initial therapy and disease recurs 6–12 months from the completion of primary treatment may be considered to have platinum sensitive disease. This group may have greatly improved survival from further chemotherapy and surgery. The DESKTOP (Descriptive Evaluation of preoperative Selection KriTeria for OPerability in recurrent OVARian cancer) studies reported that as with primary ovarian cancer complete resection of disease was associated with improved median survival (45.2 *vs* 19.7 months). Predictors for complete resection (positive AGO score) were ECOG performance status 0, FIGO stage I or II at initial diagnosis, absence of residual disease after primary surgery and absence of ascites [36, 37]. In the prospective validation study (DESKTOP-II), preoperative imaging underestimated disease spread in around half of patients and overestimated in a quarter. The DESKTOP-III study will report on outcomes in patients with platinum sensitive disease, a positive AGO score randomised to secondary cytoreduction and chemotherapy *vs* chemotherapy alone. In addition to MRI and CT, laparoscopy and FDG-PET may be used to assess sites and resectability of recurrent disease [38, 39]. Although a midline laparotomy is usually performed for the resection of recurrent ovarian cancer, conventional or robotically assisted laparoscopic surgery may be performed [40].

Intraperitoneal Chemotherapy Ports

Intraperitoneal chemotherapy ports may be placed at the same time as debulking surgery, at a subsequent laparoscopy or under radiological guidance [41]. Complications from port placement include bleeding, catheter blockage, infection and bowel perforation [42].

Novel Surgical Techniques

The introduction of new surgical instruments and techniques has been applied to ovarian cancer. Metastatic deposits may be ablated with radiofrequency, argon beam coagulation or microwave ablation [43–45]. These techniques may be applied to minimally invasive surgery or as an adjunct to conventional laparotomy. New tissue sealing and coagulation devices such as harmonic scalpel (ethicon endosurgery) and ligasure (covidien) are sometimes used an alternative to traditional haemostasis with suture and diathermy in order to reduce operating times and blood loss.

Future Directions

Ovarian cancer remains a major challenge for gynaecological oncologists and advances in surgery and chemotherapy have improved survival for ovarian cancer. Despite medical and surgical progress, most patients will die from their disease. As most treatments are therefore ultimately palliative rather than curative, it is essential that quality of life measures are recorded alongside survival. Inequities in survival for patients with advanced stage ovarian cancer persist both within and between countries that need to be addressed to ensure that patients have access to optimum therapies [46].

References

1. Griffiths CT. Surgical resection of tumor bulk in the primary treatment of ovarian carcinoma. Natl Cancer Inst Monogr. 1975;42:101–4.
2. Meigs J. Tumors of the female pelvic organs. New York: Macmillan; 1934.
3. Bristow RE, Tomacruz RS, Armstrong DK, Trimble EL, Montz FJ. Survival effect of maximal cytoreductive surgery for advanced ovarian carcinoma during the platinum era: a meta-analysis. J Clin Oncol. 2002; 20(5):1248–59.
4. Vergote I, Tropé CGC, Amant F, et al. Neoadjuvant chemotherapy or primary surgery in stage IIIC or IV ovarian cancer. N Engl J Med. 2010;363(10):943–53.
5. Covens AL. A critique of surgical cytoreduction in advanced ovarian cancer. Gynecol Oncol. 2000; 78(3 Pt 1):269–74.
6. Junor EJ, Hole DJ, Gillis CR. Management of ovarian cancer: referral to a multidisciplinary team matters. Br J Cancer. 1994;70(2):363–70.

7. Eisenkop SM, Spirtos NM, Montag TW, Nalick RH, Wang HJ. The impact of subspecialty training on the management of advanced ovarian cancer. Gynecol Oncol. 1992;47(2):203–9.
8. Elattar A, Bryant A, Winter-Roach BA, Hatem M, Naik R. Optimal primary surgical treatment for advanced epithelial ovarian cancer. Cochrane Database Syst Rev. 2011;8, CD007565.
9. Qiu L, Yang T, Shan X-H, Hu M-B, Li Y. Metastatic factors for Krukenberg tumor: a clinical study on 102 cases. Med Oncol. 2011;28(4):1514–9.
10. Eisenkop SM, Spirtos NM, Friedman RL, et al. Relative influences of tumor volume before surgery and the cytoreductive outcome on survival for patients with advanced ovarian cancer: a prospective study. Gynecol Oncol. 2003;90(2):390–6.
11. Hoskins WJ, McGuire WP, Brady MF, et al. The effect of diameter of largest residual disease on survival after primary cytoreductive surgery in patients with suboptimal residual epithelial ovarian carcinoma. Am J Obstet Gynecol. 1994;170(4):974–9; discussion 979–80.
12. Bristow RE, Duska LR, Lambrou NC, et al. A model for predicting surgical outcome in patients with advanced ovarian carcinoma using computed tomography. Cancer. 2000;89(7):1532–40.
13. Ferrandina G, Sallustio G, Fagotti A, et al. Role of CT scan-based and clinical evaluation in the preoperative prediction of optimal cytoreduction in advanced ovarian cancer: a prospective trial. Br J Cancer. 2009;101(7):1066–73.
14. Axtell AE, Lee MH, Bristow RE, et al. Multi-institutional reciprocal validation study of computed tomography predictors of suboptimal primary cytoreduction in patients with advanced ovarian cancer. J Clin Oncol. 2007;25(4):384–9.
15. Chi DS, Eisenhauer EL, Zivanovic O, et al. Improved progression-free and overall survival in advanced ovarian cancer as a result of a change in surgical paradigm. Gynecol Oncol. 2009;114(1):26–31.
16. Güenaga KF, Matos D, Wille-Jørgensen P. Mechanical bowel preparation for elective colorectal surgery. Cochrane Database Syst Rev (Online). 2011;(9): CD001544.
17. Tamussino KF, Lim PC, Webb MJ, Lee RA, Lesnick TG. Gastrointestinal surgery in patients with ovarian cancer. Gynecol Oncol. 2001;80(1):79–84.
18. Fanning J, Valea FA. Perioperative bowel management for gynecologic surgery. Am J Obstet Gynecol. 2011;205(4):309–14.
19. Wilmore DW, Kehlet H. Management of patients in fast track surgery. BMJ. 2001;322(7284):473–6 (Clinical research ed.).
20. Lv D, Wang X, Shi G. Perioperative enhanced recovery programmes for gynaecological cancer patients. Cochrane Database Syst Rev. 2010;6, CD008239.
21. Eberhart LHJ, Koch T, Ploger B, et al. Enhanced recovery after major gynaecological surgery for ovarian cancer - an objective and patient-based assessment of a traditional versus a multimodal "fast track" rehabilitation programme. [German] Beschleunigte erholung nach laparotomien bei ovarialka. Anasthesiologie Intensivmedizin. 2008;49(4):180–94.
22. Gerardi MA, Santillan A, Meisner B, et al. A clinical pathway for patients undergoing primary cytoreductive surgery with rectosigmoid colectomy for advanced ovarian and primary peritoneal cancers. Gynecol Oncol. 2008;108(2):282–6.
23. Armstrong DKD, Bundy B, Wenzel L, et al. Intraperitoneal cisplatin and paclitaxel in ovarian cancer. N Engl J Med. 2006;354(1):34–43. doi:10.1056/NEJMoa052985.
24. Markman M, Walker JL. Intraperitoneal chemotherapy of ovarian cancer: a review, with a focus on practical aspects of treatment. J Clin Oncol. 2006;24(6): 988–94.
25. Burger RA, Brady MF, Bookman MA, et al. Incorporation of bevacizumab in the primary treatment of ovarian cancer. N Engl J Med. 2011;365(26): 2473–83.
26. Perren TJ, Swart AM, Pfisterer J, et al. A phase 3 trial of bevacizumab in ovarian cancer. N Engl J Med. 2011;365(26):2484–96.
27. Rose PG, Nerenstone S, Brady MF, et al. Gynecologic Oncology Group. N Engl J Med. 2004;351(24): 2489–97.
28. Fagotti A, Ferrandina G, Fanfani F, et al. A laparoscopy-based score to predict surgical outcome in patients with advanced ovarian carcinoma: a pilot study. Ann Surg Oncol. 2006;13(8):1156–61.
29. Vergote I, De Wever I, Tjalma W, et al. Neoadjuvant chemotherapy or primary debulking surgery in advanced ovarian carcinoma: a retrospective analysis of 285 patients. Gynecol Oncol. 1998;71(3): 431–6.
30. Angioli R, Palaia I, Zullo MA, et al. Diagnostic open laparoscopy in the management of advanced ovarian cancer. Gynecol Oncol. 2006;100(3):455–61.
31. Krivak TC, Elkas JC, Rose GS, et al. The utility of hand-assisted laparoscopy in ovarian cancer. Gynecol Oncol. 2005;96(1):72–6.
32. Farghaly SA. Robotic-assisted laparoscopic anterior pelvic exenteration in patients with advanced ovarian cancer: Farghaly's technique. Eur J Gynaecol Oncol. 2010;31(4):361–3.
33. von Gruenigen VE, Frasure HE, Reidy AM, Gil KM. Clinical disease course during the last year in ovarian cancer. Gynecol Oncol. 2003;90(3):619–24.
34. Kolomainen DF, Daponte A, Barton DPJ, et al. Outcomes of surgical management of bowel obstruction in relapsed epithelial ovarian cancer (EOC). Gynecol Oncol. 2011;125(1):31–6.
35. Caceres A, Zhou Q, Iasonos A, et al. Colorectal stents for palliation of large-bowel obstructions in recurrent gynecologic cancer: an updated series. Gynecol Oncol. 2008;108(3):482–5.
36. Harter P, Bois A, Hahmann M. Surgery in recurrent ovarian cancer: the Arbeitsgemeinschaft Gynaekologische Onkologie (AGO) DESKTOP OVAR trial. Ann Surg Oncol. 2006;13(12):1702–10.

37. Harter P, Sehouli J, Reuss A, et al. Prospective validation study of a predictive score for operability of recurrent ovarian cancer: the Multicenter Intergroup Study DESKTOP II. A project of the AGO Kommission OVAR, AGO Study Group, NOGGO, AGO-Austria, and MITO. Int J Gynecol Cancer. 2011;21(2):289–95.
38. Son H, Khan SM, Rahaman J, et al. Role of FDG PET/CT in staging of recurrent ovarian cancer. Radiographics. 2011;31(2):569–83.
39. Fagotti A, Fanfani F, Rossitto C, et al. A treatment selection protocol for recurrent ovarian cancer patients: the role of FDG-PET/CT and staging laparoscopy. Oncology. 2008;75(3–4):152–8.
40. Holloway RW, Brudie LA, Rakowski JA, Ahmad S. Robotic-assisted resection of liver and diaphragm recurrent ovarian carcinoma: description of technique. Gynecol Oncol. 2011;120(3):419–22.
41. Henretta MS, Anderson CL, Angle JF, Duska LR. It's not just for laparoscopy anymore: use of insufflation under ultrasound and fluoroscopic guidance by Interventional Radiologists for percutaneous placement of intraperitoneal chemotherapy catheters. Gynecol Oncol. 2011;123(2):342–5.
42. Ivy JJ, Geller M, Pierson SM, Jonson AL, Argenta PA. Outcomes associated with different intraperitoneal chemotherapy delivery systems in advanced ovarian carcinoma: a single institution's experience. Gynecol Oncol. 2009;114(3):420–3.
43. Yu J, Liang P, Yu X, Wang Y, Gao Y. Ultrasound-guided percutaneous microwave ablation of splenic metastasis: report of four cases and literature review. Int J Hyperthermia. 2011;27(5):517–22.
44. Bristow RE, Montz FJ. Complete surgical cytoreduction of advanced ovarian carcinoma using the argon beam coagulator. Gynecol Oncol. 2001;83(1):39–48.
45. Jiao LR, Tierris I, Ayav A, et al. A new technique for spleen preservation with radiofrequency. Surgery. 2006;140(3):464–6.
46. Coleman MP, Forman D, Bryant H, et al. Cancer survival in Australia, Canada, Denmark, Norway, Sweden, and the UK, 1995–2007 (the International Cancer Benchmarking Partnership): an analysis of population-based cancer registry data. Lancet. 2011;377(9760):127–38.

Diagnosis and Management of Epithelial Ovarian Cancer with Peritoneal Metastases

11

Paul H. Sugarbaker and Cyril W. Helm

Introduction

Epithelial ovarian cancer (EOC) affects over 200,000 women and globally causes 125,000 deaths annually [1]. Within the USA, it is the ninth most common female cancer (21,000 cases annually) and the fifth most common cause of cancer death (14,600) in women [2]. Despite a favorable trend in incidence and mortality, improved treatments for EOC are needed because with current treatment only less than 50 % of women with EOC will survive 5 years [3, 4]. The lifetime risk of ovarian cancer is 1 in 70, but there are women with much higher risk especially those with germ line mutations of *BRCA1* and *BRCA2* tumor suppressor genes and certain mismatch repair genes [5].

Pathology

Malignancies of the ovary are classified according to the World Health Organization system [6] with a majority arising from the epithelium of the ovary (epithelial ovarian cancer [EOC]) [7].

P.H. Sugarbaker, MD, FACS, FRCS (✉)
Department of Center for Gastrointestinal Malignancies, Washington Cancer Institute, MedStar Washington Hospital Center, Washington, DC, USA
e-mail: paul.sugarbaker@medstar.net

C.W. Helm, MB.BChir
Northern Gynaecological Oncology Centre, Queen Elizabeth Hospital, Queen Elizabeth Avenue, Gateshead, Tyne and Wear, NE9 6SX, UK
e-mail: cwilliamhelm@gmail.com

Carcinoma arising from the peritoneum (primary peritoneal) and fallopian tube is histologically and clinically similar to EOC and is treated in identical fashion [8, 9]. In some patients, high-grade carcinoma may actually be arising from the fallopian tube [10]. Currently, it is estimated that of all EOC, 91.8 % arise from the ovary, 5.3 % the peritoneum, and 2.8 % the fallopian tube [11]. In the remainder of this chapter, EOC will include these three types of carcinoma as one (EOC). The common histological subtypes of EOC are serous, endometrioid, mucinous, clear cell, and Brenner (transitional cell) [6].

It is important to differentiate between ovarian malignancy that is truly invasive and those that are low malignant potential (LMP), sometimes called "borderline" or "atypical proliferative tumors" [6]. LMP tumors are a distinct type of ovarian tumors occurring at a younger age and acting with a less aggressive tendency and with an improved prognosis. The 10-year relative overall survival for stage I, II, III, and IV is 97, 90, 88, and 69 %, respectively [12]. International Federation of Gynecology and Obstetrics (FIGO) data showed an overall 5-year survival of 87.3 % compared with 49.7 % for invasive EOC [4]. However, because of the indolent natural history of LMP tumors, recurrence after 5 years and a late death even 20 years after diagnosis may occur. In general, LMP tumors do not respond to systemic chemotherapy although it may be used in those tumors associated with invasive peritoneal implants or advanced disease [12]. LMP tumors will not be considered further in this chapter.

S.A. Farghaly (ed.), *Advances in Diagnosis and Management of Ovarian Cancer*,
DOI 10.1007/978-1-4614-8271-0_11,

Staging of Ovarian Cancer

Primary peritoneal carcinoma is an EOC that is a true "peritoneal surface malignancy" in that it is thought to arise from the peritoneum itself. All EOC metastasize by exfoliation of cells into the abdominal and pelvic cavity. The cancer cells or small free-floating nodules implant and progress in a characteristic pattern on peritoneal surfaces. Also, the disease progresses by direct extension to neighboring organs, to retroperitoneal lymph nodes, and less frequently by dissemination into the blood stream. All three types of EOC are staged by both the tumor, node, metastasis (TNM) [13, 14] and FIGO systems [15]. FIGO stage III includes disease that has spread from the ovaries with visible peritoneal implants outside the pelvis (IIIB and IIIC) as well as retroperitoneal lymph node involvement (IIIC). EOC most often presents in an advanced stage with peritoneal metastases and direct extension to pelvic structures. The stages most likely to be associated with peritoneal metastases are FIGO stage IIIB and C which represent 60 % of cases of EOC [4]. This would include TNM stage T3b, T3c, and/or any T:N1, and any IV. Despite remaining confined to the peritoneal cavity for much of its natural history, patients with peritoneal metastases, especially large volume disease, have a poor outcome [16].

Symptoms of Primary Disease

Unfortunately, EOC remains asymptomatic until the ovaries become greatly enlarged or peritoneal metastases cause pain or result in ascites. Even then, symptoms are relatively nonspecific including pelvic/abdominal pain, urinary frequency and urgency, increased abdominal girth, bloating, indigestion, reflux, early satiety, and pain with intercourse [17]. Attempts have been made to identify and validate a symptom index in order to identify women at risk, but the value of this is disputed [18–20].

Laboratory and Radiologic Studies with Primary Disease

While cancer antigen 125 (CA-125) is elevated in most patients with advanced disease, it is not specific for EOC; CA-125 may be elevated in many other conditions [21–23]. Even in the presence of confirmed EOC, CA-125 cannot differentiate between localized and diffuse tumor [24]. However, serial measurement of CA-125 is useful for monitoring for recurrent disease provided that it was elevated prior to treatment and normalized during treatment [25]. In this setting, it has a sensitivity of 79–95 % and a positive predictive value approaching 100 % [26].

Ultrasound is the imaging modality of choice for the initial investigation of an adnexal mass. It can detect metastatic spread such as ascites and intraperitoneal masses including liver and splenic metastases and retroperitoneal masses. It is not an accurate test for investigating the extent of peritoneal dissemination [27].

In cases with suspect extra-ovarian disease, additional imaging is required in the form of computed tomography (CT), magnetic resonance imaging (MRI), ^{18}F-FDG (fluorodeoxyglucose) positron emission tomography (PET), or combined PET/CT to define the extent of disease and assess operability. Each modality has advantages and disadvantages, but they all share a lack of accuracy for the detection of small peritoneal metastases.

Spiral CT [28] has low sensitivity for peritoneal implants less than 1 cm, particularly in the omentum and on the small bowel mesentery [29]. CT may be more reliable for detecting persistent and recurrent disease and to monitor response to therapy [30]. It has an accuracy of 70–90 % in preoperative staging [31] with a reported sensitivity of 40–93 % for detecting recurrent disease [26].

Preoperative assessment to identify patients whose disease cannot be optimally cytoreduced would enable these patients to avoid unnecessary surgery. Although studies have investigated the value of CT for this purpose [32–36], it appears that the determinants vary widely between institutions reflecting factors such as surgical philosophy and the level of surgical expertise available [37, 38]. Thus, the use of CT in determining resectability varies widely between institutions.

MRI is as useful in the staging of EOC as CT [36, 39], and gadolinium-enhanced MRI has advantages over both non-contrast-enhanced MRI and CT [40]. While MRI does not involve radiation exposure, it is more expensive, time consuming, and demanding for patients [40].

PET imaging evaluates the biologic activity of tumors, generating an estimate of metabolic tumor activity that is not possible with CT or MRI [41]. The accuracy of PET in recurrent ovarian cancer is approximately 80 % [26]. Similar to CT and MRI, it has a lower range of nodule detection of approximately 1 cm and is ineffective for identifying microscopic tumor [26]. PET does not provide precise anatomic location of tumors it identifies making it less than ideal for evaluating the feasibility of surgical resection. It usually does not detect ascites or mucinous malignancies [40].

To overcome these limitations, combined PET and CT (PET/CT) images acquired separately were developed. This has allowed more precise intraperitoneal localization of ovarian and other cancers [42–44]. PET/CT is also of value in detecting and localizing unsuspected lesions outside of the peritoneal cavity that alter the surgical approach to patients with peritoneal metastases (PM) [24, 45]. In view of this, when PM are suspected but scans are negative, direct visualization of the peritoneal cavity by laparoscopy or open surgery may be necessary.

Surgical Management of Ovarian Cancer

The surgical intervention in EOC with peritoneal metastases may occur with initial treatment (frontline), at interval debulking surgery following neoadjuvant chemotherapy, or with recurrence. The major treatment modalities are cytoreductive surgery (CRS), perioperative including hyperthermic intraperitoneal chemotherapy, and long-term combined intravenous and intraperitoneal chemotherapy. It has been established that improved outcome is associated with small-volume residual disease following cytoreductive surgery [46, 47]. Therefore, the goal of surgery must be to remove all visible evidence of disease or at least, leave the amount of residual disease [48–50]. In the past, CRS that left residual cancerous lesions up to 2 cm in greatest dimension was considered "optimal." However, the precise definition of optimal cytoreduction has been open to wide differences of opinion which have changed considerably over time [51]. It is now established that leaving no visible disease should always be the surgical goal at all time points for EOC surgery except for palliation [50, 52].

Multiple different surgical procedures may be necessary to achieve complete cytoreduction because EOC can be widespread within the abdominal and pelvic cavity. In the past, disease involving upper abdominal structures such as the undersurface of the diaphragm, liver surface or parenchyma, porta hepatis, pancreas, and spleen were considered obstacles to the achievement of optimal CRS. It has been shown that the resection of tumor from these sites does improve survival whether this is achieved by the gynecologic oncologists or surgical oncologists [53]. The actual sites of intra-abdominal disease not amenable to safe resection vary according to surgical expertise and practice. However, the sites most likely to preclude complete resection include multiple parenchymal liver metastases, extensive disease in the porta hepatis, retroperitoneal adenopathy behind and superior to the pancreas, and extensive disease involving proximal small bowel and small bowel mesentery.

Selection Criteria for a Comprehensive Treatment Plan

Cytoreductive surgery and perioperative intraperitoneal chemotherapy represent an innovative strategy for the management of EOC. It is used for frontline treatment, interval cytoreduction, or with recurrent disease. It requires a knowledgeable selection of patients, a strong commitment from the surgical team, and institutional support.

Selection of patients is based on two well-defined criteria: First, the ability of the patient to survive an extensive surgical procedure with acceptable morbidity and mortality and, second, no evidence of intraoperative findings that would result in a futile surgical procedure. Patients of advanced age, poor performance status, malnourished, or with medical conditions that would decrease the likelihood of postoperative survival should not be operated. Also, patients with systemic metastases, multiple sites of bowel obstruction, common bile duct obstruction, or ureteral obstruction should not be submitted to this comprehensive treatment.

Comprehensive management requires dedication from a surgeon who must have broad surgical knowledge, a thorough understanding of perioperative chemotherapy, unusual technical skills, and the stamina to endure long procedures. Realizing that these interventions are extensive and thereby costly, institutional backing is important. An effort to educate other physicians involved in this treatment, as well as nurses and ancillary personnel, should be undertaken. Standardized orders for chemotherapy as part of a well-defined clinical pathway are necessary to coordinate the actions of the clinical staff. The steep learning curve that characterizes this treatment strategy makes it essential to design a careful plan and to regularly critically evaluate all adverse events.

Quantitative Prognostic Indicators

The three assessments helpful for patient selection in order to treat patients most likely to benefit are the prior surgical score (PSS), the peritoneal cancer index (PCI), and the completeness of cytoreduction score (CC). These scores are determined from 13 abdominopelvic regions. Two transverse planes and two sagittal planes are used to divide the abdomen into nine abdominopelvic regions (AR 0–8). The upper transverse plane is located at the lowest aspect of the costal margin. Regions 9 and 10 define the upper and lower portions of the jejunum, and regions 11 and 12 define the upper and lower portions of the ileum.

Surgical trauma promotes the implantation and progression of cancer nodules on peritoneal surfaces. Prior surgeries may modify the natural history of ovarian cancer by inducing cancer growth in crucial anatomic sites located beyond the peritoneal layer. Patients with no prior abdominopelvic surgery or biopsy only received a PSS of 0, those with up to one abdominopelvic region dissected received a PSS of 1, those with two to five ARs received a PSS of 2, and those with six or more regions dissected received a PSS of 3.

The PCI is a quantitative prognostic indicator determined after abdominal exploration and complete separation of intestinal adhesions (Fig. 11.1). This index adds a lesion size parameter to the ARs so that a numerical score estimating the extent of carcinomatosis is available. The PCI is an accurate prognostic indicator for ovarian cancer [54].

CC is a quantitative prognostic indicator determined once the surgical resection has been completed. A patient receives a CC-0 score when no visible peritoneal carcinomatosis remains after cytoreduction, CC-1 is recorded when tumor nodules persist after cytoreduction but they measure less than 0.25 cm, and CC-2 when remaining tumor measures between 0.25 and 2.5 cm. When tumor nodules are greater than 2.5 cm or there is confluence of unresectable tumor, a CC-3 score is given to the patient. Many prior studies in ovarian cancer have shown that the extent of disease remaining after cytoreduction is directly related to the survival [47–54].

Surgical Techniques Used to Complete Cytoreduction in Selected Patients

The goal of CRS is to reduce the tumor burden within the abdomen and pelvis to its absolute minimal volume. The best result is a patient who

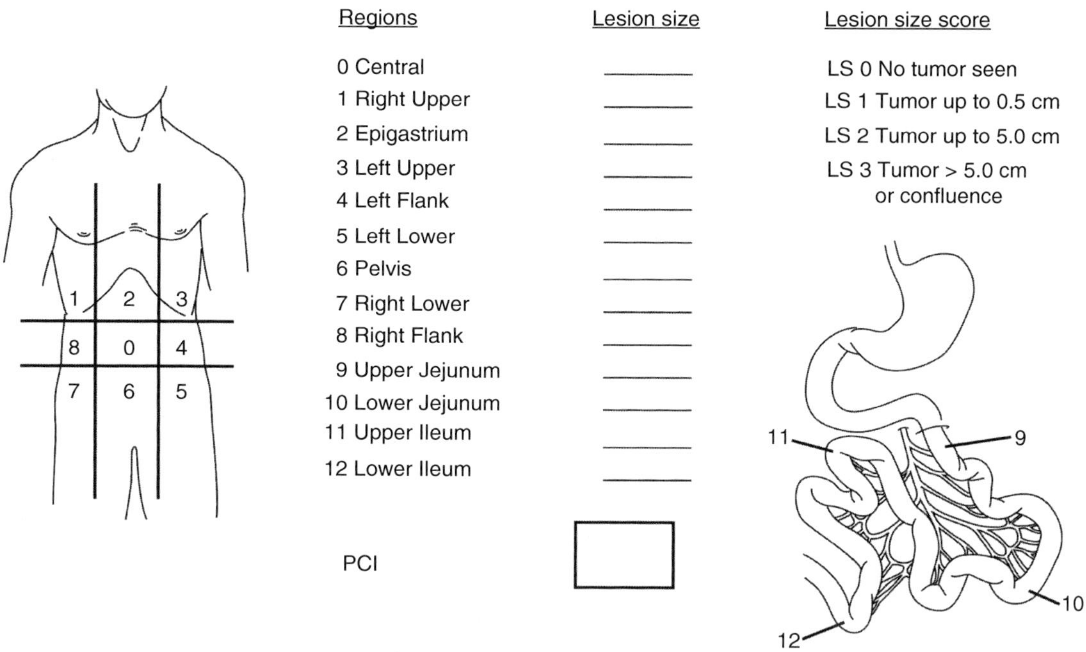

Fig. 11.1 The peritoneal cancer index uses the distribution of cancer implants throughout the abdomen and pelvis combined with a lesion size of these nodules in order to quantitate the disease upon abdominal exploration

is visibly free of disease at the close of the procedure. The surgery combines a series of peritonectomy procedures and visceral resections. The peritonectomy procedures include anterior parietal peritonectomy, stripping of right and left hemidiaphragm, pelvic peritonectomy, and omental bursa peritonectomy. Visceral resections include hysterectomy and oophorectomy, greater and lesser omentectomy, splenectomy, right colectomy, and rectosigmoid colectomy.

Construction of the Surgical Field to Provide Simultaneous Exposure of the Abdomen and Pelvis

A self-retaining retractor (Thompson Surgical Instruments, Traverse City, Michigan) is positioned so that continuous retraction of all parts of the abdominal incision occurs (Fig. 11.2). The retraction system must be securely anchored to the operating table to provide for continuous unencumbered visualization of a large operative field. An incision starting above the xiphisternal junction and continuing down the pubis through the midline is constructed. An ellipse is created around the umbilicus to allow for the peritoneal plane to be clearly exposed throughout the extent of the abdominal incision. The fascia is divided through the linea alba from the xiphoid bone to the pubic bone. If there has been prior midline abdominal incision, it is widely excised. Routinely, the xiphoid is completely resected at the xiphisternal junction as part of the specimen. With the fascia divided, the parietal peritoneum remains intact.

Parietal Peritoneal Stripping from the Anterior Abdominal Wall

A single entry into the peritoneal cavity in the middle portion of the incision allows the surgeon to assess the parietal peritoneum and the small bowel surfaces. If cancer nodules are palpated on the parietal peritoneum larger than those covering the small bowel and its mesentery, a decision for a complete dissection is made. Except for the small defect in the peritoneum required for this peritoneal exploration, the remainder of the peritoneum is kept intact to facilitate the peritonectomy.

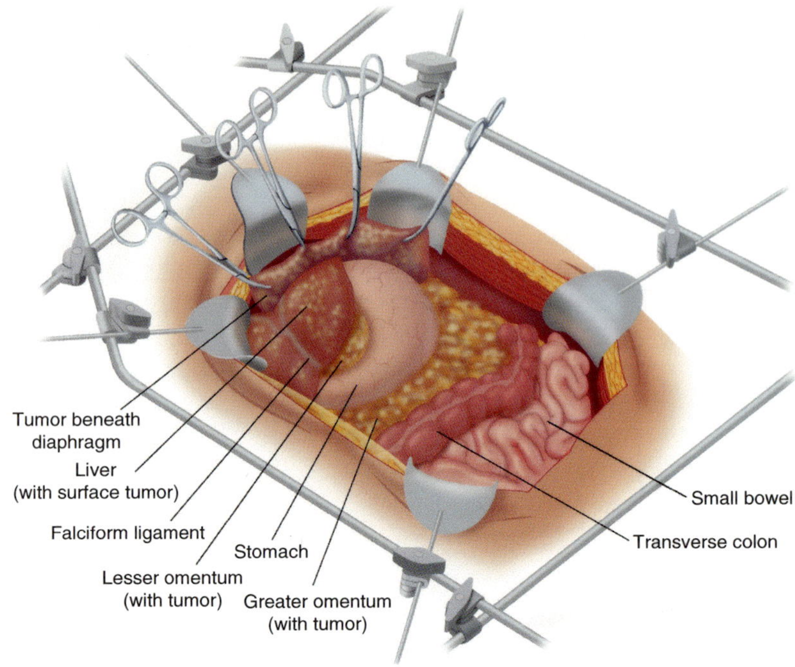

Fig. 11.2 A fixed retractor is used to provide exposure of the entire abdomen so that peritonectomy procedures on the anterior abdominal wall, beneath the hemidiaphragms, and within the pelvis can proceed in an efficient manner (From Sugarbaker PH. An overview of peritonectomy, visceral resections, and perioperative chemotherapy for peritoneal surface malignancy. In: Sugarbaker PH. (ed.) Cytoreductive Surgery and Perioperative Chemotherapy for Peritoneal Surface Malignancy. Woodbury, CT: Textbook and Video Atlas. Cine-Med Publishing; 2012. pp. 1–30)

Stripping the Visceral Peritoneum from the Surface of the Bladder

After dissecting generously the peritoneum on the right and left sides of the bladder, the apex of the bladder (preferably the urachus) is localized and placed on strong traction using a Babcock clamp. The peritoneum with the underlying fatty tissues is stripped away from the muscular surface of the bladder. Broad traction on the entire anterior parietal peritoneal surface and frequent saline irrigation reveals the point for tissue transection that is precisely located between the bladder musculature and its adherent fatty tissue. This dissection is continued inferiorly down to the cervix in the female or to the seminal vesicles in the male.

Parietal Peritoneal Dissection to the Paracolic Sulcus and Beyond

The self-retaining retraction system is steadily advanced more deeply into the abdominal cavity. Firm broad traction on the peritoneum at the point of dissection facilitates accurate dissection. The peritoneum strips readily from the undersurface of the hemidiaphragm. The dissection joins the right and left subphrenic peritonectomy superiorly and the complete pelvic peritonectomy inferiorly. As the dissection proceeds beyond the peritoneum overlying the paracolic sulcus (line of Toldt), the dissection becomes more rapid because of the loose connections of the peritoneum to the underlying fatty tissue at this anatomic site.

When the anterior parietal peritonectomy has been completed, removal of this large peritoneal layer eradicates cancer implants from the posterior aspect of the anterior abdominal wall. Complete exploration of the abdomen and pelvis proceeds.

Peritoneal Stripping from Beneath the Left Hemidiaphragm

To begin peritonectomy of the left upper quadrant, the peritoneum is progressively stripped off the posterior rectus sheath (Fig. 11.3). Broad traction must be exerted on the tumor specimen throughout the left upper quadrant. Strong traction combined

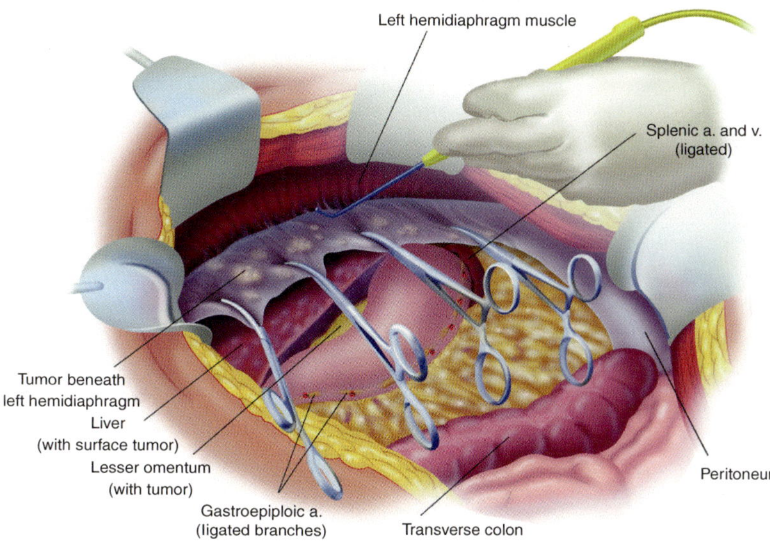

Fig. 11.3 Left upper quadrant peritonectomy (From Sugarbaker PH. An overview of peritonectomy, visceral resections, and perioperative chemotherapy for peritoneal surface malignancy. In: Sugarbaker PH. (ed.) Cytoreductive Surgery and Perioperative Chemotherapy for Peritoneal Surface Malignancy. Woodbury, CT: Textbook and Video Atlas. Cine-Med Publishing; 2012. pp. 1–30)

with ball-tipped electrosurgical dissection allows separation of the peritoneum with tumor from all normal tissue in the left upper quadrant including the diaphragmatic muscle, the left adrenal gland, and the superior aspect of perirenal fat. The splenic flexure of the colon is released from the peritoneum of the left abdominal gutter and moved medially.

Greater Omentectomy and Splenectomy with Completion of the Left Subphrenic Peritonectomy

To free the mid-abdomen of a large volume of tumor, the greater omentectomy–splenectomy is performed. The greater omentectomy is elevated and then separated from the transverse colon using electrosurgery. The omental tissue on the anterior aspect of the transverse mesocolon is also resected. The gastroepiploic vessels on the greater curvature of the stomach are ligated and divided. Also, the short gastric vessels are transected. This freely exposes the splenic artery and vein at the tail of the pancreas. These vessels are ligated in continuity and proximally suture ligated taking care not to traumatize pancreas parenchyma. This allows the greater curvature of the stomach to be reflected to the right from the pylorus to the gastroesophageal junction.

Peritoneal Stripping from Beneath the Right Hemidiaphragm

Peritoneum is stripped away from the right posterior rectus sheath to begin the peritonectomy in the right upper quadrant of the abdomen. Strong traction on the specimen is used to elevate the rolled muscular edge of the hemidiaphragm into the operative field. Again, ball-tipped electrosurgery on pure cut is used to dissect at the interface of tumor and normal tissue. Coagulation current is used to divide the blood vessels as they are encountered and before they bleed.

Cholecystectomy, Lesser Omentectomy, and Peritonectomy of the Omental Bursa

The gallbladder is removed in a routine fashion from its fundus toward the cystic artery and cystic duct (Fig. 11.4). Blunt dissection of the cystic artery and cystic duct away from the common duct and right hepatic artery distinguishes these structures from the surrounding tumor and fatty tissue. These structures are ligated and divided.

To strip the peritoneum from the anterior aspect of the hepatoduodenal ligament, its peritoneal reflection to the liver surface is divided. Special care is taken not to injure the left hepatic

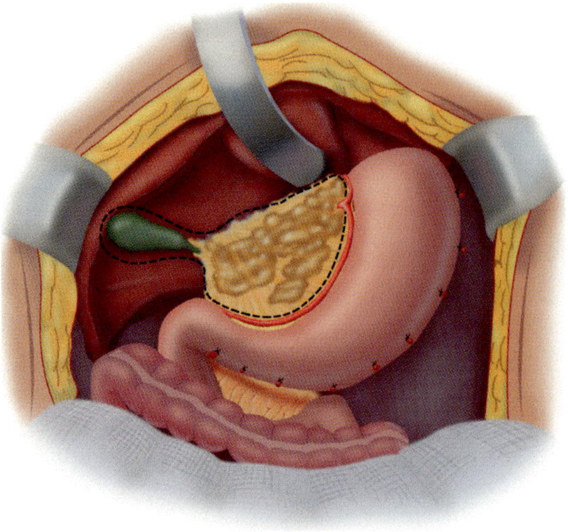

Fig. 11.4 Cholecystectomy, lesser omentectomy, and peritonectomy of the omental bursa (From Sugarbaker PH. An overview of peritonectomy, visceral resections, and perioperative chemotherapy for peritoneal surface malignancy. In: Sugarbaker PH. (ed.) Cytoreductive Surgery and Perioperative Chemotherapy for Peritoneal Surface Malignancy. Woodbury, CT: Textbook and Video Atlas. Cine-Med Publishing; 2012. pp. 1–30)

artery, which is usually the most superficial of the portal structures. The peritoneum, often layered by tumor nodules, is firmly grasped using a Russian forceps and peeled away from the common bile duct and hepatic artery.

Resection of the Hepatogastric Ligament and Lesser Omentum

The left lateral segment of the liver is retracted left to right to expose the hepatogastric ligament in its entirety. A circumferential release of this ligament from the fissure between the left lateral portion of the liver and segment 1 occurs first. The arcade of right gastric artery to left gastric artery along the lesser curvature of the stomach must be skeletonized. After electrosurgically dividing the peritoneum on the lesser curvature of the stomach, digital dissection with extreme pressure from the surgeon's thumb and index finger separates lesser omental fat and tumor from the vascular arcade. As much of the anterior vagus nerve is spared as is possible with patience and persistence. The tumor and fatty tissue surrounding the right and left gastric arteries are split away from the vascular arcade. In this manner the specimen is centralized over the major branches of the left gastric artery. With strong traction on the specimen, the lesser omentum is released from the left gastric artery and vein.

Resection of Rectosigmoid Colon, Uterus, Ovaries, and Cul-de-sac of Douglas

To being the rectosigmoid colon resection, a linear stapler is used to divide the sigmoid colon just above the limits of the pelvic tumor; this is usually at the junction of sigmoid and descending colon. The vascular supply of the distal portion of the bowel is traced back to its origin on the aorta. The inferior mesenteric artery and vein are ligated, suture ligated, and divided. This allows one to pack all the viscera, including the proximal descending colon into the upper abdomen.

Ball-tipped electrosurgery is used to dissect at the limits of the pelvic peritonectomy (Fig. 11.5). The surgeon works in a centripetal fashion. Extraperitoneal ligation of the uterine arteries is performed just above the ureter and close to the base of the bladder. In women, the bladder is moved gently off the cervix and the vagina is entered. The vaginal cuff anterior and posterior to the cervix is transected using ball-tipped electrosurgery, and the rectovaginal septum is entered. Ball-tipped electrosurgery is used to divide the perirectal fat beneath the peritoneal reflection. This ensures that all tumors that occupy the peritoneum within the cul-de-sac are removed intact with the specimen. The anterior rectal musculature is skeletonized using ball-tipped electrosurgery. Preservation of the lower half of the rectum will allow for a larger stool reservoir and diminish frequent bowel movements. A stapler is used to close off the rectal stump, and the rectum is sharply divided above the stapler.

Secure Vaginal Closure and Colorectal Anastomosis

Additional sutures are placed to close the apex of the vagina (Fig. 11.6). These sutures are left long so that they may be used to elevate the vaginal cuff and clearly expose the stump of the rectum.

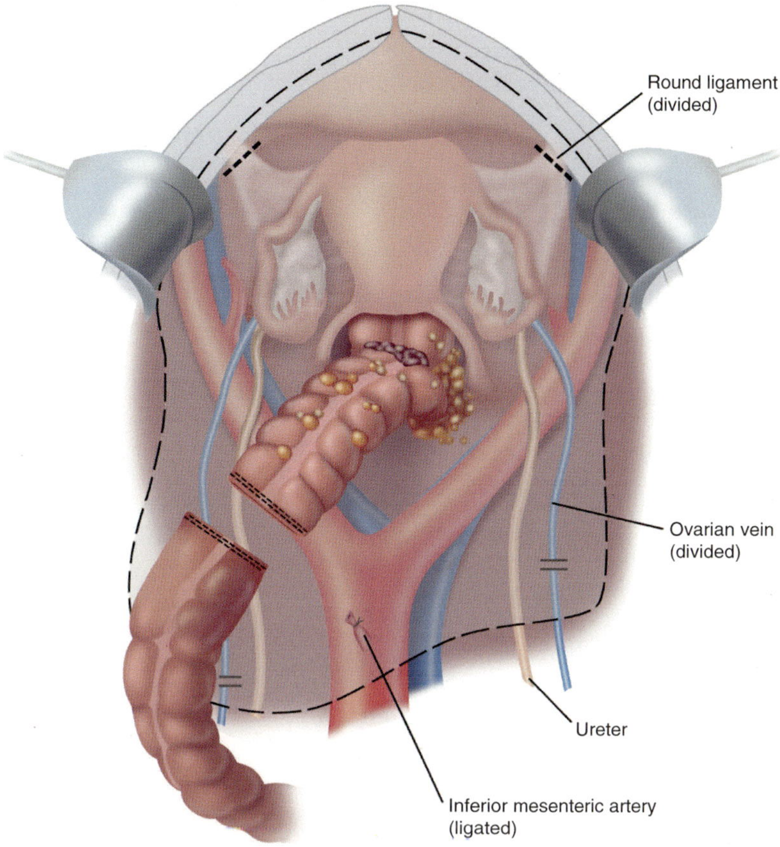

Fig. 11.5 Rectosigmoidectomy and complete peritonectomy (From Sugarbaker PH. An overview of peritonectomy, visceral resections, and perioperative chemotherapy for peritoneal surface malignancy. In: Sugarbaker PH. (ed.) Cytoreductive Surgery and Perioperative Chemotherapy for Peritoneal Surface Malignancy. Woodbury, CT: Textbook and Video Atlas. Cine-Med Publishing; 2012. pp. 1–30)

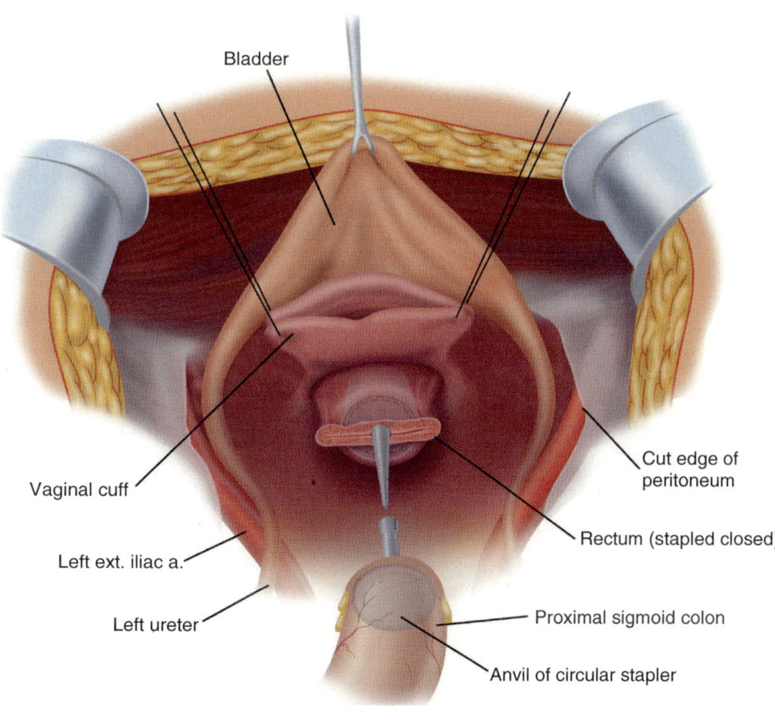

Fig. 11.6 Reconstruction after rectosigmoid colon resection and complete pelvic peritonectomy. The vagina is closed prior to the hyperthermic intraperitoneal chemotherapy. The low-stapled colorectal anastomosis is performed after the chemotherapy lavage is complete (From Sugarbaker PH. An overview of peritonectomy, visceral resections, and perioperative chemotherapy for peritoneal surface malignancy. In: Sugarbaker PH. (ed.) Cytoreductive Surgery and Perioperative Chemotherapy for Peritoneal Surface Malignancy. Woodbury, CT: Textbook and Video Atlas. Cine-Med Publishing; 2012. pp. 1–30)

Rationale for Hyperthermic Intraperitoneal Chemotherapy and Early Postoperative Intraperitoneal Chemotherapy

After completion of the cytoreduction when no visible cancer remains, it is invariably true that invisible to the naked eye, an immense number of cancer cells will remain within the peritoneal cavity. Tumor manipulation, transected lymphatic ducts leaking tumor cells throughout the procedure, and small tumor nodules remaining on the abdominal and pelvic surfaces of organs not amenable to peritonectomy procedures, namely, small bowel, make necessary the implementation of some method that will eradicate residual tumor cells. Another well-known site for persistent disease is the suture lines that are an ideal site for cancer cell implants. Tumor cell entrapment occurs on these raw surfaces with fibrin accumulating and tissues compressed together by stitches or staples. Suture lines are at high risk for recurrence if constructed before the hyperthermic intraperitoneal chemotherapy (HIPEC).

Technique for Hyperthermic Intraperitoneal Chemotherapy

An abdominopelvic reservoir is constructed by tenting up the skin edges on a fixed retractor that allows hand distribution of the chemotherapy agent and total containment. The gloved hand guarantees that the perfusate reaches all surfaces within the peritoneal cavity, such as the space between the bowel loops, the space behind the liver, and the pelvic cavity.

In order to keep the temperature at a constant 42 °C, a hyperthermia pump forces the solution through a heat exchanger. Then it proceeds into the abdominopelvic cavity through an inflow catheter. The hyperthermic perfusate is drained from the abdomen through four closed drains going back to the heat exchanger and closing the circuit. The inflow catheter and the closed suction drains are secured watertight with purse-string sutures on the skin of the abdomen to avoid leaks and spillage. The chemotherapy solution circulates for 90 min at 42 °C.

Table 11.1 Intraoperative bidirectional chemotherapy orders

1. Add cisplatin (50 mg/m^2) ________ mg to 2 l of 1.5 % dextrose peritoneal dialysis solution. Add doxorubicin (15 mg/m^2) ________ mg to same 2 l of 1.5 % dextrose peritoneal dialysis solution
2. Add ifosfamide (1,300 mg/m^2) ________ mg to 1-l normal saline. Begin continuous IV infusion over 90 min simultaneous with IP chemotherapy
3. Add mesna disulfide (260 mg/m^2) ________ mg in 100 ml 0.9 % sodium chloride to be given IV as a bolus 15 min prior to ifosfamide infusion
4. Add mesna disulfide (260 mg/m^2) ________ mg in 100 ml 0.9 % sodium chloride to be given IV as a bolus 4 h after ifosfamide infusion
5. Add mesna disulfide (260 mg/m^2) ________ mg in 100 ml 0.9 % sodium chloride to be given IV as a bolus 8 h after ifosfamide infusion
6. Send all the above to operating room # _______ at _______ o'clock on ___________(Date) for a 90-min treatment

After the 90 min of HIPEC with manual distribution, the surgeon may assume that fibrin and tissue debris and the microscopic residual disease they contain have been eradicated. At this time, all the anastomosis and any additional reconstruction can occur. Closed-suction drains and an inflow catheter are properly positioned for subsequent early postoperative intraperitoneal chemotherapy (EPIC) with paclitaxel. Standardized orders for bidirectional intraperitoneal chemotherapy are given in Table 11.1. Cisplatin and doxorubicin are given by intraperitoneal administration and ifosfamide by intravenous continuous infusion [55, 56] (Fig. 11.7).

Technique for Early Perioperative Intraperitoneal Chemotherapy

In the first 5 postoperative days, the patient receives normothermic intraperitoneal paclitaxel (20–40 mg/m^2/day), with the goal of consolidating the EPIC treatments. The extremely favorable area under the

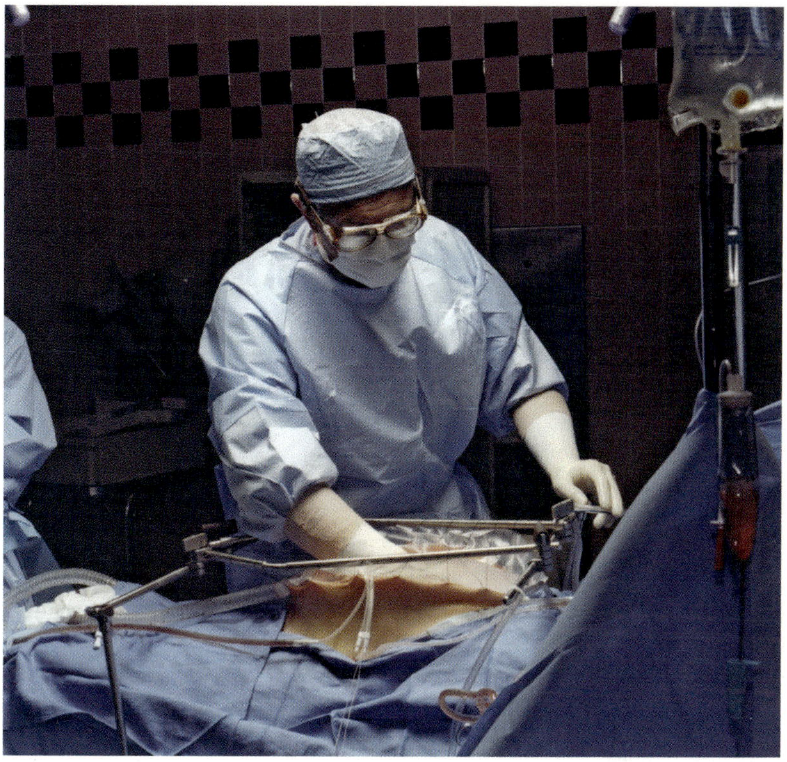

Fig. 11.7 Hyperthermic intraperitoneal chemotherapy (HIPEC) proceeds by constructing a reservoir from the abdominal space. The skin edges are elevated on a self-retaining retractor, and a plastic sheet covers the open abdomen. A cruciate incision in this plastic sheet allows free access of the surgeon's double-gloved hand. Uniform distribution of heat and chemotherapy is maintained throughout the 90 min of the HIPEC treatment

Table 11.2 Early postoperative intraperitoneal chemotherapy orders

1. Paclitaxel ________ mg (20–40 mg/m^2 × ________m^2) (maximum dose: 80 mg) in________ml 6 % Hespan® (B. Braun, Irvine, CA) via the Tenckhoff catheter or IP port daily Start date:________________ Stop date: __________________(For daily doses >500 ml total volume, pharmacy will split dose equally into two bags)
2. Instill as rapidly as possible via the Tenckhoff catheter or IP port. Dwell for 23 h. Drain from Jackson-Pratt drains for one hour prior to the next instillation
3. Continue to drain the abdominal cavity by Jackson-Pratt drains after the last dose of IP chemotherapy
4. During the initial 6 h after chemotherapy instillation, patient's bed should be kept flat. The patient should be on the right side during instillation. Turn ½ hour post-instillation onto the left side and continue to change sides at ½ hour intervals for 6 h
5. Monitor with a pulse oximeter during the first 6 h of each intraperitoneal chemotherapy

curve ratio and the remarkable drug penetration of up to 80 cell layers deserve mention. Standardized orders for EPIC are given in Table 11.2.

Results of Comprehensive Treatment in Advanced Primary and Recurrent Ovarian Cancer

In patients who have failed the standard treatments of primary ovarian cancer, the survival is short, with an estimated median survival of 9 months. The median survival of 28 patients with advanced primary and recurrent epithelial ovarian cancer who had an attempt at complete cytoreduction at the Washington Cancer Institute was 45.8 months [57]. Further analysis by Look and colleagues of the clinical features that affected survival showed that extent of prior surgery and completeness of cytoreduction were independent factors significantly affecting survival. Those patients with extensive prior surgery, that is, with three or more abdominopelvic regions subjected to surgical dissection, were less likely to receive a complete cytoreduction, and their survival was significantly shorter. Patients with a low prior surgical score who had less than three abdominopelvic regions previously dissected had a median survival of 6.5 years, compared to 1.5 years for those patients with a higher PSS ($p<0.001$). Patients with an adequate cytoreduction had a median survival of 55.9 months; suboptimal cytoreduction showed an 8-month survival ($p=0.037$).

Tentes and colleagues reported on the peritoneal cancer index as a quantitative prognostic indicator in 60 women with ovarian cancer [54]. Those patients with a lower PCI than ten had a median survival of 80 months and a 5-year survival of 65 %, while those patients with a PCI greater than ten had a median survival of 38 months and a 5-year survival rate of 29 % ($p=0.0253$).

Recently, Bijelic and colleagues published a systematic review analyzing 14 studies that reported on cytoreduction and HIPEC [58]. Ten studies reported a positive impact on survival, and in four, survival was not analyzed. Morbidity ranged from 5 to 36 % and the median mortality was 3 %.

Conclusions

This highly specialized treatment needs to be performed by qualified surgeons who are knowledgeable about perioperative chemotherapy administration as well as the complications of this aggressive approach. Accepting the fact that there might be a selection bias, the results with this comprehensive treatment are encouraging. Multi-institutional trials are in progress to further validate these results in patients with recurrent ovarian cancer. Until results of these trials are available, the strong rationale, the initial favorable results by competent groups, and the demonstrated safety justify the current use of CRS and HIPEC for EOC [59].

References

1. Parkin DM, Bray F, Ferlay J, Pisani P. Global cancer statistics, 2002. CA Cancer J Clin. 2005;55(2):74–108.
2. American Cancer Society. Cancer facts and digures 2010, Available at: http://www.cancer.org/Research/CancerFactsFigures/CancerFactsFigures/cancer-facts-and-figures-2010. Accessed 7 Oct 2010.
3. Horner MJ, Ries LAG, Krapcho M, et al. eds. SEER cancer statistics review, 1975–2006. Bethesda: National Cancer Institute, http://seer.cancer.gov/csr/1975_2006/, based on November 2008 SEER data submission, posted to the SEER web site, 2009. Accessed 7 Oct 2010.
4. Heintz AP, Odicino F, Maisonneuve P, et al. Carcinoma of the ovary. FIGO 6th annual report on the results of treatment in gynecological cancer. Int J Gynaecol Obstet. 2006;95 Suppl 1:S161–92.
5. Tavassoli FA, Devilee P. (eds.) Pathology and genetics of tumours of the breast and female genital organs. World health organization classification of tumours. Lyon: IARC Press; 2003.
6. Seidman JD, Russell P, Kurman RJ. Surface epithelial tumors of the ovary. In: Kurman RJ, editor. Blaustein's pathology of the female genital tract. 5th ed. New York: Springer; 2002. p. 791–904.
7. Barda G, Menczer J, Chetrit A, et al. Comparison between primary peritoneal and epithelial ovarian carcinoma: a population-based study. Am J Obstet Gynecol. 2004;190(4):1039–45.
8. Gadducci A, Landoni F, Sartori E, et al. Analysis of treatment failures and survival of patients with fallopian tube carcinoma: a cooperation task force (CTF) study. Gynecol Oncol. 2001;81(2):150–9.
9. Tuma RS. Origin of ovarian cancer may have implications for screening. J Natl Cancer Inst. 2010;102(1):11–3.
10. Goodman MT, Shvetsov YB. Incidence of ovarian, peritoneal, and fallopian tube carcinomas in the United States, 1995–2004. Cancer Epidemiol Biomarkers Prev. 2009;18(1):132–9.
11. Prat J, Ribe A, Gallardo A. Hereditary ovarian cancer. Hum Pathol. 2005;36(8):861–70.
12. Trimble CL, Kosary C, Trimble EL. Long-term survival and patterns of care in women with ovarian tumors of low malignant potential. Gynecol Oncol. 2002;86(1):34–7.
13. AJCC. Fallopian tube carcinoma. AJCC cancer staging handbook. 2009th ed. New York: Springer; 2009. p. 501–6.
14. AJCC. Ovary and primary peritoneal carcinoma. AJCC cancer staging handbook. 7th ed. New York: Springer; 2009. p. 493–506.
15. FIGO. Current FIGO staging for cancer of the vagina, fallopian tube, ovary, and gestational trophoblastic neoplasia. Int J Gynaecol Obstet. 2009;105:3–4.
16. Bergman F. Carcinoma of the ovary. A clinicopathological study of 86 autopsied cases with special reference to mode of spread. Acta Obstet Gynecol Scand. 1966;45(2):211–31.
17. Friedman GD, Skilling JS, Udaltsova NV, Smith LH. Early symptoms of ovarian cancer: a case–control study without recall bias. Fam Pract. 2005;22(5):548–53.
18. Goff BA, Mandel LS, Drescher CW, et al. Development of an ovarian cancer symptom index: possibilities for earlier detection. Cancer. 2007;109(2):221–7.

19. Andersen MR, Goff BA, Lowe KA, et al. Use of a symptom index, CA125, and HE4 to predict ovarian cancer. Gynecol Oncol. 2010;116(3):378–83.
20. Rossing MA, Wicklund KG, Cushing-Haugen KL, Weiss NS. Predictive value of symptoms for early detection of ovarian cancer. J Natl Cancer Inst. 2010;102(4):222–9.
21. Bast Jr RC, Feeney M, Lazarus H, et al. Reactivity of a monoclonal antibody with human ovarian carcinoma. J Clin Invest. 1981;68(5):1331–7.
22. Bast Jr RC, Klug TL, St John E, et al. A radioimmunoassay using a monoclonal antibody to monitor the course of epithelial ovarian cancer. N Engl J Med. 1983;309(15):883–7.
23. Jacobs I, Bast RC. The CA 125 tumour-associated antigen: a review of the literature. Hum Reprod. 1989;4(1):1–12.
24. Lenhard MS, Burges A, Johnson TRC, et al. PET-CT in recurrent ovarian cancer: impact on treatment planning. Anticancer Res. 2008;28(4C):2303–8.
25. Rustin GJ, Quinn M, Thigpen T, Rustin GJ, Quinn M, Thigpen T, et al. Re: new guidelines to evaluate the response to treatment in solid tumors (ovarian cancer). J Natl Cancer Inst. 2004;96(6): 487–8.
26. Bristow RE, del Carmen MG, Pannu HK, et al. Clinically occult recurrent ovarian cancer: patient selection for secondary cytoreductive surgery using combined PET/CT. Gynecol Oncol. 2003;90(3): 519–28.
27. Loyer EM, Whitman GJ, Fenstermacher MJ. Imaging of ovarian carcinoma. Int J Gynecol Cancer. 1999;9(5):351–61.
28. Coakley FV. Staging ovarian cancer: role of imaging. Radiol Clin North Am. 2002;40(3):609–36.
29. Nelson RC, Chezmar JL, Hoel MJ, Buck DR, Sugarbaker PH. Peritoneal carcinomatosis: preoperative CT with intraperitoneal contrast material. Radiology. 1992;182(1):133–8.
30. Kawamoto S, Urban BA, Fishman EK. CT of epithelial ovarian tumors. Radiographics. 1999;19:S85–102; quiz S263-104.
31. Forstner R, Hricak H, White S. CT and MRI of ovarian cancer. Abdom Imaging. 1995;20(1):2–8.
32. Forstner R, Hricak H, Occhipinti KA, et al. Ovarian cancer: staging with CT and MR imaging. Radiology. 1995;197(3):619–26.
33. Meyer JI, Kennedy AW, Friedman R, Ayoub A, Zepp RC. Ovarian carcinoma: value of CT in predicting success of debulking surgery. Am J Roentgenol. 1995;165(4):875–8.
34. Bristow RE, Duska LR, Lambrou NC, et al. A model for predicting surgical outcome in patients with advanced ovarian carcinoma using computed tomography. Cancer. 2000;89(7):1532–40.
35. Dowdy SC, Mullany SA, Brandt KR, Huppert BJ, Cliby WA. The utility of computed tomography scans in predicting suboptimal cytoreductive surgery in women with advanced ovarian carcinoma. Cancer. 2004;101(2):346–52.
36. Qayyum A, Coakley FV, Westphalen AC, et al. Role of CT and MR imaging in predicting optimal cytoreduction of newly diagnosed primary epithelial ovarian cancer. Gynecol Oncol. 2005;96(2):301–6.
37. Axtell AE, Lee MH, Bristow RE, et al. Multi-institutional reciprocal validation study of computed tomography predictors of suboptimal primary cytoreduction in patients with advanced ovarian cancer. J Clin Oncol. 2007;25(4):384–9.
38. Eisenkop SM, Spirtos NM, Lin WC. "Optimal" cytoreduction for advanced epithelial ovarian cancer: a commentary. Gynecol Oncol. 2006;103(1):329–35.
39. Kurtz AB, Tsimikas JV, Tempany CM, et al. Diagnosis and staging of ovarian cancer: comparative values of Doppler and conventional US, CT, and MR imaging correlated with surgery and histopathologic analysis–report of the Radiology Diagnostic Oncology Group. Radiology. 1999;212(1):19–27.
40. Kubik-Huch RA, Dorffler W, von Schulthess GK, et al. Value of (18F)-FDG positron emission tomography, computed tomography, and magnetic resonance imaging in diagnosing primary and recurrent ovarian carcinoma. Eur Radiol. 2000;10(5):761–7.
41. Ak I, Stokkel MP, Pauwels EK. Positron emission tomography with 2-[18F]fluoro-2-deoxy-D-glucose in oncology. Part II. The clinical value in detecting and staging primary tumours. J Cancer Res Clin Oncol. 2000;126(10):560–74.
42. Schroder W, Zimny M, Rudlowski C, Bull U, Rath W. The role of 18F-fluoro-deoxyglucose positron emission tomography (18F-FDG PET) in diagnosis of ovarian cancer. Int J Gynecol Cancer. 1999;9(2): 117–22.
43. Charron M, Beyer T, Bohnen NN, et al. Image analysis in patients with cancer studied with a combined PET and CT scanner. Clin Nucl Med. 2000;25(11): 905–10.
44. Makhija S, Howden N, Edwards R, et al. Positron emission tomography/computed tomography imaging for the detection of recurrent ovarian and fallopian tube carcinoma: a retrospective review. Gynecol Oncol. 2002;85(1):53–8.
45. Risum S, Hogdall C, Loft A, et al. Does the use of diagnostic PET/CT cause stage migration in patients with primary advanced ovarian cancer? Gynecol Oncol. 2010;116(3):395–8.
46. Munnell E. The changing prognosis and treatment in cancer of the ovary. Am J Obstet Gynecol. 1968; 100:790–5.
47. Griffiths CT. Surgical resection of tumor bulk in the primary treatment of ovarian carcinoma. Natl Cancer Inst Monogr. 1975;42:101–4.
48. Hoskins WJ, Bundy BN, Thigpen JT, Omura GA. The influence of cytoreductive surgery on recurrence-free interval and survival in small-volume stage III epithelial ovarian cancer: a Gynecologic Oncology Group study. Gynecol Oncol. 1992;47(2):159–66.
49. Bristow RE, Tomacruz RS, Armstrong DK, Trimble EL, Montz FJ. Survival effect of maximal cytoreductive surgery for advanced ovarian carcinoma during

the platinum era: a meta-analysis. J Clin Oncol. 2002;20(5):1248–59.
50. Chi DS, Eisenhauer EL, Lang J, et al. What is the optimal goal of primary cytoreductive surgery for bulky stage IIIC epithelial ovarian carcinoma (EOC)? Gynecol Oncol. 2006;103(2):559–64.
51. Eisenkop SM, Spirtos NM. What are the current surgical objectives, strategies, and technical capabilities of gynecologic oncologists treating advanced epithelial ovarian cancer? Gynecol Oncol. 2001;82: 489–97.
52. Eisenkop SM, Friedman RL, Wang HJ. Complete cytoreductive surgery is feasible and maximizes survival in patients with advanced epithelial ovarian cancer: a prospective study. Gynecol Oncol. 1998;69(2): 103–8.
53. Eisenhauer EL, Abu-Rustum NR, Sonoda Y, et al. The addition of extensive upper abdominal surgery to achieve optimal cytoreduction improves survival in patients with stages IIIC-IV epithelial ovarian cancer. Gynecol Oncol. 2006;103(3):1083–90.
54. Tentes AA, Tripsiannis G, Markakidis SK, et al. Peritoneal cancer index: a prognostic indicator of survival in advanced ovarian cancer. Eur J Surg Oncol. 2003;29(1):69–73.
55. Van der Speeten K, Stuart OA, Mahteme H, Sugarbaker PH. Heat targeting of perioperative intravenous ifosfamide. Int J Surg Oncol. 2011; Volume 2011, Article ID 185092, 9 pages. doi:10.1155/2011/185092.
56. Zylberberg B, Dormont D, Madelenat P, Darai E. First-line intraperitoneal cisplatin-paclitaxel and intravenous ifosfamide in stage IIIc ovarian epithelial cancer. Eur J Gynaecol Oncol. 2004;25:327–32.
57. Look M, Chang D, Sugarbaker PH. Long-term results of cytoreductive surgery for advanced and recurrent epithelial ovarian cancers and papillary serous carcinoma of the peritoneum. Int J Gynecol Cancer. 2003;13:764–70.
58. Bijelic L, Jonson A, Sugarbaker PH. Systematic review of cytoreductive surgery and heated intraoperative intraperitoneal chemotherapy for treatment of peritoneal carcinomatosis in primary and recurrent ovarian cancer. Ann Oncol. 2007;18:1943–50.
59. Yan TD, Zappa L, Edwards G, Alderman R, Marquardt CE, Sugarbaker PH. Perioperative outcomes of cytoreductive surgery and perioperative intraperitoneal chemotherapy for non-appendiceal peritoneal carcinomatosis from a prospective database. J Surg Oncol. 2007;96:102–12.

Targeted Molecular Therapy for Patients with Ovarian Cancer

12

Samir A. Farghaly

Introduction

Over 230,000 women are diagnosed with ovarian cancer each year worldwide, and this disease is responsible for an estimated 140,000 deaths per year worldwide. The American Cancer Society estimates that in 2013, about 22,240 new cases of ovarian cancer will be diagnosed and 15,500 women will die of ovarian cancer in the USA. Ovarian cancer is the most common cause of death from cancers of the female genital tract [1, 2]. The high case fatality rate results from the frequent diagnosis of epithelial ovarian cancer at an advanced stage: 75 % of all cases are diagnosed as stage III or IV, where the disease has spread throughout the abdomen [3, 4]. Patients with advanced-stage disease have a 5-year survival of 29 %. There are only a limited number of chemotherapeutic agents with reasonable effectiveness against epithelial ovarian cancer. Most patients develop recurrent disease, which commonly acquires chemoresistance. The identification of the genes and their protein products in ovarian cancer that contribute to the malignant phenotype has increased our knowledge of human tumorigenesis. There are several cell surface receptors, signaling pathways, and nuclear proteins, which are possible targets for molecular therapeutic approach. Targeting specific cellular mechanisms associated with ovarian tumorigenesis and progression may serve to improve oncologic outcome and limit toxicity in patients with ovarian cancer. The standard therapy involves a combination of optimal cytoreductive surgery with chemotherapy that consists of a platinum agent and a taxane compound [5]. The response rate of the standard regimen for ovarian cancer exceeds 80 %, but about 70 % of patients with advanced ovarian cancer experience recurrence within 5 years, and they die because their cancer disease becomes resistant to platinum and taxane [6, 7]. Most of these patients are subsequently treated with other agents, such as liposomal doxorubicin, gemcitabine, topotecan, or etoposide. The overall response rates to these other drugs are 10–25 % [8]. So, targeted molecular therapy is needed to improve oncologic outcome for patients with advanced and recurrent ovarian cancer. The ideal molecular target ought to be differentially expressed by the tumor, have a potential chemosensitive molecular site, and be necessary for the viability of the cancer cell. The molecular heterogeneity of ovarian cancer compared with other disease sites has made the successful transfer of molecular agents into the ovarian cancer treatment feasible [9]. Ovarian cancer has been recognized to possess a multitude of molecular abnormalities any of which may play a role in ovarian cancer proliferation and survival. The understanding of the complex

S.A. Farghaly, MD, PhD
Department of Obstetrics and Gynecology,
The Weill Cornell Medical College/
Weill Cornell Graduate School of Medical Sciences,
and The New York Presbyterian Hospital- Weill
Cornell Medical Center, Cornell University,
New York, NY, USA
e-mail: samirfarghaly@yahoo.com

S.A. Farghaly (ed.), *Advances in Diagnosis and Management of Ovarian Cancer*,
DOI 10.1007/978-1-4614-8271-0_12, © Springer Science+Business Media New York 2014

pathways of growth deregulation in gynecologic cancers has provided us with a basis for the application and testing of novel therapies [10, 11].

Antiangiogenic Therapy

Rationale

There are several reasons for using antiangiogenic therapy. First, all solid tumors require increased tumor angiogenesis to facilitate growth and metastasis, and therefore, inhibitors may have activity across a variety of malignancies. Second, the development of resistance is rare, because the primary target is normal endothelial cells. Third, side effects are relatively mild and limited.

One of the major mediators of tumor angiogenesis is VEGF. In ovarian cancer, microvessel density, intratumoral VEGF, and VEGF receptor (VEGFR) expression have been associated with a poor prognosis, suggesting that angiogenesis should be considered a target for novel therapies. It is established that VEGF and several antiangiogenic mediators, including platelet-derived growth factor and fibroblast growth factor (FDF), serve as mediators of tumor angiogenesis (Fig. 12.1). VEGF was noted to be overexpressed in primary ovarian neoplasms and in the ascites and plasma of ovarian cancer patients. VEGF was characterized and was found to inhibit tumor growth in vivo in several cancers, including rhabdomyosarcoma, glioblastoma multiforme, leiomyosarcoma, and prostate cancer [5].

Antiangiogenic Agents

Bevacizumab

Bevacizumab is a recombinant, humanized, monoclonal immunoglobulin G1 antibody targeted at VEGF-A, which is approved for the treatment of metastatic colorectal cancer, non-squamous non-small cell lung cancer, glioblastoma, and metastatic renal cell carcinoma [12]. This antibody binds to and neutralizes all forms of VEGF-A, which suppresses growth of tumors and inhibits progression of metastatic disease [13, 14]. Also, anti-VEGF drugs enhance the effects of chemotherapeutic agents by improving the structure and function of tumor vessels [15]. Two phase II studies of bevacizumab monotherapy conducted

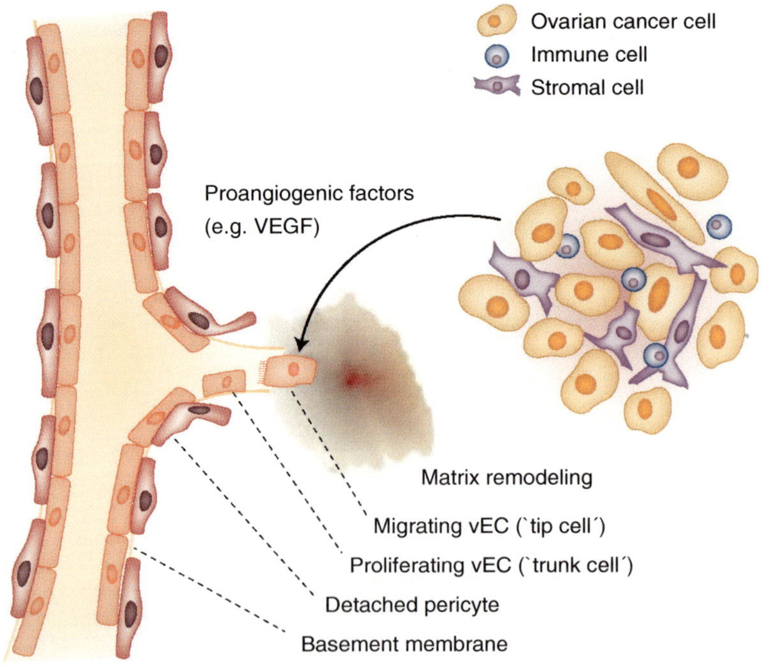

Fig. 12.1 Mediators of tumor angiogenesis

on patients with recurrent ovarian or primary peritoneal cancers found response rates of 15.9–21.0 % [16, 17]. Also in one of those studies, gastrointestinal perforation (GIP) was observed in 5 of 44 (11.4 %) patients who had been treated with three or more regimens [17]. Bevacizumab was evaluated combined with first-line chemotherapy (paclitaxel+carboplatin) for ovarian cancer [18, 19]. Two phase III studies, the Gynecologic Oncology Group (GOG) 218 and the International Collaborative Group for Ovarian Neoplasia (ICON) 7, examined the combined effects with bevacizumab and standard chemotherapy (paclitaxel+carboplatin) in a first-line/adjuvant chemotherapy setting and results are shown in (Table 12.1) [20, 21]. The Ovarian Cancer Education Awareness Network (OCEANS) trial evaluated the efficacy of bevacizumab in combination with carboplatin and gemcitabine in patients with recurrent, platinum-sensitive ovarian, primary peritoneal, or fallopian tube cancers after frontline, platinum-based therapy [22]. In this study, PFS for the bevacizumab arm was significantly longer than for the placebo arm (median PFS, 12.4 vs. 8.4 months). Grade 3 or higher hypertension and proteinuria occurred more frequently in the bevacizumab arm. A multicenter, open-label, randomized, two-arm, phase III trial, AURELIA, was conducted on patients with ovarian, primary peritoneal, or fallopian tube

Table 12.1 Phase III trials of bevacizumab in ovarian cancer

Trial	Patients	Treatment	Median PFS (M)	Median OS (M)	Selected adverse events	Reference
First line						
GOG 218	1873					[20]
Arm 1	625	CP	10.3	39.3	1.2 % GI events (G ≥2), 7.2 % HT (G ≥2), 5.8 % VTE (any grade)	
Arm 2	625	CP+Bev	11.2	38.7	2.8 % GI events (G ≥2), 16.5 % HT (G ≥2)***, 5.3 % VTE (any grade)	
Arm 3	623	CP+Bev → Bev	14.1*	39.7	2.6 % GI events (G ≥2), 22.9 % HT (G ≥2)***, 6.7 % VTE (any grade)	
ICON7	1528					[21]
Arm 1	764	CP	17.4		1.3 % GI events, 0.3 % HT, 1.7 % VTE	
Arm 2	764	CP+Bev → Bev	19.8*		2.1 % GI events, 6.2 % HT, 4.3 % VTE	
Second line						
OCEANS	484					[22]
Arm 1	242	CG	8.4	35.2	0.4 % HT, 0.9 % proteinuria, 2.6 % VTE	
Arm 2	242	CG+Bev	12.4*	33.3	17.4 % HT***, 8.5 % proteinuria***, 4.0 VTE	
AURELIA	361					[23]
Arm 1	182	Chemotherapy alone	12.6		2.2 % TEE	
Arm 2	179	Chemotherapy + Bev	30.9**		2.8 % TEE	

Investigator selected chemotherapy (pegylated liposomal doxorubicin, topotecan, or weekly paclitaxel)
PFS progression-free survival, *M* months, *OS* overall survival, *GOG* Gynecologic Oncology Group, *ICON* International Collaborative Group for Ovarian Neoplasia, *CP* carboplatin plus paclitaxel, *Bev* bevacizumab, *CG* carboplatin plus gemcitabine, *GI events* gastrointestinal events, *G* grade, *HT* hypertension, *VTE* venous thrombosis, *TEE* thromboembolic events
*$P<0.0001$, **$P<0.001$, ***$P<0.05$ versus chemotherapy alone
[a]Selected adverse events (grade ≥3), except for GOG 218 trial

cancers resistant to platinum [23]. It was observed in this study that chemotherapy plus bevacizumab significantly improved PFS (median PFS, 6.7 vs. 3.4 months) and overall response rate (30.9 vs. 12.6 %) compared to chemotherapy alone. Hypertension ≥ grade 2 (11.1 vs. 3.9 %) and proteinuria (6.4 vs. 0.5 %) occurred more frequently in the bevacizumab arm. GIP was observed in 1 % patients in the bevacizumab arm.

Cediranib

Cediranib is a potent inhibitor of tyrosine kinase of VEGFR-1, VEGFR-2, and VEGFR-3 and c-Kit that competes for the ATP-binding site within the receptor kinase domain [24, 25]. In a phase II studies, patients with recurrent ovarian, fallopian tube, or peritoneal cancers were treated with cediranib, and 17.4 % of patients showed a partial response [26]. Grade 3 hypertension was observed in 46 % of patients. No GIP or fistulas were observed.

Pazopanib

Pazopanib inhibits tyrosine kinase of VEGFR-1, VEGFR-2, VEGFR-3, and PDGFR-α, PDGFR-β, and c-Kit. It has been approved for renal cell carcinoma and soft tissue sarcoma [27]. A CA-125 response was observed in 31 % of patients with median response duration of 113 days during a phase II trial of pazopanib for the treatment of recurrent ovarian, fallopian tube, and primary peritoneal carcinomas [28]. The most common adverse events, noted in this trial, were elevated grade 3 alanine aminotransferase and γ-glutamyl transpeptidase, fatigue, and diarrhea.

Classical Transgene Delivery

Over the past several years, there has been an increased understanding of the mechanisms behind transgene delivery. Efficient full gene (s) delivery to a mammalian cell involves several steps: delivery of genes to target cells, cellular entry, endosome escape, and integration into the nucleus [28, 29]. No single gene transfer system has been developed that can effectively fulfill the requirements for all of the features noted above. A combination of multifunctional nonviral gene transfer systems may satisfy the requirements for efficient gene delivery. Cationic gene carriers can facilitate the cellular entry of DNA by interacting with the negatively charged cell surface [29, 30]. Endosomal escape is achieved by including components that induce membrane fusion at low pH or block pH lowering inside the endosome in the DNA-carrier complex. PEI is a cationic polymer that serves as an effective vehicle for in vivo gene delivery in many tissues. It facilitates effective DNA binding and protection, combined with the capability to escape the endosome due to its proton buffering ability with resultant osmotic swelling and endosomal disruption [30]. PEI has been shown to be an efficient transfection agent for ovarian carcinoma cells by intraperitoneal injection [31]. Several studies indicated that PEI-mediated transgene expression was dose dependent and transient, with maximal transgene expression observed during 48 h immediately following transfection [32]. DNA was detectable in very small amounts after 72 h, indicating probable degradation and clearance [31]. This would indicate that development of nonviral gene transfer technologies that can support chromosomal integration and persistent gene expression in vivo is desirable. Transposon-mediated DNA delivery systems have shown to allow the development of a new generation of vectors for human gene therapy and mammalian [33]. Transposon-based systems have been proven to be effective integrating nonviral vectors that can mediate long-term in vivo transgene expression [34]. It has been shown that SB transposons are an efficient intratumoral gene transfer vector for glioblastoma multiforme and was delivered using PEI as gene transfer reagent. The investigators of these two studies observed a marked antitumor activity as reflected by reduced tumor vessel density, inhibition of tumor growth, and tumor elimination in up to 50 % of nude mice [35, 36]. In other studies, a more active transposon used [37–42], combined with PEI to deliver HSV-TK gene into ovarian cancer xenografts. Further studies are needed to determine how PB transposon performs in vivo in the long term. In addition, the potential safety issues from insertional disruption/deregulation in genome needed to be addressed.

DNA Vectors

Adenoviruses are well-understood vectors for gene therapy. Human adenovirus serotype 5 (Ad5) is a reasonable vector to use, as it is not associated with a serious disease [43]. It has several advantages: it is well characterized, it is not restricted to infecting only dividing cells, and it can be grown in high titers with relative biologic stability allowing it to be administered systemically. Early clinical trials utilizing no replicative adenoviruses demonstrated the feasibility and potential utility of adenoviral-based gene therapy strategies for the treatment of malignancy. *While the initial adenoviral-based trials utilized no replicative vectors, subsequent studies investigated the potential of conditionally replicative adenoviruses (CRAd) for the treatment of cancer. These viral agents are designed to infect cancer cells specifically, replicate selectively within these cells, and then to spread* laterally to other cancer cells. A key element of CRAd development is to replicate in cancer cells selectively, without damaging normal host cells. CRAds have thus been engineered to selectively replicate within tumor cells using two broad strategies. The first employs deletion of part of the E1A or E1B genome to prevent replication in normal cells but allow replication in tumor cells with genetic defects that complement the deleted viral genome functions. The second employs a tumor-selective promoter (TSP) to drive the expression of genes involved in viral replication selectively in tumor cells. An example of the first strategy is the E1B-negative adenovirus (*dl*1520), Onyx-015 [44–51]. In this approach, the *E1B-55 k* gene of Onyx-015 was deleted, resulting in a virus that would replicate selectively within p53-deficient tumor cells. These viruses expressed the E1A protein, which overrode the block imposed by p53 in infected cells, resulting in apoptosis of normal cells, in addition to tumor cells. ONYX-015 demonstrated notable results in both in vitro and in vivo studies but had limited effects in human clinical trials for ovarian cancer. Bischoff et al. demonstrated that ONYX-015 was capable of efficient, selective replication in p53-deficient human tumor cells [52]. Heise et al. demonstrated in vivo correlation in three nude mouse–human ovarian carcinomatosis xenograft models [53]. Clinical studies of patients with head and neck cancer demonstrated safety and efficacy, but Vasey et al. failed to demonstrate similar results in ovarian cancer patients. Fifteen of the 16 study patients were taken off of the study because they developed progressive disease [54].

Enhancing Vector Infectivity

The major limitation of gene-based therapies lies within the vector systems. As the majority of patients have been previously exposed to Ad5, there is high level of immunity to the virus with preformed antibodies. In addition, primary tumor cells have low levels of the coxsackie and adenovirus receptor (CAR) relative to their cell line counterparts [55–57]. For the adenovirus vector to facilitate expression of the therapeutic gene in target cells, three steps must occur: first, the adenovirus must attach to the above receptors, second it must be internalized into the cell, and third it has to transfer the gene to the nucleus where it can be expressed. The adenovirus binds to the primary high-affinity CAR receptor and to the integrins $\alpha\upsilon\beta3$ and $\alpha\upsilon\beta5$ using two capsid proteins, the fiber and penton base, respectively. The carboxy-terminal (C-terminal) knob domain of the adenovirus fiber protein is the ligand for attachment to CAR [58–60]. It has been demonstrated that adenovirus infection is dependent upon the C-terminal knob [61]. After attachment the adenovirus is internalized using receptor-mediated endocytosis. This is reliant upon the interaction of the Arg–Gly–Asp (RGD) sequences in the penton base with the integrins $\alpha\upsilon\beta3$ and $\alpha\upsilon\beta5$ [62]. After internalization, the virus enters the cytosol via a pH-induced conformational change. The virus then localizes to the nuclear pore and is translocated into the nucleus of the host cell. One method of improving adenoviral tropism in low CAR-expressing cells such as ovarian cancer cells is by replacing the serotype knob in order to utilize a different receptor other than CAR. It has been shown that the knob domain of serotype 3 binds to CD46 and possibly CD80 and CD86, instead of CAR [63–65]. The 5/3 mutated adenovirus incorporates the alternate fiber knob domain from serotype 3 increasing the cytopathicity of a CRAd [66]. In another study, Ad5/3 has been shown to enhance tumor cell destruction in an orthotopic murine model of ovarian cancer [67] by a Δ24 CRAd with the Ad5/3 fiber chimera. Another method to improve transduction of the adenovirus is by utilizing fiber peptide modifications [67]. Ad fiber protein can enhance transduction in ovarian cancer cells by overcoming the low CAR expression. However, this method has been limited by the fact that the addition of more than 27 amino acids or more to the C-terminal end of the fiber will inhibit trimer formation [68]. X-ray crystallography showed that the HI loop is exposed on the fiber knob of the adenovirus and will allow the addition of up to 83 amino acids without affecting replication [69]. Incorporation of the RGD motif into the HI loop as compared to the C-terminus exhibited an increased level of gene transfer in in vitro studies [70, 71], and it also retargeted viruses to ovarian cancer cells that were previously resistant to adenovirus infection [56]. These tropism modifications have been incorporated into the context of CRAds, and infectivity enhancements have been achieved [72].

Achieving Selectivity with Tumor-Specific Promoters

The use of tumor-specific promoters (TSPs) is a strategy to drive viral E1 expression increasing tumor specificity. This strategy showed improved efficacy and tumor specificity [73]. TSPs have also been incorporated into CRAds. This CRAd demonstrated efficient replication and oncolysis in vitro and therapeutic efficacy in murine models of ovarian cancer [73]. Other TSP examples include CXCR4 and survivin. *CXCR4* is a chemokine receptor gene that plays a role in progression and metastasis in ovarian cancer cells. A CRAd modified to include a CXCR4 TSP (CRAd–CXCR4.RGD) has demonstrated improved viral infectivity and tumor specificity in both established ovarian cancer cell lines and in primary ovarian cancer tissue samples [49]. Survivin is a protein that inhibits apoptosis, allowing the survival and progression of cancer cells [74]. In addition, CRAd showed a decreased hepatic uptake [75].

Armed CRAds

CRAds killing ability can be enhanced by constructing an "armed" entity [76]. Several aspects must be considered when constructing an "armed" CRAd. The adenoviral genome can only encapsulate approximately 105 % of the wild genome, or 38 kb; therefore the size of any insert is limited [77]. In addition, the efficacy of the virus is dependent upon replication, and the insertion of a transgene should not interfere with this critical feature. CRAds can be armed with a variety of transgenes that directly enhance the killing of the cancer cell. The most commonly used transgenes that affect cell killing are the "suicide genes" that encode prodrug-converting enzymes that convert nontoxic prodrugs into toxic metabolites. These metabolites then diffuse away from the expressing cell and kill neighboring cells as a "bystander effect." An early example of this system is the herpes simplex virus thymidine kinase/ganciclovir (HSV-TK/GCV), which replaces the *E1B-55 k* gene with HSV-*tk*. This system is very dependent on the *E1B-55 k* gene as well as the amount of ganciclovir given. Another system is CD-5-FC that converts prodrug 5-FC into 5-fluorouracil (5-FU) which can be incorporated into both RNA and DNA, making it toxic to both dividing and nondividing cells [78]. CRAds constructed with short hairpin RNAs directed against vascular endothelial growth factor (VEGF) and/or interleukin 8 have also demonstrated improved antitumor efficacy [56, 57]. Immunomodulatory transgenes are designed to stimulate the immune system into recruiting immune cells to the site of the tumor and to enhance the cells' proliferation and activation. Examples of immunomodulatory CRAds include CRAds armed with TNFα, IFN-γ, and IL-4 [79–84].

Incorporating Imaging into CRAds

An ideal noninvasive monitoring system would emit a signal that directly correlated with the level of viral replication, would be associated with the packaging of the virions to allow detection, and would be continued in viral progeny. To be effective, the system would have to minimally disrupt the replication and spread of the virus. An early approach at noninvasive imaging included positron emission tomography (PET)-directed thymidine kinase as a reporter of oncolytic herpes simplex replication [85]. There are three broad categories of reporters used to monitor the systemic distribution of CRAds in vivo. The first category consists of secreted reporters that are soluble proteins not existent in low levels in serum. [86]. The second category of reporters allows the cells to be directly visualized by arming the CRAds with imaging molecules [64–67]. A third system consists of reporters that have been incorporated into the viral capsid. This allows visualization of the viral particle itself [68]. For example, the expression of human somatostatin receptor subtype 2 (SSTR) can be followed by intravenous administration of radiolabeled somatostatin [87].

Cellular Delivery of CRAds

Therapeutic agents often have decreased efficacy in vivo compared to in vitro studies due to physiologic variants. The accurate delivery of these agents to the target tissue can enhance their therapeutic efficiency and decrease toxicity. There are several delivery systems including liposomes, microspheres, synthetic polymers, and protein DNA complexes [88, 89]. Human mesenchymal stem cells have been utilized to improve the delivery of an Ad 5/3 CXCR4 CRAd to pulmonary metastasis in a murine model of advanced breast cancer [90].

Immunotherapy Therapy for Ovarian Cancer

The available scientific data suggest that immunotherapy for ovarian cancer (OC) could be effective. Ovarian cancer cells express tumor-associated antigens against which specific immune responses have been detected. The tumor immune surveillance plays an important role in clinical outcomes in OC, as manifested by the correlation between survival and tumor infiltration with $CD3^+$ T cells.

Animal studies and human clinical trials have demonstrated that therapeutically induced tumor-specific immunity is an efficient methodology to treat human cancer based on facts that support this concept. Tumors generally can prevent tumor-specific immunity from eliminating tumors by inducing tumor-specific tolerance or inflammation. The effective immunotherapy for ovarian cancer will have to surmount these obstacles for optimal effectiveness.

Cancer Vaccines

Vaccines have been the main approach to ovarian cancer immunotherapy, as with many other types [91–94]. Vaccines have limited efficacy as monotherapy in patients with advanced and recurrent ovarian cancer. Some studies' results provide encouragement for vaccine development and optimization for use. Sabbatini et al. [95] noted that patients vaccinated with monovalent or heptavalent vaccines against carbohydrate epitopes experienced significantly longer time to progression and higher progression-free survival rates. Also, vaccination with anti-idiotype ACA-125 resulted in CA-125-specific antibodies and was associated with prolonged survival [96]. Carcinoembryonic antigen–MUC-1–TRICOM poxviral-based vaccines were used in 16 patients, including three of them being ovarian cancer patients. Immune responses to MUC-1 and/or carcinoembryonic antigen were seen after vaccination in nine patients. A patient with clear-cell ovarian cancer and symptomatic ascites had a radiographically and biochemically clinical response [97]. The limitation in vaccine development in ovarian cancer is due to the lack of well-characterized rejection antigens and by notable molecular heterogeneity of the disease. HER2 is a rejection antigen, and it may also serve as a rejection antigen in ovarian cancer [98, 99]. Vaccination against HER2 has resulted in sustained antigen-specific T cell, humoral immunity, and epitope spreading in patients with ovarian cancer [100]. NY-ESO-1 is a bona fide ovarian cancer rejection antigen, and it is expressed in less than 30 % of ovarian cancers [101, 102]. A viable alternative to vaccines are whole-tumor antigen vaccines created using tumor cells, autologous tumor lysate, or tumor-derived RNA [103–105]. The advantages of these vaccines are the opportunity to induce immunity to a personalized and broad range of antigens, which could minimize the development of tumor escape variants; the inclusion of yet unidentified tumor rejection antigens; no HLA haplotype restriction; and the simultaneous administration of MHC class I and class II epitopes which could prove beneficial for immunologic memory. In a meta-analysis, it was found that 8.1 % of patients vaccinated with whole-tumor antigen had notable clinical responses, while 3.6 % of patients vaccinated with molecularly defined tumor antigens had objective clinical responses ($P<.001$, χ^2 test) [106]. An intracavitary delivery of a viral oncolysate vaccine generated with ovarian cancer cell lines infected with influenza A virus showed objective clinical responses [107, 108]. Delivery of autologous tumor cells infected with Newcastle disease virus showed the same response [109]. HSV-infected tumor cells used directly or pulsed on dendritic cells have been shown to stimulate marked antitumor immune response in the mouse, which was better than utilizing ultraviolet-irradiated tumor cells [110–112]. Using mature dendritic cells (DCs) with whole autologous tumor lysate, 50 % of patients demonstrated remission inversion [113]. The use of DC/tumor cell fusion demonstrated to be able to induce antitumor cytotoxic T-lymphocyte activity in vitro [114]. There is a concern about the use of whole-tumor vaccination which relates to the inclusion of a large number of self-antigens, as it could drive tolerogenic responses (i.e., expand Treg) rather than cytotoxic lymphocyte responses. It has been shown that DCs can be polarized ex vivo with the use of interferons, Toll-like receptor agonists, or p38 mitogen-activated protein kinase inhibitors to stimulate cytotoxic lymphocytes and Th17. [115]. The limitation of cancer vaccines is due to the fact that it is unable to elicit an overwhelming T-cell response. In addition, it has been shown that immune modulation through blockade of the endothelin B receptor markedly increases the efficacy of weak vaccines by reversing the inhibitory function of tumor endothelium and enabling homing of tumor-reactive T cells [106, 116]. Moreover, it was observed that, depletion of Treg is a critical maneuver to enhance vaccine therapy [117].

Adoptive T-Cell Therapy

The advantages of TIL-based adoptive therapy include the presence of spontaneously occurring T cells with avidity against tumor which have escaped thymic deletion, the use of a polyclonal population of T cells, and the natural selection of patients whose tumor microenvironment is already conducive to T-cell homing. Incremental lymphodepletion through high-dose nonmyeloablating chemotherapy and added whole-body radiation was studied. Regression of metastatic tumors was observed, with 16 % complete response and 72 % objective response rates in recent reports with maximal lymphodepletion and radiation [118, 119]. In another study, it was shown that adoptive immunotherapy is a viable methodology and can control tumors of all sizes [120]. It was reported that patients who received adjuvant therapy with adoptive transfer of tumor-derived lymphocytes expanded ex vivo with IL-2 had a 3-year disease-free survival rate of 82.1 %, and the control group had 54.5 % [121, 122]. In melanoma trials, it was shown that TILs persisted 2 months after infusion in patients who exhibited tumor regression and were characterized by a less differentiated phenotype ($CD27^+$ $CD28^+$ $CD45RA^+$ but $CD62L^-$ $CCR7^-$) and longer telomeres [123–127]. It has been argued that the use of memory rather than effector cells may be more efficacious for adoptive transfer [128], and this was confirmed by mouse models [129]. June et al. [130] described the development of a next-generation K562-based aAPC platform capable of expressing multiple gene inserts, including human lymphocyte antigen (HLA) -A2, CD64 CD80, CD83, CD86, CD137L (4-1BBL), and CD252 (Ox40L), and several T-cell supporting cytokines. Rosenberg et al. [119] have demonstrated the clinical feasibility, safety, and preliminary efficacy of redirecting T cells of patients with melanoma using a TCR specific to the melanoma antigen MART-1. Adoptive transfer of TCR-transduced cells in 15 patients resulted in durable engraftment at levels exceeding 10 % of peripheral blood lymphocytes for at least 2 months after the infusion. In addition, high levels of circulating engineered cells at 1 year after infusion was observed in two patients who demonstrated regression of metastatic melanoma lesions. TCR-based engineering represents a reasonable strategy for ovarian cancer therapy as TCRs recognize HLA-A2 restricted epitopes from known ovarian cancer antigens such as NY-ESO-1 and p53 [131–134]. Optimization through selection of naturally occurring or recombinant high-affinity receptors, engineering to prevent recombination with endogenous TCR, and the use of lentiviral vectors have been developed [135]. Genetic modification to recognize antigens in an MHC-unrestricted fashion through the use of chimeric antigen receptors (CARs), fusion genes encoding an extracellular domain that specifically binds to tumor epitopes through a single-chain variable fragment (scFv) antibody, linked to intracellular signaling modules that mediate T-cell activation has been developed [130, 136, 137]. The tumor binding function of CARs is usually accomplished by the inclusion of a scFv antibody, containing the V_H and V_L chains joined by a peptide linker of about 15 residues in length. The universal targeting vectors can be constructed, as the scFvs bind to native cell surface epitopes and bypass the requirement for MHC restriction [138, 139]. Several CARs targeting diverse tumors have been developed [130, 140, 141, 142, 143], and some of the ovarian tumor antigens and CAR investigated in vitro and in vivo in T lymphocytes are FBP [144, 145], MUC-1 [145], HER2, and mesothelin [146].

Antibody-Based Immunomodulation

Modulating immune checkpoints by activation of effector cells, depletion of Tregs, or activation of professional APCs could improve the therapeutic efficacy of vaccines or adoptively transferred T cells. The development of functional antibodies has enabled effective immune modulation as shown in Fig. 12.2.

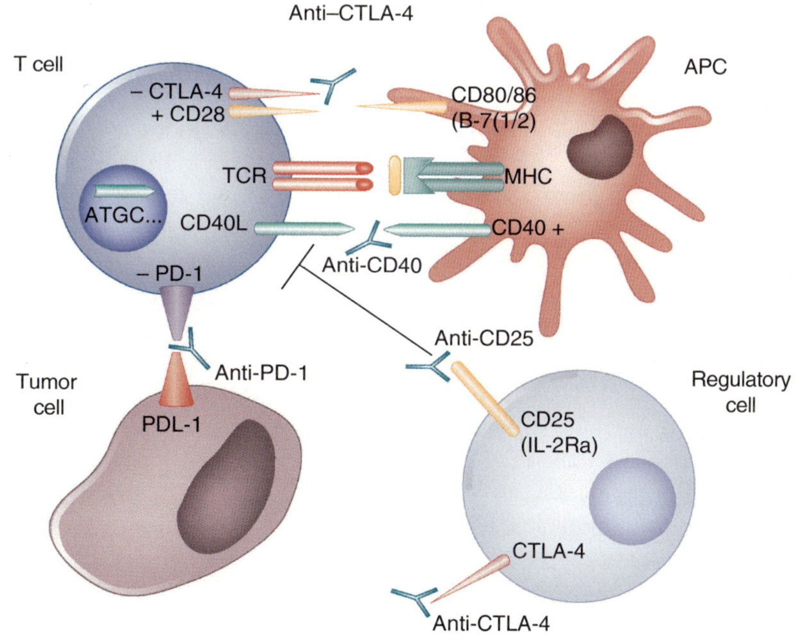

Fig. 12.2 Improved therapeutic efficacy of vaccines or adoptively transferred T cells can be achieved by modulating immune checkpoints, including activation of effector cells by blocking CTLA4 or PD-1; depletion of regulatory T cells by use of low-dose oral or intravenous cyclophosphamide or through targeting the interleukin-2 (IL-2) receptor **α** chain, also known as CD25; or activation of professional antigen-presenting cells (*APCs*) by stimulation with CD40 ligands

Dendritic Cell Activation

The main mechanism of immune stimulation by CD40 ligands is the activation of DCs resulting in increased survival, upregulation of molecules, and secretion of critical cytokines for T-cell priming. This promotes antigen presentation, priming, and cross-priming of $CD4^+$ and $CD8^+$ effector T cells. It was observed that agonistic anti-CD40 antibody is well used in combination with vaccines or Toll-like receptor agonists [147, 148], as it can accelerate the deletion of tumor-specific cytotoxic lymphocytes [149]. It was noted that ovarian cancers express the CD40 receptor [150–154] and respond to CD40 agonists with apoptosis and growth inhibition in vitro and in vivo [153, 155, 156].

Effector T-Cell Activation

T-cell activation is triggered through the T-cell receptor by recognition of the cognate antigen complexed with MHC. CTLA-4 blockade activates CD4 and $CD8^+$ T effector cells by removing an inhibitory checkpoint on proliferation and function [157], and combination of direct enhancement of Teff cell function and inhibition of Treg activity is important for mediating the therapeutic effects of anti-CTLA-4 antibodies during cancer immunotherapy [158].

Most of clinical data to date have emerged from studies in patients with melanoma [159], where CTLA-4 blockade has yielded notable responses. It has been shown in patients with ovarian carcinoma, previously vaccinated with granulocyte–macrophage colony-stimulating factor modified, irradiated autologous tumor cells (GVAX) and received ipilimumab (1 month to 3 years after GVAX), that tumor regression correlated with the $CD8^+$/Treg ratio [160]. PD-1 is a negative regulator of lymphocyte activation, which binds PD-L1 and PD-L2 ligands. PD-L1 is expressed on many tissues. Ovarian carcinoma cells, tumor-infiltrating tolerogenic DCs, and myeloid-derived suppressor cells express PD-L1 [161, 162]. It was observed that expression of PD-L1 by tumors conferred resistance to immunotherapy in mice [163], while antibodies blocking PD-L1 or PD-1 enhanced the efficacy of immune therapy [163, 164]. A phase I study using PD-1-blocking antibody showed the antibody to be safe and well tolerated in patients with hematologic malignancies [165].

Treg Depletion

$CD4^+$ $CD25^+$ $Foxp3^+$ Treg is responsible for maintaining peripheral tolerance by inhibiting T-cell activity. A number of Treg-depleting strategies have been investigated. [119, 166–170]. One of these strategies was the use of low-dose oral or intravenous cyclophosphamide [118, 171]. It was shown that the use of anti-CD25 monoclonal antibody before vaccination led to complete tumor rejection and establishment of extended immunity with no side effects [118, 172]. Also, it was observed that administration of anti-CD25 resulted in transient reduction in $CD4^+$ $CD25^+$ Treg in patients with metastatic melanoma [173]. Denileukin diftitox, a fusion protein of IL-2 and diphtheria toxin that targets CD25-expressing cells was used in patients with melanoma, ovarian cancer, and renal cell carcinoma [174–177]. It was observed that these conjugates were immunogenic and induced neutralizing antibodies. In addition, daclizumab, which is humanized immunoglobulin G1-kappa monoclonal antibody that binds specifically to CD25 [178] has been used in autoimmune disorders [179, 180], acute graft-versus-host disease [181], and in patients with cancer with $CD25^+$ T-cell malignancies [182]. The advantage of daclizumab is that it is well tolerated and has a half-life of 20 days [183]. Moreover, daclizumab was found to be compatible with effective vaccination [184]. As above, the assumption is that innovative immunotherapeutic strategies offer the promise of enhancing host antitumor responses which may improve clinical outcomes in women with ovarian cancer. While many preliminary phase I/II studies have demonstrated induction of antitumor responses, currently there is no clinically effective antigen-specific active immunotherapy available for patients with ovarian cancer.

Ongoing investigation may help to define the role of immunotherapy alone or in combination with other treatment strategies in the treatment of ovarian cancer patients. These trials may determine a role for immunotherapy in the treatment of ovarian cancer.

Epithelial Growth Factor Receptor Targeting Therapy

The epithelial growth factor receptor (EGFR; also known as Her or ErbB) family of receptor tyrosine kinases has been shown to have oncogenic characteristics in several human cancers. It was suggested that members of the EGFR family, such as ErbB3, may have a role in promoting the growth and proliferation of human ovarian cancer cells. The EGFR family of receptor tyrosine kinases consists of four closely related family members: EGFR (Her1), ErbB2 (Her2), ErbB3 (Her3), and ErbB4 (Her4) [185]. These cytoplasmic membrane-bound receptors share a common extracellular ligand-binding domain and a single transmembrane domain, followed by an intracellular tyrosine kinase domain and a C-terminal non-catalytic signaling tail. Signaling through these receptors is typically mediated by homodimerization or heterodimerization with other family members. Binding of the ligand with the extracellular domain of its corresponding receptor induces a structural reconfiguration of the receptor, promoting exposure of dimerization domain [186, 187]. The EGFR family members can be activated by unphysiological stimuli (e.g., oxidative stress, UV, and γ-irradiation), by other receptor tyrosine kinases (MET, insulin-like growth factor-1 receptor, or tyrosine kinase receptor B), or by G protein-coupled receptors and adhesion proteins [188].

Epithelial Growth Factor Receptor (Her1)/ErbB2 (Her2) in Ovarian Cancer

Siwak et al., *in a review* [189], noted that epithelial growth factor receptor amplification and activating mutations have been reported in a small percentage of ovarian cancer cases (4–22 and <4 %, respectively). The EGFR overexpression rate varies from 9 to 62 %. Increased EGFR expression has been correlated with poorer patient outcomes. Several small molecule inhibitors that block EGFR kinase activity (e.g., gefitinib and erlotinib) have been explored. There are two phase II clinical trials on gefitinib (Iressa or ZD1839) as a single agent in treating platinum-refractory or -resistant ovarian cancer. No complete response was observed in either trial. In one trial, 37 % of the patients had stable disease for over 2 months while none of the patients had a partial or complete response. In the second trial, 4 out of 27 patients had progression-free disease for over 6 months, and one of these four patients had an objective response. Erlotinib (Tarceva, OSI Pharmaceuticals, Long Island, NY, USA), another small molecule inhibitor of EGFR, demonstrated a 6 % partial response rate in a multicenter phase II trial with EGFR-positive ovarian cancer patients with taxane- and/or platinum-refractory or -resistant disease. In a phase II study, 56 patients demonstrated no improvement in pathological CR rates compared with historical experience with erlotinib added to carboplatin and paclitaxel in the first-line therapy for ovarian cancer [189]. An additional study comparing the combination of erlotinib and the antiangiogenic agent bevacizumab also did not show any improvement compared with bevacizumab alone. Also, vandetanib, a small molecule inhibitor of VEGFR and EGFR signaling, did not demonstrate significant clinical benefit in recurrent ovarian cancer [190]. Monoclonal antibodies that bind directly to the extracellular domain of EGFR to block EGFR activation or reduce surface EGFR levels have also been tested. The objective clinical response of these therapeutic antibodies, such as cetuximab (Erbitux, ImClone LLC, Bridgewater, NJ, USA) and matuzumab (EMD7200), in ovarian cancer was limited [188]. Early studies suggested that Her2 overexpression in ovarian cancer was a frequent event; but, other studies using techniques validated in breast cancer suggest that Her2 overexpression and amplification frequency in ovarian cancer is a rarer event [191]. Overexpression of Her2 has been associated with poor prognosis in some studies but not others. This discrepancy may be explained by differences in the criteria and methods used to assess Her2 overexpression. A phase II trial with trastuzumab (Herceptin, Genentech, Inc., South San Francisco, CA, USA), a humanized anti-Her2 monoclonal antibody, reported a low (7 %) partial response rate with only a 2-month progression-free interval in recurrent ovarian cancers overexpressing Her2 [192]. In a phase II multicenter open-label trial, CI-1033 (Canertinib, Pfizer, Inc., New York City, NY, USA), an irreversible pan-EGFR family inhibitor, was shown to have no activity in unscreened patients who have failed previous platinum-based chemotherapy [193]. A phase I trial combining carboplatin and lapatinib (Tykerb, Tyverb, GlaxoSmithKline, plc, London, UK), an EGFR–Her2 dual inhibitor, was performed in unscreened patients with platinum-sensitive recurrent ovarian cancer [194]. In this trial, 27 % of patients had a partial response and another 27 % had stable disease.

ErbB3 (Her3) in Ovarian Cancer

ErbB3 has been reported to be amplified [193, 196] and overexpressed in epithelial ovarian cancers (197; 196, 198, 199, 200). Overexpression of ErbB3 has been reported to correlate with poorer overall prognosis [197]. Several truncated ErbB3 isoforms composed of the extracellular domains of the protein have been described in ovarian cancer cell lines, but the functional significance of these remains unclear [198]. In addition, ErbB3 has been recently characterized as having a marked role in mediating resistance to EGFR, and Her2-directed therapies in other solid malignancies [199]. Sergina et al. [200] demonstrated that in gefitinib-resistant Her2-overexpressing breast cancer cell lines, ErbB3 activation is increased, through increased localization of ErbB3 to the cytoplasmic membrane. Engelman et al. [201] demonstrated that ErbB3 activation by MET amplification could overcome resistance to gefitinib in EGFR-mutant non-small cell lung cancer cell lines. Inhibition of AKT has been demonstrated to upregulate ErbB3 expression and phosphorylation, so that ErbB3 may have a role in mediating resistance to PI3K/AKT pathway inhibitors [202]. A humanized monoclonal antibody that binds to the extracellular domain of Her2 and blocks its heterodimerization with ErbB3 and other EGFR family members, pertuzumab (2C4), has been studied. Pertuzumab treatment demonstrated a 4.3 % partial response in platinum-refractory and -resistant patients. The median progression-free survival in the eight pHer2+ patients (tumors demonstrated positively for pHer2 by an ELISA assay) was 20.9 weeks as compared with 5.8 weeks in the pHer2 patients ($P=0.14$), [203]. In a clinical trial conducted using the combination of pertuzumab with gemcitabine versus gemcitabine alone for ovarian cancer patients [204], there was no significant difference seen in the outcome between the two arms. However, a subset analysis demonstrated a potential benefit in progression-free survival to gemcitabine plus pertuzumab in patients with low ErbB3 expression by mRNA (hazard ratio 0.32; 95 % CI 0.17–0.59; $P=0.0002$). Signaling through the ErbB3 pathway has been reported to correlate with expression of its natural ligand, neuregulin-1 (NRG1) in both ovarian cancer cell lines and in primary human ovarian cancer cells [205]. Moreover, expression of NRG1 has been observed in 30–83 % of ovarian carcinomas [205, 206].

ErbB4 (Her4) in Ovarian Cancer

The role of ErbB4 in cancer is not clearly understood. Conflicting reports regarding the potential transforming activity of ErbB4 have been published, which may partly reflect the unique mechanism of ErbB4 signaling. ErbB4 is spliced into multiple isoforms, some of which are further processed by tumor necrosis factor-α-converting enzyme and γ-secretase to generate a soluble ErbB4 intracellular domain that has a BH3 homologous region that can distribute to both the nucleus and the cytoplasm [207]. Nuclear-localized ErbB4 intracellular domain may act as a transcription co-activator, whereas the cytoplasmic/mitochondria-localized ErbB4 intracellular domain may act as a BH3-only protein and induce apoptosis in tumor cells [207]. In breast cancer, cytoplasmic ErbB4 independently predicted for improved patient survival [207]. ErbB4 somatic mutations have been detected in 19 % of melanoma patients [208] and in several cancer types, but at a lower frequency: 1–5 % [209]. It has been shown that ErbB4 is weakly expressed in adult ovarian surface epithelium [210]. In addition, early studies suggested that ErbB4 expression is either absent or decreased in some ovarian cancers when compared with normal ovarian tissues [210, 211]. In several studies, using either IHC, RT-PCR, or Western blotting techniques have demonstrated the presence of ErbB4 in a high percentage of ovarian tumors [212, 213], and RT-PCR has detected at least four different ErbB4 splice variants in both established and primary ovarian cancer cell lines [212]. Gilmour et al. [212] reported that tumors of serous histology tend to express higher levels of ErbB4 than that of the endometrioid subtype, and Steffensen et al. [214] found that ErbB4 expression is significantly higher in epithelial ovarian cancer tumors as compared with borderline/benign ovarian tumors or normal ovaries. Somatic mutations in the intronic regions of ErbB4 have been detected in ovarian cancers [213]. The clinical significance of ErbB4 in ovarian cancer is currently unknown. It is noteworthy that established ovarian cancer cell lines that express high ErbB4 protein level have all been derived from platinum-refractory tumors, raising the possibility that ErbB4 expression may be related to platinum therapy resistance [212].

Poly (Adenosine Diphosphate Ribose) Polymerase (PARP) Inhibition Therapy

It was reported that *BRCA1*-deficient and *BRCA2-deficient* cells were sensitive to poly (adenosine diphosphate ribose) polymerase (PARP) inhibition when compared to wild-type or heterozygous mutant cells [215, 216]. These findings highlighted the clinical potential of PARP inhibitors to treat patients with *BRCA1/2*-associated breast and ovarian cancers. The activity of PARP inhibitors has been examined in selected subsets of breast cancer and epithelial ovarian cancer.

PARP Family of Enzymes

PARPs are a family of enzymes which catalyze poly adenosine diphosphate (ADP)-ribosylation of target proteins in a wide variety of eukaryotes [217]. PARP1 is the most abundant and well-characterized PARP enzyme, accounting for more than 90 % of ADP-ribosylation occurring in cells [218, 219]. PARP1 and PARP2 are the only PARP enzymes that are activated by DNA damage and that facilitate DNA repair [220, 221]. It was shown that mice generated to lack either PARP1 or PARP2 has hypersensitivity to ionizing radiation and alkylating agents [222, 223]. Improved understanding of the biology and function of the other PARPs may aid interpretation of the mechanism of PARP inhibition and long-term therapy implication.

PARP1 Role in DNA Repair

PARP1 plays a critical role in the repair of DNA single-strand breaks (SSB) via the base excision repair (BER) pathway. DNA damage due to peroxidation, irradiation, and DNA-damaging chemicals such as chemotherapy stimulates the catalytic activity of PARP1 [224–227]. PARP1 is recruited to the damaged DNA by two zinc finger motifs in the DNA-binding domain of PARP1 binding to DNA SSB, thus activating the BER machinery to repair the SSB [221, 228]. PARP1 has also been implicated in the two major pathways for the repair of DNA double-strand breaks (DSB): homologous recombination (HR) and nonhomologous end joining [NHEJ]) [229]. Genomic instability was observed in HR-deficient cells treated with PARP inhibitors [230].

Structure of Common PARP Inhibitors

AZD2281 (olaparib) and ABT-888 (veliparib) are both p.o. formulations. AZD2281 has an IC for PARP1 of 5 nmol/L, and ABT-888 inhibits PARP1 and PARP2 with a K_i of 5.2 and

2.9 nmol/L, respectively [231–233]. BSI-201 (iniparib) was described as having PARP inhibitory activity, but iniparib does not appear to inhibit PARP1 and 2 [234, 235].

Use of PARP Inhibitors in BRCA1/2 Mutations

Carriers of germline mutations in *BRCA1* or *BRCA2* are at a high risk of developing breast cancer (85 % lifetime risk) and ovarian cancer (54 % lifetime risk) and are also predisposed to developing pancreatic, prostate, and male breast cancer [236–239]. *BRCA1* and *BRCA2* are classified as tumor suppressor genes, as the wild-type *BRCA1* and *2* alleles are lost in the tumor, with the retention of the mutant allele [229]. *It has been shown that BRCA1* is important for DNA repair, transcriptional regulation, and chromatin remodeling [240]. The function of *BRCA2* appears to be limited to DNA recombination and repair processes [241, 242]. Cells deficient in either *BRCA1* or *BRCA2* repair these lesions using alternative mechanisms, alternative homology-directed repair pathway, and SSA and potentially by the error-prone microhomology-mediated sub-pathway of NHEJ [230, 243–245]. In *BRCA1*-deficient cells, both GC and SSA are impaired, and DSBs are repaired by the error-prone NHEJ pathway [243, 246, 247]. *In BRCA2 deficiency*, repair by GC is impaired. Synthetic lethality occurs when the combination of two genetic alterations result

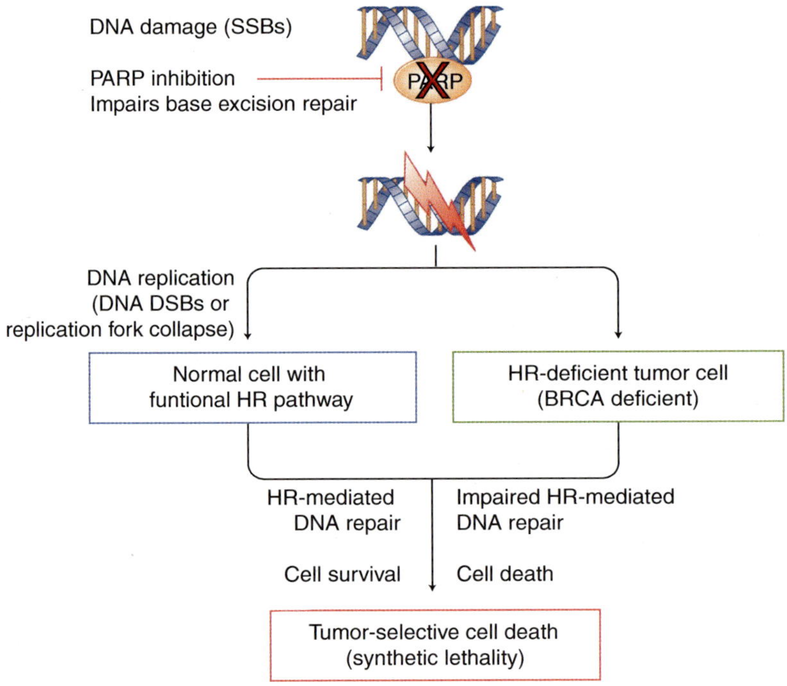

Fig. 12.3 Inhibition of base excision repair (BER) is responsible for poly ADP ribose polymerase (PARP) inhibitor-induced lethality in homologous recombination (HR)-defective cells. The original model for explaining the antitumor effects of PARP inhibitors in BRCA-deficient tumors postulates a synthetic lethal interaction between PARP inhibition and DNA repair defects in BRCA-deficient tumor cells. PARP inhibition prevents cells from responding to endogenous DNA damage through BER. This result in persistent DNA single-strand breaks (SSB), which lead to fork collapse and the increased formation of double-strand breaks (DSB) when they encounter a DNA replication fork. Under normal circumstances, DSB are repaired by the error-free gene conversion pathway. However, in the setting of BRCA deficiency, DSB are more likely to be repaired by error-prone repair mechanisms, resulting in chromosome aberrations and cell death. *GC* gene conversion, *NHEJ* non-homologous end joining, *SSA* single-strand annealing, *XRCC1* X-ray repair cross-complementing 1 enzyme Fig. 12.1. Mediators of tumor angiogenesis

in a lethal phenotype [248]. The original model for explaining the antitumor effects of PARP inhibitors in *BRCA-deficient* tumors postulated a synthetic lethal interaction between PARP inhibition and the DNA repair defects present in *BRCA*-deficient tumor cells (Fig. 12.3). The inhibition of PARP1 prevents cells from responding to endogenous DNA damage through BER, which results in persistent DNA SSB and, in turn, leads to DNA replication fork collapse and increased formation of DSB [249, 250].

Efficacy of PARP Inhibition Therapy in BRCA-Deficient Tumors

The mechanism of PARP inhibitor-induced cytotoxicity appears to be more complex than it was thought. Patel et al. [230] demonstrated that downregulation of X-ray repair cross-complementing 1 enzyme in *BRCA2*-deficient cells failed to produce synthetic lethality. According to the BER-dependent model, if accumulated DNA damage were responsible for mediating PARP inhibitor action, HR-deficient cells would be expected to depend on alternate DSB repair pathways such as NHEJ for survival. It has been shown that PARP inhibitor-induced genomic instability is driven by the activation of NHEJ and that disabling NHEJ using genetic and pharmacological approaches impaired the genomic instability and lethality of PARP inhibition in HR-deficient cells [230]. These findings support an NHEJ-dependent model whereby PARP inhibition leads to defective BER and the aberrant activation of NHEJ in HR-deficient cells.

References

1. Bhoola S, Hoskins WJ. Diagnosis and management of epithelial ovarian cancer. Obstet Gynecol. 2006;107:1399–410.
2. Cannistra SA. Cancer of the ovary. N Engl J Med. 2004;351:2519–29.
3. Piccart MJ, Bertelsen K, Stuart G, et al. Long-term follow-up confirms a survival advantage of the paclitaxel-cisplatin regimen over the cyclophosphamide-cisplatin combination in advanced ovarian cancer. Int J Gynecol Cancer. 2003;13 Suppl 2:144–8.
4. Tummala MK, McGuire WP. Recurrent ovarian cancer. Clin Adv Hematol Oncol. 2005;3:723–36.
5. Bristow RE, Tomacruz RS, Armstrong DK, et al. Survival effect of maximal cytoreductive surgery for advanced ovarian carcinoma during the platinum era: a meta-analysis. J Clin Oncol. 2002;20:1248–59.
6. Heintz AP, Odicino F, Maisonneuve P, et al. Carcinoma of the ovary. FIGO 26th annual report on the results of treatment in gynecological cancer. Int J Gynaecol Obstet. 2006;95 Suppl 1:S161–92.
7. Markman M, Markman J, Webster K, et al. Duration of response to second-line, platinum-based chemotherapy for ovarian cancer: implications for patient management and clinical trial design. J Clin Oncol. 2004;22:3120–5.
8. Agarwal R, Kaye SB. Ovarian cancer: strategies for overcoming resistance to chemotherapy. Nat Rev Cancer. 2003;3:502–16.
9. Darcy KM, Schilder RJ. Relevant molecular markers and targets. Gynecol Oncol. 2006;103:S6–13.
10. Bookman MA. Biologic therapies for gynecologic cancer. Curr Opin Oncol. 1995;7:478–84.
11. Bookman MA. Biological therapy of ovarian cancer: current directions. Semin Oncol. 1998;25:381–96.
12. Kim KJ, Li B, Houck K, et al. The vascular endothelial growth factor proteins: identification of biologically relevant regions by neutralizing monoclonal antibodies. Growth Factors. 1992;7:53–64.
13. Kim KJ, Li B, Winer J, et al. Inhibition of vascular endothelial growth factor-induced angiogenesis suppresses tumour growth in vivo. Nature. 1993;362:841–4.
14. Jain RK. Normalization of tumor vasculature: an emerging concept in antiangiogenic therapy. Science. 2005;307:58–62.
15. Burger RA, Sill MW, Monk BJ, et al. Phase II trial of bevacizumab in persistent or recurrent epithelial ovarian cancer or primary peritoneal cancer: a Gynecologic Oncology Group Study. J Clin Oncol. 2007;25:5165–71.
16. Cannistra SA, Matulonis UA, Penson RT, et al. Phase II study of bevacizumab in patients with platinum-resistant ovarian cancer or peritoneal serous cancer. J Clin Oncol. 2007;25:5180–6.
17. Micha JP, Goldstein BH, Rettenmaier MA, et al. A phase II study of outpatient first-line paclitaxel, carboplatin, and bevacizumab for advanced-stage epithelial ovarian, peritoneal, and fallopian tube cancer. Int J Gynecol Cancer. 2007;17:771–6.
18. Penson RT, Dizon DS, Cannistra SA, et al. Phase II study of carboplatin, paclitaxel, and bevacizumab with maintenance bevacizumab as first-line chemotherapy for advanced mullerian tumors. J Clin Oncol. 2010;28:154–9.
19. Burger RA, Brady MF, Bookman MA, et al. Incorporation of bevacizumab in the primary treatment of ovarian cancer. N Engl J Med. 2011;365:2473–83.

20. Perren TJ, Swart AM, Pfisterer J, et al. A phase 3 trial of bevacizumab in ovarian cancer. N Engl J Med. 2011;365:2484–96.
21. Aghajanian C, Blank SV, Goff BA, et al. OCEANS: a randomized, double-blind, placebo-controlled phase iii trial of chemotherapy with or without bevacizumab in patients with platinum-sensitive recurrent epithelial ovarian, primary peritoneal, or fallopian tube cancer. J Clin Oncol. 2012;30:2039–45.
22. Pujade-Lauraine E, Hilpert F, Weber B, et al. AURELIA: a randomized phase III trial evaluating bevacizumab (BEV) plus chemotherapy (CT) for platinum (PT)-resistant recurrent ovarian cancer (OC). J Clin Oncol. 2012;30, LBA5002.
23. Heckman CA, Holopainen T, Wirzenius M, et al. The tyrosine kinase inhibitor cediranib blocks ligand-induced vascular endothelial growth factor receptor-3 activity and lymphangiogenesis. Cancer Res. 2008;68:4754–62.
24. Wedge SR, Kendrew J, Hennequin LF, et al. AZD2171: a highly potent, orally bioavailable, vascular endothelial growth factor receptor-2 tyrosine kinase inhibitor for the treatment of cancer. Cancer Res. 2005;65:4389–400.
25. Matulonis UA, Berlin S, Ivy P, et al. Cediranib, an oral inhibitor of vascular endothelial growth factor receptor kinases, is an active drug in recurrent epithelial ovarian, fallopian tube, and peritoneal cancer. J Clin Oncol. 2009;27:5601–6.
26. Sonpavde G, Hutson TE. Pazopanib: a novel multitargeted tyrosine kinase inhibitor. Curr Oncol Rep. 2007;9:115–9.
27. Friedlander M, Hancock KC, Rischin D, et al. A phase II, open-label study evaluating pazopanib in patients with recurrent ovarian cancer. Gynecol Oncol. 2010;119:32–7.
28. Min SH, Lee DC, Lim MJ, Park HS, Kim DM, Cho CW, Yoon do Y, Yeom YI. A composite gene delivery system consisting of polyethylenimine and an amphipathic peptide KALA. J Gene Med. 2006;8(12):1425–34.
29. Audouy S, Hoekstra D. Cationic lipid-mediated transfection in vitro and in vivo (review). Mol Membr Biol. 2001;18(2):129–43.
30. Lungwitz U, Breunig M, Blunk T, Gopferich A. Polyethylenimine-based non-viral gene delivery systems. Eur J Pharm Biopharm. 2005;60(2):247–66.
31. Louis MH, Dutoit S, Denoux Y, Erbacher P, Deslandes E, Behr JP, Gauduchon P, Poulain L. Intraperitoneal linear polyethylenimine (L-PEI)-mediated gene delivery to ovarian carcinoma nodes in mice. Cancer Gene Ther. 2006;13(4):367–74.
32. Dolivet G, Merlin JL, Barberi-Heyob M, Ramacci C, Erbacher P, Parache RM, Behr JP, Guillemin F. In vivo growth inhibitory effect of iterative wild-type p53 gene transfer in human head and neck carcinoma xenografts using glucosylated polyethylenimine nonviral vector. Cancer Gene Ther. 2002;9(8):708–14.
33. Hackett PB, Ekker SC, Largaespada DA, McIvor RS. Sleeping beauty transposon-mediated gene therapy for prolonged expression. Adv Genet. 2005;54:189–232.
34. Yant SR, Meuse L, Chiu W, Ivics Z, Izsvak Z, Kay MA. Somatic integration and long-term transgene expression in normal and haemophilic mice using a DNA transposon system. Nat Genet. 2000;25(1):35–41.
35. Ohlfest JR, Demorest ZL, Motooka Y, Vengco I, Oh S, Chen E, Scappaticci FA, Saplis RJ, Ekker SC, Low WC. Combinatorial antiangiogenic gene therapy by nonviral gene transfer using the sleeping beauty transposon causes tumor regression and improves survival in mice bearing intracranial human glioblastoma. Mol Ther. 2005;12(5):778–88.
36. Ohlfest JR, Lobitz PD, Perkinson SG, Largaespada DA. Integration and long-term expression in xenografted human glioblastoma cells using a plasmid-based transposon system. Mol Ther. 2004;10(2):260–8.
37. Ding S, Wu X, Li G, Han M, Zhuang Y, Xu T. Efficient transposition of the piggyBac (PB) transposon in mammalian cells and mice. Cell. 2006;122(3):473–83.
38. Feschotte C. The piggyBac transposon holds promise for human gene therapy. Proc Natl Acad Sci U S A. 2006;103(41):14981–2.
39. Morales ME, Mann VH, Kines KJ, Gobert GN, Fraser Jr MJ, Kalinna BH, Correnti JM, Pearce EJ, Brindley PJ. piggyBac transposon mediated transgenesis of the human blood fluke, Schistosoma mansoni. FASEB J. 2007;21(13):3479–89.
40. Wilson MH, Coates CJ, George Jr AL. PiggyBac transposon-mediated gene transfer in human cells. Mol Ther. 2007;15(1):139–45.
41. Wu SC, Meir YJ, Coates CJ, Handler AM, Pelczar P, Moisyadi S, Kaminski JM. piggyBac is a flexible and highly active transposon as compared to sleeping beauty, Tol2, and Mos1 in mammalian cells. Proc Natl Acad Sci U S A. 2006;103(41):15008–13.
42. Chu RL, Post DE, Khuri FR, Van Meir EG. Use of replicating oncolytic adenoviruses in combination therapy for cancer. Clin Cancer Res. 2004;15:5299–312.
43. Kirn D. Oncolytic virotherapy for cancer with the adenovirus dl1520 (ONYX-015): results of phase I and II trials. Expert Opin Biol Ther. 2001;1:525–38.
44. Geoerger B, Grill J, Opolon P, Morizet J, Aubert G, Terrier-Lacombe MJ, Bressac De-Paillerets B, Barrois M, Feunteun J, Kim DH, Vassal G. Oncolytic activity of the E1B-55 kDa-deleted adenovirus ONYX-015 is independent of cellular p53 status in human malignant glioma xenografts. Cancer Res. 2002;62:764–72.
45. Rogulski KR, Freytag SO, Zhang K. In vivo antitumor activity of ONYX-015 is influenced by p53 status and is augmented by radiotherapy. Cancer Res. 2000;60:1193–6.
46. Aghi M, Rabkin S. Viral vectors as therapeutic agents for glioblastoma. Curr Opin Mol Ther. 2005;7:419–30.
47. Reid T, Warren R, Kirn D. Intravascular adenoviral agents in cancer patients: lessons from clinical trials. Cancer Gene Ther. 2002;9:979–86.

48. Ganly D, Kirn G, Eckhardt G. A phase I study of ONYX-015, an E1B attenuated adenovirus, administered intratumorally to patients with recurrent head and neck cancer. Clin Cancer Res. 2000;6: 798–806.
49. Khuri FR, Nemunaitis J, Ganly I. A controlled trial of intratumoral ONYX-015, a selectively-replicating adenovirus, in combination with cisplatin and 5-fluorouracil in patients with recurrent head and neck cancer. Nat Med. 2000;6:879–85.
50. Nemunaitis J, Ganly I, Khuri F. Selective replication and oncolysis in p53 mutant tumors with ONYX-015, an E1B-55kD gene-deleted adenovirus, in patients with advanced head and neck cancer: a phase II trial. Cancer Res. 2000;60:6359–66.
51. Bischoff JR, Kirn D, Williams A, Heise C, Horn S, Muna M, Ng L, Nye NA, Sampson-Johannes A, Fattaey A, McCormick F. An adenovirus mutant that replicates selectively in p53-deficient human tumor cells. Science. 1996;274:373–6.
52. Heise C, Ganly I, Kirn YT, Sampson-Johannes A, Brown R, Kirn D. Efficacy of a replication-selective adenovirus against ovarian carcinomatosis is dependent on tumor burden, viral replication and p53 status. Gene Ther. 2000;7:1925–9.
53. Vasey PA, Schulman LN, Campo S, Davis J, Gore M, Johnston S, Kirn DH, O'Neill V, Siddiqui N, Seiden MV, Kaye SB. Phase I trial of intraperitoneal injection of the EiB-55kD gene-deleted adenovirus ONYX-015 (dl1520) given on days 1 through 5 every 3 weeks in patients with recurrent/refractory epithelial ovarian cancer. J Clin Oncol. 2002;15:1562–9.
54. Dmitriev I, Krasnykh V, Miller CR, Wang M, Kashentseva E, Mikheeva G, Belousova N, Curiel DT. An adenovirus with genetically modified fibers demonstrates expanded tropism via utilization of a coxsackievirus and adenovirus receptor-independent cell entry mechanism. J Virol. 1998;72:9706–13.
55. Vanderkwaak JT, Wang M, Gomez-Navarro J, Rancourt C, Dmitriev I, Krasnyk V, Barnes M, Siegal GP, Alvarez RD, Curiel DT. An advanced generation of adenoviral vectors selectively enhances gene transfer for ovarian cancer gene therapy approaches. Gynecol Oncol. 1999;74:227–34.
56. Blackwell JL, Li H, Gomez-Navarro J, Dmitriev I, Krasnykh V, Richter CA, Shaw DR, Alvarez RD, Curiel DT, Strong TV. Using a tropism-modified adenoviral vector to circumvent inhibitory factors in ascites fluid. Hum Gene Ther. 2000;11:1657–69.
57. Louis N, Fender P, Barge A, Kitts P, Chroboczek J. Cell-binding domain of adenovirus serotype 2 fiber. J Virol. 1994;68:4104–6.
58. Bergelson JM, Cunningham JA, Droguett G, Droguett G, Kurt-Jones EA, Krithivas A, Hong JS, Horwitz MS, Crowell RL, Finberg RW. Isolation of a common receptor for Coxsackie B viruses and adenoviruses 2 and 5. Science. 1997;275:1320–3.
59. Hong SS, Karayan L, Tournier J, Curiel DT, Boulanger PA. Adenovirus type 5 fiber knob binds to MHC class I alpha2domain at the surface of the human epithelial and B lymphoblastoid cells. EMBO J. 1997;16: 2294–306.
60. Henry LJ, Xia D, Wilke ME, Deisenhofer J, Gerard RD. Characterization of the knob domain of the adenovirus type 5 fiber protein expressed in *Escherichia coli*. J Virol. 1994;68:5239–46.
61. Wickam TJ, Mathias P, Deresh DA, Nemerow GR. Integrins alpha v beta 3 and alpha v beta 5 promote adenovirus internalization but not virus attachment. Cell. 1993;73:309–19.
62. Stevenson SC, Rollence M, White B, Weaver L, McClelland A. Human adenoviruses serotypes 3 and 5 bind to two different cellular receptors via the fiber head domain. J Virol. 1995;69:2850–7.
63. Short JJ, Pereboev AV, Kawakami Y, Vasu C, Holterman MJ, Curiel DT. Adenovirus serotype 3 utilizes CD80 (B7.1) and CD86 (B7.2) as cellular attachment receptors. Virology. 2004;322:349–59.
64. Sirena D, Lillenfeld B, Eisenhut M, Kalin S, Boucke K, Beerli RR, Vogt L, Ruedl C, Bachmann MF, Greber UF, Hemmi S. The human membrane cofactor CD46 is a receptor for species B adenovirus serotype 3. J Virol. 2004;78:4454–62.
65. Krasnykh VN, Mikheeva MV, Douglas JT, Curiel DT. Generations of recombinant adenovirus vectors with modified fibers for altering viral tropism. J Virol. 1996;70:6839–46.
66. Raki M, Kanerva A, Ristimaki A, Desmond RA, Chen DT, Ranki T, Sarkioja M, Kangasniemi L, Hemminki A. Combination of gemcitabine and Ad5/3-Delta24, a tropism modified conditionally replicating adenovirus, for the treatment of ovarian cancer. Gene Ther. 2005;12:1198–205.
67. Yoshida Y, Sadata A, Zhang W, Saito K, Shinoura N, Hamada H. Generation of fiber-mutant recombinant adenoviruses for gene therapy of malignant gliomas. Hum Gene Ther. 1998;102:1807–14.
68. Wickham TJ, Tzeng E, Shears II LL, Roelvink PW, Li Y, Lee GM, Brough DE, Lizonova A, Kovesdi I. Increased in vitro and in vivo gene transfer by adenovirus vectors containing chimeric fiber proteins. J Virol. 1997;71:8221–9.
69. Belousova N, Krendelchtchikova V, Curiel DT, Krasnyk V. Modulation of adenovirus vector tropism via incorporation of polypeptide ligands into the fiber protein. J Virol. 2002;76:8621–31.
70. Wu H, Dmitriev I, Kashentseva E, Seki T, Wang M, Curiel DT. Construction and characterization of adenovirus serotype 5 packaged with serotype 3 hexon. J Virol. 2002;76:12775–82.
71. Koizumi N, Moizuguchi H, Utoguchi N, Watanbe Y, Hayakawa T. Generation of fiber-modified adenovirus vectors containing heterologous peptides in both the HI loop and C terminus of the fiber knob. J Gene Med. 2003;5:267–76.
72. Page JG, Tian B, Schweikart K, Taomaszewski J, Harris R, Broadt T, Polley-Nelson J, Noker PE, Wang M, Makhija S, Aurigemma R, Curiel DT, Alvarez RD. Identifying the safety profile of a novel infectivity-enhanced conditionally replicative adenovirus,

Ad5-delta24-RGD in anticipation of a phase I trial for recurrent ovarian cancer. Am J Obstet Gynecol. 2007;196(389):el–9.
73. Rein DT, Breidenbach M, Kirby TO, Han T, Siegal GP, Bauerschmitz GJ, Wang M, Nettlebeck DM, Tsuruta Y, Yamamoto M, Dall P, Hemminki A, Curiel DT. A fiber-modified, secretory leukoprotease inhibitor promoter-based conditionally replicating adenovirus for treatment of ovarian cancer. Clin Cancer Res. 2005;11:1327–35.
74. Rocconi RP, Zhu ZB, Stoff-Khalili M, Rivera AA, Lu B, Wang M, Alvarez RD, Curiel DT, Makhija SK. Treatment of ovarian cancer with a novel dual targeted conditionally replicative adenovirus (CRAd). Gynecol Oncol. 2007;105:113–21.
75. Zhu ZB, Makhija SK, Lu B, Wang M, Kaliberova L, Liu B, Rivera AA, Nettlebeck DM, Mahasreshti PJ, Leath CA, Barker S, Yamaoto M, Li F, Alvarez RD, Curiel DT. Transcriptional targeting of tumors with a novel tumor-specific survivin promoter. Cancer Gene Ther. 2004;11:256–62.
76. Zhu ZB, Lu B, Park M, Makhija SK, Numnum TM, Kendrick JE, Wang M, Tsuruta Y, Fisher P, Alvarez RD, Zhou F, Siegal GP, Wu H, Curiel DT. Development of an optimized conditionally replicative adenoviral vector for ovarian cancer. Int J Oncol. 2008;32(6):1179–88.
77. Hermiston T. Gene delivery from replication-selective viruses: arming guided missiles in the war against cancer. J Clin Invest. 2000;105:1169–72.
78. Bett AJ, Prevec L, Graham FL. Packaging capacity and stability of human adenovirus type 5 vectors. J Virol. 1993;67:5911–21.
79. Wildner O, Morris JC, Vahanian NN, Ford Jr H, Ramsey WJ, Blaese RM. Adenoviral vectors capable of replication improve the efficacy of HSVtk/GCV suicide gene therapy of cancer. Gene Ther. 1999;6:57–62.
80. Akbulut H, Zhang L, Tang Y, Deisseroth A. Cytotoxic effect of replication-competent adenoviral vectors carrying L-plastin promoter regulated E1A and cytosine deaminase genes in cancers of the breast, ovary, and colon. Cancer Gene Ther. 2003;10:388–95.
81. Yoo JY, Kim JH, Kwon YG, Kim EC, Kim NK, Choi HJ, Yun CO. VEGF-specific short hairpin RNA-expressing oncolytic adenovirus-mediated adenovirus elicits potent inhibition of angiogenesis and tumor growth. Mol Ther. 2007;15:295–302.
82. Yoo JY, Kim JH, Kim J, Huang JHM, Zhang SN, Kang YA, Kim H, Yun CO. Short hairpin RNA-expressing oncolytic adenovirus-mediated inhibition of IL-8: effects on antiangiogenesis and tumor growth inhibition. Gene Ther. 2008;15:635–51.
83. Kurihara T, Brough DE, Kovesdi I, Kufe DW. Selectivity of a replication-competent adenovirus for human breast carcinoma cells expressing the MUC1 antigen. J Clin Invest. 2000;106:763–71.
84. Su C, Peng L, Sham J, Wang X, Zhang Q, Chua D, Liu C, Ciu X, Xue H, Wu H, Yang Q, Zhang B, Liu X, Wu M, Qian Q. Immune gene–viral therapy with triplex efficacy mediated by oncolytic adenovirus carrying an interferon-gamma gene yields efficient antitumor activity in immunodeficient and immunocompetent mice. Mol Ther. 2006;13:918–27.
85. Post DE, Sandberg EM, Kyle MM, Devi NS, Brat DJ, Xu Z, Tighiouart M, Van Meir EG. Targeted cancer gene therapy using a hypoxia inducible factor dependent oncolytic adenovirus armed with interleukin-4. Cancer Res. 2007;67:6872–81.
86. Bennett JJ, Tjuvajev J, Johnson P, Doubrovin M, Akhurst T, Malholtra S, Hackman T, Balatoni J, Finn R, Larson SM, Federoff H, Blasberg R, Fong R. Positron emission tomography for herpes virus infection: implications for oncolytic viral treatments of cancer. Nat Med. 2001;7:859–63.
87. Kanerva A, Zinn KR, Peng KW, Ranki T, Kangasniemi L, Chaudhuri TR, Desmond RA, Wang M, Takayama K, Hakkarainen T, Alfthan H, Stenman UH, Curiel DT, Hemminki A. Noninvasive dual modality in vivo monitoring of the persistence and potency of a tumor targeted conditionally replicating adenovirus. Gene Ther. 2005;12:87–94.
88. Bhaumik S, Gambhir SS. Optical imaging of Renilla luciferase reporter gene expression in living mice. Proc Natl Acad Sci U S A. 2002;99:377–82.
89. Patel AR, Vavia PR. Preparation and in vivo evaluation of SMEDDS (self-microemulsifying drug delivery system) containing fenofibrate. AAPS J. 2007;26:344–52.
90. Vasir JK, Labhasetwar V. Biodegradable nanoparticles for cytosolic delivery of therapeutics. Adv Drug Deliv Rev. 2007;59:718–28.
91. Stoff-Khalili MA, Rivera AA, Mathis JM, Banerjee NS, Moon AS, Hess A, Rocconi RP, Numnum TM, Everts M, Chow LT, Douglas JT, Siegal GP, Zhu ZB, Bender HG, Dall P, Stoff A, Pereboeva L, Curiel DT. Mesenchymal stem cells as a vehicle for targeted delivery of CRAds to lung metastases of breast carcinoma. Breast Cancer Res Treat. 2007;105:157–67.
92. Kim SH, June CH, et al. Immunotherapy opportunities in ovarian cancer. Expert Rev Anticancer Ther. 2008;8:243–57.
93. Hung CF, Wu TC, Monie A, et al. Antigen-specific immunotherapy of cervical and ovarian cancer. Immunol Rev. 2008;222:43–69.
94. Odunsi K, Sabbatini P. Harnessing the immune system for ovarian cancer therapy. Am J Reprod Immunol. 2008;59:62–74.
95. Sabbatini P, Odunsi K. Immunologic approaches to ovarian cancer treatment. J Clin Oncol. 2007;25:2884–93.
96. Sabbatini P, Spriggs D, Aghajanian C, et al. Consolidation strategies in ovarian cancer: observations for future clinical trials. Gynecol Oncol. 2010;116:66–71.
97. Reinartz S, Kohler S, Schlebusch H, et al. Vaccination of patients with advanced ovarian carcinoma with the anti-idiotype ACA125: immunological response and survival (phase Ib/II). Clin Cancer Res. 2004;10:1580–7.

98. Gulley JL, Arlen PM, Tsang KY, et al. Pilot study of vaccination with recombinant CEA-MUC-1-TRICOM poxviral-based vaccines in patients with metastatic carcinoma. Clin Cancer Res. 2008;14:3060–9.
99. Peoples GE, Goedegebuure PS, Smith R, et al. Breast and ovarian cancer-specific cytotoxic T lymphocytes recognize the same HER2/neu-derived peptide. Proc Natl Acad Sci U S A. 1995;92:432–6.
100. Disis ML, Bernhard H, Jaffee EM. Use of tumour-responsive T cells as cancer treatment. Lancet. 2009;373:673–83.
101. Disis ML, Goodell V, Schiffman K, et al. Humoral epitope-spreading following immunization with a HER-2/neu peptide based vaccine in cancer patients. J Clin Immunol. 2004;24:571–8.
102. Diefenbach CS, Gnjatic S, Sabbatini P, et al. Safety and immunogenicity study of NY-ESO-1b peptide and montanide ISA-51 vaccination of patients with epithelial ovarian cancer in high-risk first remission. Clin Cancer Res. 2008;14:2740–8.
103. Odunsi K, Qian F, Matsuzaki J, et al. Vaccination with an NY-ESO-1 peptide of HLA class I/II specificities induces integrated humoral and T cell responses in ovarian cancer. Proc Natl Acad Sci U S A. 2007;104:12837–42.
104. Chianese-Bullock KA, Irvin Jr WP, Petroni GR, et al. A multipeptide vaccine is safe and elicits T-cell responses in participants with advanced stage ovarian cancer. J Immunother. 2008;31:420–30.
105. Tsuda N, Mochizuki K, Harada M, et al. Vaccination with predesignated or evidence-based peptides for patients with recurrent gynecologic cancers. J Immunother. 2004;27:60–72.
106. Chu CS, Kim SH, June CH, Coukos G. Immunotherapy opportunities in ovarian cancer. Expert Rev Anticancer Ther. 2008;8(2):243–57.
107. Buckanovich RJ, Facciabene A, Kim S, et al. Endothelin B receptor mediates the endothelial barrier to T cell homing to tumors and disables immune therapy. Nat Med. 2008;14:28–36.
108. Ioannides CG, Platsoucas CD, Freedman RS. Immunological effects of tumor vaccines: II. T cell responses directed against cellular antigens in the viral oncolysates. In Vivo. 1990;4:17–24.
109. Ioannides CG, Platsoucas CD, Patenia R, et al. T-cell functions in ovarian cancer patients treated with viral oncolysates: I. Increased helper activity to immunoglobulins production. Anticancer Res. 1990;10:645–53.
110. Schirrmacher V. Clinical trials of antitumor vaccination with an autologous tumor cell vaccine modified by virus infection: improvement of patient survival based on improved antitumor immune memory. Cancer Immunol Immunother. 2004;54:587–98.
111. Benencia F, Courreges MC, Fraser NW, et al. Herpes virus oncolytic therapy reverses tumor immune dysfunction and facilitates tumor antigen presentation. Cancer Biol Ther. 2008;7:1194–205.
112. Benencia F, Courreges MC, Conejo-Garcia JR, et al. Direct vaccination with tumor cells killed with ICP4-deficient HSVd120 elicits effective antitumor immunity. Cancer Biol Ther. 2006;5:867–74.
113. Benencia F, Courreges MC, Coukos G. Whole tumor antigen vaccination using dendritic cells: comparison of RNA electroporation and pulsing with UV-irradiated tumor cells. J Transl Med. 2008;6:21.
114. Hernando JJ, Park TW, Kubler K, et al. Vaccination with autologous tumour antigen-pulsed dendritic cells in advanced gynaecological malignancies: clinical and immunological evaluation of a phase I trial. Cancer Immunol Immunother. 2002;51:45–52.
115. Gong J, Nikrui N, Chen D, et al. Fusions of human ovarian carcinoma cells with autologous or allogeneic dendritic cells induce antitumor immunity. J Immunol. 2000;165:1705–11.
116. Cannon MJ, O'Brien TJ. Cellular immunotherapy for ovarian cancer. Expert Opin Biol Ther. 2009;9:677–88.
117. Kandalaft LE, Facciabene A, Buckanovich RJ, et al. Endothelin B receptor, a new target in cancer immune therapy. Clin Cancer Res. 2009;15:4521–8.
118. Benencia F, Coukos G. T regulatory cell depletion can boost DC-based vaccines. Cancer Biol Ther. 2005;4.
119. Rosenberg SA, Yang JC, Restifo NP. Cancer immunotherapy: moving beyond current vaccines. Nat Med. 2004;10:909–15.
120. Dudley ME, Wunderlich JR, Yang JC, et al. Adoptive cell transfer therapy following non-myeloablative but lymphodepleting chemotherapy for the treatment of patients with refractory metastatic melanoma. J Clin Oncol. 2005;23:2346–57.
121. Rosenberg SA, Dudley ME. Adoptive cell therapy for the treatment of patients with metastatic melanoma. Curr Opin Immunol. 2009;21:233–40.
122. Aoki Y, Takakuwa K, Kodama S, et al. Use of adoptive transfer of tumor-infiltrating lymphocytes alone or in combination with cisplatin-containing chemotherapy in patients with epithelial ovarian cancer. Cancer Res. 1991;51:1934–9.
123. Fujita K, Ikarashi H, Takakuwa K, et al. Prolonged disease-free period in patients with advanced epithelial ovarian cancer after adoptive transfer of tumor-infiltrating lymphocytes. Clin Cancer Res. 1995;1:501–7.
124. Gattinoni L, Finkelstein SE, Klebanoff CA, et al. Removal of homeostatic cytokine sinks by lymphodepletion enhances the efficacy of adoptively transferred tumor-specific CD8+ T cells. J Exp Med. 2005;202:907–12.
125. Huang J, Kerstann KW, Ahmadzadeh M, et al. Modulation by IL-2 of CD70 and CD27 expression on CD8+ T cells: importance for the therapeutic effectiveness of cell transfer immunotherapy. J Immunol. 2006;176:7726–35.
126. Powell Jr DJ, Dudley ME, Robbins PF, et al. Transition of late-stage effector T cells to CD27+

CD28+ tumor-reactive effector memory T cells in humans after adoptive cell transfer therapy. Blood. 2005;105:241–50.
127. Shen X, Zhou J, Hathcock KS, et al. Persistence of tumor infiltrating lymphocytes in adoptive immunotherapy correlates with telomere length. J Immunother. 2007;30:123–9.
128. Zhou J, Shen X, Huang J, et al. Telomere length of transferred lymphocytes correlates with in vivo persistence and tumor regression in melanoma patients receiving cell transfer therapy. J Immunol. 2005;175:7046–52.
129. Perret R, Ronchese F. Memory T cells in cancer immunotherapy: which CD8 T-cell population provides the best protection against tumours? Tissue Antigens. 2008;72:187–94.
130. June CH, Blazar BR, Riley JL. Engineering lymphocyte subsets: tools, trials and tribulations. Nat Rev Immunol. 2009;9:704–16.
131. Morgan RA, Dudley ME, Wunderlich JR, et al. Cancer regression in patients after transfer of genetically engineered lymphocytes. Science. 2006;314:126–9.
132. Theoret MR, Cohen CJ, Nahvi AV, et al. Relationship of p53 overexpression on cancers and recognition by anti-p53 T cell receptor-transduced T cells. Hum Gene Ther. 2008;19:1219–32.
133. Riley JL, June CH, Blazar BR. Human T regulatory cell therapy: take a billion or so and call me in the morning. Immunity. 2009;30:656–65.
134. Parkhurst MR, Joo J, Riley JP, et al. Characterization of genetically modified T-cell receptors that recognize the CEA:691–699 peptide in the context of HLA-A2.1 On human colorectal cancer cells. Clin Cancer Res. 2009;15:169–80.
135. Robbins PF, Li YF, El-Gamil M, et al. Single and dual amino acid substitutions in TCR CDRs can enhance antigen-specific T cell functions. J Immunol. 2008;180:6116–31.
136. Sadelain M, Riviere I, Brentjens R. Targeting tumours with genetically enhanced T lymphocytes. Nat Rev Cancer. 2003;3:35–45.
137. Walker RE, Bechtel CM, Natarajan V, et al. Long-term in vivo survival of receptor-modified syngeneic T cells in patients with human immunodeficiency virus infection. Blood. 2000;96:467–74.
138. Brocker T, Karjalainen K. Adoptive tumor immunity mediated by lymphocytes bearing modified antigen-specific receptors. Adv Immunol. 1998;68:257–69.
139. Gross G, Waks T, Eshhar Z. Expression of immunoglobulin-T-cell receptor chimeric molecules as functional receptors with antibody-type specificity. Proc Natl Acad Sci U S A. 1989;86:10024–8.
140. Pinthus JH, Waks T, Kaufman-Francis K, et al. Immuno-gene therapy of established prostate tumors using chimeric receptor-redirected human lymphocytes. Cancer Res. 2003;63:2470–6.
141. Sadelain M, Brentjens R, Riviere I. The promise and potential pitfalls of chimeric antigen receptors. Curr Opin Immunol. 2009;21:215–23.
142. Hinrichs CS, Borman ZA, Cassard L, et al. Adoptively transferred effector cells derived from naive rather than central memory CD8+ T cells mediate superior antitumor immunity. Proc Natl Acad Sci U S A. 2009;106:17469–74.
143. Suhoski MM, Golovina TN, Aqui NA, et al. Engineering artificial antigen-presenting cells to express a diverse array of co-stimulatory molecules. Mol Ther. 2007;15:981–8.
144. Wang G, Chopra RK, Royal RE, et al. A T cell-independent antitumor response in mice with bone marrow cells retrovirally transduced with an antibody/Fc-gamma chain chimeric receptor gene recognizing a human ovarian cancer antigen. Nat Med. 1998;4:168–72.
145. Parker LL, Do MT, Westwood JA, et al. Expansion and characterization of T cells transduced with a chimeric receptor against ovarian cancer. Hum Gene Ther. 2000;11:2377–87.
146. Wilkie S, Picco G, Foster J, et al. Retargeting of human T cells to tumor-associated MUC1: the evolution of a chimeric antigen receptor. J Immunol. 2008;180:4901–9.
147. Carpenito C, Milone MC, Hassan R, et al. Control of large, established tumor xenografts with genetically retargeted human T cells containing CD28 and CD137 domains. Proc Natl Acad Sci U S A. 2009;106:3360–5.
148. Elgueta R, Benson MJ, de Vries VC, et al. Molecular mechanism and function of CD40/CD40L engagement in the immune system. Immunol Rev. 2009;229:152–72.
149. Scarlett UK, Cubillos-Ruiz JR, Nesbeth YC, et al. In situ stimulation of CD40 and toll-like receptor 3 transforms ovarian cancer-infiltrating dendritic cells from immunosuppressive to immunostimulatory cells. Cancer Res. 2009;69:7329–37.
150. Kedl RM, Jordan M, Potter T, et al. CD40 stimulation accelerates deletion of tumor-specific CD8(+) T cells in the absence of tumor-antigen vaccination. Proc Natl Acad Sci U S A. 2001;98:10811–6.
151. Melichar B, Patenia R, Gallardo S, et al. Expression of CD40 and growth-inhibitory activity of CD40 ligand in ovarian cancer cell lines. Gynecol Oncol. 2007;104:707–13.
152. Hakkarainen T, Hemminki A, Pereboev AV, et al. CD40 is expressed on ovarian cancer cells and can be utilized for targeting adenoviruses. Clin Cancer Res. 2003;9:619–24.
153. Gallagher NJ, Eliopoulos AG, Agathangelo A, et al. CD40 activation in epithelial ovarian carcinoma cells modulates growth, apoptosis, and cytokine secretion. Mol Pathol. 2002;55:110–20.
154. Ciaravino G, Bhat M, Manbeian CA, et al. Differential expression of CD40 and CD95 in ovarian carcinoma. Eur J Gynaecol Oncol. 2004;25:27–32.
155. Toutirais O, Gervais A, Cabillic F, et al. Effects of CD40 binding on ovarian carcinoma cell growth and cytokine production in vitro. Clin Exp Immunol. 2007;149:372–7.

156. Ghamande S, Hylander BL, Oflazoglu E, et al. Recombinant CD40 ligand therapy has significant antitumor effects on CD40-positive ovarian tumor xenografts grown in SCID mice and demonstrates an augmented effect with cisplatin. Cancer Res. 2001;61:7556–62.
157. Korman AJ, Peggs KS, Allison JP. Checkpoint blockade in cancer immunotherapy. Adv Immunol. 2006;90:297–339.
158. Peggs KS, Quezada SA, Korman AJ, et al. Principles and use of anti-CTLA4 antibody in human cancer immunotherapy. Curr Opin Immunol. 2006;18: 206–13.
159. Fong L, Small EJ. Anti-cytotoxic T-lymphocyte antigen-4 antibody: the first in an emerging class of immunomodulatory antibodies for cancer treatment. J Clin Oncol. 2008;26:5275–83.
160. Hodi FS, Butler M, Oble DA, et al. Immunologic and clinical effects of antibody blockade of cytotoxic T lymphocyte-associated antigen 4 in previously vaccinated cancer patients. Proc Natl Acad Sci U S A. 2008;105:3005–10.
161. Curiel TJ, Wei S, Dong H, et al. Blockade of B7–H1 improves myeloid dendritic cell-mediated antitumor immunity. Nat Med. 2003;9:562–7.
162. Liu SM, Meng Q, Zhang QX, et al. Expression and significance of B7–H1 and its receptor PD-1 in human gastric carcinoma (Chinese). Zhonghua Zhong Liu Za Zhi. 2008;30:192–5.
163. Hirano F, Kaneko K, Tamura H, et al. Blockade of B7–H1 and PD-1 by monoclonal antibodies potentiates cancer therapeutic immunity. Cancer Res. 2005;65:1089–96.
164. Blank C, Mackensen A. Contribution of the PD-L1/PD-1 pathway to T-cell exhaustion: an update on implications for chronic infections and tumor evasion. Cancer Immunol Immunother. 2007;56:739–45.
165. Berger R, Rotem-Yehudar R, Slama G, et al. Phase I safety and pharmacokinetic study of CT-011, a humanized antibody interacting with PD-1, in patients with advanced hematologic malignancies. Clin Cancer Res. 2008;14:3044–51.
166. Dudley ME, Wunderlich JR, Robbins PF, et al. Cancer regression and autoimmunity in patients after clonal repopulation with antitumor lymphocytes. Science. 2002;298:850–4.
167. Machiels JP, Reilly RT, Emens LA, et al. Cyclophosphamide, doxorubicin, and paclitaxel enhance the antitumor immune response of granulocyte/macrophage-colony stimulating factor-secreting whole-cell vaccines in HER-2/neu tolerized mice. Cancer Res. 2001;61:3689–97.
168. Berd D, Sato T, Maguire Jr HC, et al. Immunopharmacologic analysis of an autologous, hapten-modified human melanoma vaccine. J Clin Oncol. 2004;22:403–15.
169. Klebanoff CA, Khong HT, Antony PA, et al. Sinks, suppressors and antigen presenters: How lymphodepletion enhances T cell-mediated tumor immunotherapy. Trends Immunol. 2005;26:111–7.
170. Berd D, Maguire Jr HC, Mastrangelo MJ. Induction of cell-mediated immunity to autologous melanoma cells and regression of metastases after treatment with a melanoma cell vaccine preceded by cyclophosphamide. Cancer Res. 1986;46:2572–7.
171. MacLean GD, Reddish MA, Koganty RR, et al. Antibodies against mucin-associated sialyl-Tn epitopes correlate with survival of metastatic adenocarcinoma patients undergoing active specific immunotherapy with synthetic STn vaccine. J Immunother Emphasis Tumor Immunol. 1996;19:59–68.
172. Prasad SJ, Farrand KJ, Matthews SA, et al. Dendritic cells loaded with stressed tumor cells elicit long-lasting protective tumor immunity in mice depleted of CD4+CD25+ regulatory T cells. J Immunol. 2005;174:90–8.
173. Powell Jr DJ, Attia P, Ghetie V, et al. Partial reduction of human FOXP3+ CD4 T cells in vivo after CD25-directed recombinant immunotoxin administration. J Immunother. 2008;31:189–98.
174. Dannull J, Su Z, Rizzieri D, et al. Enhancement of vaccine-mediated antitumor immunity in cancer patients after depletion of regulatory T cells. J Clin Invest. 2005;115:3623–33.
175. Barnett B, Kryczek I, Cheng P, et al. Regulatory T cells in ovarian cancer: biology and therapeutic potential. Am J Reprod Immunol. 2005;54:369–77.
176. Mahnke K, Schonfeld K, Fondel S, et al. Depletion of CD4+CD25+ human regulatory T cells in vivo: Kinetics of Treg depletion and alterations in immune functions in vivo and in vitro. Int J Cancer. 2007;120:2723–33.
177. Rasku MA, Clem AL, Telang S, et al. Transient T cell depletion causes regression of melanoma metastases. J Transl Med. 2008;6:12.
178. Waldmann TA. Daclizumab (anti-Tac, Zenapax) in the treatment of leukemia/lymphoma. Oncogene. 2007;26:3699–703.
179. Kreijveld E, Koenen HJ, Klasen IS, et al. Following anti-CD25 treatment, a functional CD4+ CD25+ regulatory T-cell pool is present in renal transplant recipients. Am J Transplant. 2007;7:249–55.
180. Nussenblatt RB, Fortin E, Schiffman R, et al. Treatment of noninfectious intermediate and posterior uveitis with the humanized anti-Tac mAb: A phase I/II clinical trial. Proc Natl Acad Sci U S A. 1999;96:7462–6.
181. Przepiorka D, Kernan NA, Ippoliti C, et al. Daclizumab, a humanized anti-interleukin-2 receptor alpha chain antibody, for treatment of acute graft-versus-host disease. Blood. 2000;95:83–9.
182. Lehky TJ, Levin MC, Kubota R, et al. Reduction in HTLV-I proviral load and spontaneous lymphoproliferation in HTLV-I-associated myelopathy/tropical spastic paraparesis patients treated with humanized anti-Tac. Ann Neurol. 1998;44:942–7.
183. Vincenti F, Nashan B, Light S. Daclizumab: outcome of phase III trials and mechanism of action: double therapy and the triple therapy study groups. Transplant Proc. 1998;30:2155–8.

184. Rech AJ, Vonderheide RH. Clinical use of anti-CD25 antibody daclizumab to enhance immune responses to tumor antigen vaccination by targeting regulatory T cells. Ann N Y Acad Sci. 2009;1174:99–106.
185. Yarden Y. The EGFR family and its ligands in human cancer. Signalling mechanisms and therapeutic opportunities. Eur J Cancer. 2001;37 Suppl 4:S3–8.
186. Ellis LM, Hicklin DJ. VEGF-targeted therapy: mechanisms of anti-tumour activity. Nat Rev Cancer. 2008;8:579–91.
187. Ogiso H, Ishitani R, Nureki O, Fukai S, Yamanaka M, Kim JH, Saito K, Sakamoto A, Inoue M, Shirouzu M, Yokoyama S. Crystal structure of the complex of human epidermal growth factor and receptor extracellular domains. Cell. 2002;110:775–87.
188. Siwak DR, Carey M, Hennessy BT, Nguyen CT, McGahren Murray MJ, Nolden L, Mills GB. Targeting the epidermal growth factor receptor in epithelial ovarian cancer: current knowledge and future challenges. J Oncol. 2010;2010:568938.
189. Blank SV, Christos P, Curtin JP, Goldman N, Runowitcz CD, Sparano JA, Liebes L, Chen HX, Muggia FM. Erlotinib added to carboplatin and paclitaxel as first-line treatment of ovarian cancer: a phase II study based on surgical reassessment. Gynecol Oncol. 2010;119:451–6.
190. Annunziata CM, Walker AJ, Minasian L, Yu M, Kotz H, Wood BJ, Calvo K, Choyke P, Kimm D, Steinberg SM, Kohn EC. Vandetanib, designed to inhibit VEGFR2 and EGFR signaling, had no clinical activity as monotherapy for recurrent ovarian cancer and no detectable modulation of VEGFR2. Clin Cancer Res. 2010;16:664.
191. Farley J, Fuchiuji S, Darcy KM, Tian C, Hoskins WJ, McGuire WP, Hanjani P, Warshal D, Greer BE, Belinson J, Birrer MJ. Associations between ERBB2 amplification and progression-free survival and overall survival in advanced stage, suboptimally-resected epithelial ovarian cancers: a Gynecologic Oncology Group Study. Gynecol Oncol. 2009;113:341–7.
192. Bookman MA, Darcy KM, Clarke-Pearson D, Boothby RA, Horowitz IR. Evaluation of monoclonal humanized anti-HER2 antibody, trastuzumab, in patients with recurrent or refractory ovarian or primary peritoneal carcinoma with overexpression of HER2: a phase II trial of the Gynecologic Oncology Group. J Clin Oncol. 2003;21:283–90.
193. Campos S, Hamid O, Seiden MV, Oza A, Plante M, Potkul RK, Lenehan PF, Kaldjian EP, Varterasian ML, Jordan C, Charbonneau C, Hirte H. Multicenter, randomized phase II trial of oral CI-1033 for previously treated advanced ovarian cancer. J Clin Oncol. 2005;23:5597–604.
194. Kimball KJ, Numnum TM, Kirby TO, Zamboni WC, Estes JM, Barnes MN, Matei DE, Koch KM, Alvarez RD. A phase I study of lapatinib in combination with carboplatin in women with platinum sensitive recurrent ovarian carcinoma. Gynecol Oncol. 2008;111:95–101.
195. Tsuda H, Birrer MJ, Ito YM, Ohashi Y, Lin M, Lee C, Wong WH, Rao PH, Lau CC, Berkowitz RS, Birrer MJ, Mok SC. Identification of DNA copy number changes in microdissected serous ovarian cancer tissue using a cDNA microarray platform. Cancer Genet Cytogenet. 2004;155:97–107.
196. Simpson BJ, Weatherill J, Miller EP, Lessells AM, Langdon SP, Miller WR. c-erbB-3 protein expression in ovarian tumours. Br J Cancer. 1995;71:758–62.
197. Tanner B, Hasenclever D, Stern K, Schormann W, Bezler M, Hermes M, Brulport M, Bauer A, Schiffer IB, Gebhard S, Schmidt M, Steiner E, Sehouli J, Edelmann J, Läuter J, Lessig R, Krishnamurthi K, Ullrich A, Hengstler JG. ErbB-3 predicts survival in ovarian cancer. J Clin Oncol. 2006;24:4317–23.
198. Lee H, Maihle NJ. Isolation and characterization of four alternate c-erbB3 transcripts expressed in ovarian carcinoma-derived cell lines and normal human tissues. Oncogene. 1998;16:3243–52.
199. Lafky JM, Wilken JA, Baron AT, Maihle NJ. Clinical implications of the ErbB/epidermal growth factor (EGF) receptor family and its ligands in ovarian cancer. Biochim Biophys Acta. 2008;1785:232–65.
200. Sergina NV, Rausch M, Wang D, Blair J, Hann B, Shokat KM, Moasser MM. Escape from HER-family tyrosine kinase inhibitor therapy by the kinase-inactive HER3. Nature. 2007;445:437–41.
201. Engelman JA, Zejnullahu K, Mitsudomi T, Song Y, Hyland C, Park JO, Lindeman N, Gale CM, Zhao X, Christensen J, Kosaka T, Holmes AJ, Rogers AM, Cappuzzo F, Mok T, Lee C, Johnson BE, Cantley LC, Jänne PA. MET amplification leads to gefitinib resistance in lung cancer by activating ERBB3 signaling. Science. 2007;316:1039–43.
202. Chandarlapaty S, Sawai A, Scaltriti M, Rodrik-Outmezguine V, Grbovic-Huezo Ol Serra V, Majumder PK, Baselga J, Rosen N. AKT inhibition relieves feedback suppression of receptor tyrosine kinase expression and activity. Cancer Cell. 2011;19(1):58–71.
203. Gordon MS, Matei D, Aghajanian C, Matulonis UA, Brewer M, Fleming GF, Hainsworth JD, Garcia AA, Pegram MD, Schilder RJ, Cohn DE, Roman L, Derynck MK, Ng K, Lyons B, Allison DE, Eberhard DA, Pham TQ, Dere RC, Karlan BY. Clinical activity of pertuzumab (rhuMAb 2C4), a HER dimerization inhibitor, in advanced ovarian cancer: potential predictive relationship with tumor HER2 activation status. J Clin Oncol. 2006;24:4324–32.
204. Makhija S, Amler LC, Glenn D, Ueland FR, Gold MA, Dizon DS, Paton V, Lin CY, Januario T, Ng K, Strauss A, Kelsey S, Sliwkowski MX, Matulonis U. Clinical activity of gemcitabine plus pertuzumab in platinum-resistant ovarian cancer, fallopian tube cancer, or primary peritoneal cancer. J Clin Oncol. 2010;28:1215–23.

205. Sheng Q, Liu X, Fleming E, Yuan K, Piao H, Chen J, Moustafa Z, Thomas RK, Greulich H, Schinzel A, Zaghlul S, Batt D, Ettenberg S, Meyerson M, Schoeberl B, Kung AL, Hahn WC, Drapkin R, Livingston DM, Liu JF. An activated ErbB3/NRG1 autocrine loop supports in vivo proliferation in ovarian cancer cells. Cancer Cell. 2010;17:298–310.
206. Gilmour LM, Macleod KG, McCaig A, Sewell JM, Gullick WJ, Smyth JF, Langdon SP. Neuregulin expression, function, and signaling in human ovarian cancer cells. Clin Cancer Res. 2002;8:3933–42.
207. Jones FE. HER4 intracellular domain (4ICD) activity in the developing mammary gland and breast cancer. J Mammary Gland Biol Neoplasia. 2008;13:247–58.
208. Prickett TD, Agrawal NS, Wei X, Yates KE, Lin JC, Wunderlich JR, Cronin JC, Cruz P, Rosenberg SA, Samuels Y. Analysis of the tyrosine kinome in melanoma reveals recurrent mutations in ERBB4. Nat Genet. 2009;41:1127–32.
209. Rudloff U, Samuels Y. A growing family: adding mutated Erbb4 as a novel cancer target. Cell Cycle. 2010;9:1487–503.
210. Srinivasan R, Poulsom R, Hurst HC, Gullick WJ. Expression of the c-erbB-4/HER4 protein and mRNA in normal human fetal and adult tissues and in a survey of nine solid tumour types. J Pathol. 1998;185:236–45.
211. Scoccia B, Lee YM, Niederberger C, Ilekis JV. Expression of the ErbB family of receptors in ovarian cancer. J Soc Gynecol Investig. 1998;5:161–5.
212. Gilmour LM, Macleod KG, McCaig A, Gullick WJ, Smyth JF, Langdon SP. Expression of erbB-4/HER-4 growth factor receptor isoforms in ovarian cancer. Cancer Res. 2001;61:2169–76.
213. Pejovic T, Pande NT, Mori M, Mhawech-Fauceglia P, Harrington C, Mongoue-Tchokote S, Dim D, Andrews C, Beck A, Tarumi Y, Djilas J, Cappuccini F, Caballero O, Huang J, Levy S, Tsiamouri A, Cain J, Bagby GC, Strausberg RL, Simpson AJ, Odunsi KO. Expression profiling of the ovarian surface kinome reveals candidate genes for early neoplastic changes. Transl Oncol. 2009;2:341–9.
214. Steffensen KD, Waldstrom M, Andersen RF, Olsen DA, Jeppesen U, Knudsen HJ, Brandslund I, Jakobsen A. Protein levels and gene expressions of the epidermal growth factor receptors, HER1, HER2, HER3 and HER4 in benign and malignant ovarian tumors. Int J Oncol. 2008;33:195–204.
215. Bryant HE, Schultz N, Thomas HD, et al. Specific killing of BRCA2-deficient tumours with inhibitors of poly(ADP-ribose) polymerase. Nature. 2005;434:913–7.
216. Farmer H, McCabe N, Lord CJ, et al. Targeting the DNA repair defect in BRCA mutant cells as a therapeutic strategy. Nature. 2005;434:917–21.
217. Krishnakumar R, Kraus WL. The PARP side of the nucleus: molecular actions, physiological outcomes, and clinical targets. Mol Cell. 2010;39:8–24.
218. Ferraris DV. Evolution of poly(ADP-ribose) polymerase-1 (PARP-1) inhibitors. From concept to clinic. J Med Chem. 2010;53:4561–84.
219. Schreiber V, Dantzer F, Ame JC, de Murcia G. Poly(ADP-ribose): novel functions for an old molecule. Nat Rev Mol Cell Biol. 2006;7:517–28.
220. Papeo G, Forte B, Orsini P, et al. Poly(ADP-ribose) polymerase inhibition in cancer therapy: are we close to maturity? Expert Opin Ther Pat. 2009;19:1377–400.
221. Zaremba T, Curtin NJ. PARP inhibitor development for systemic cancer targeting. Anticancer Agents Med Chem. 2007;7:515–23.
222. Ame JC, Rolli V, Schreiber V, et al. PARP-2, a novel mammalian DNA damage-dependent poly(ADP-ribose) polymerase. J Biol Chem. 1999;274:17860–8.
223. Yelamos J, Schreiber V, Dantzer F. Toward specific functions of poly(ADP-ribose) polymerase-2. Trends Mol Med. 2008;14:169–78.
224. Menissier de Murcia J, Ricoul M, Tartier L, et al. Functional interaction between PARP-1 and PARP-2 in chromosome stability and embryonic development in mouse. EMBO J. 2003;22:2255–63.
225. Szabo C, Zingarelli B, O'Connor M, Salzman AL. DNA strand breakage, activation of poly(ADP-ribose) synthetase, and cellular energy depletion are involved in the cytotoxicity of macrophages and smooth muscle cells exposed to peroxynitrite. Proc Natl Acad Sci U S A. 1996;93:1753–8.
226. de Murcia JM, Niedergang C, Trucco C, et al. Requirement of poly(ADP-ribose) polymerase in recovery from DNA damage in mice and in cells. Proc Natl Acad Sci U S A. 1997;94:7303–7.
227. Bowman KJ, White A, Golding BT, Griffin RJ, Curtin NJ. Potentiation of anti-cancer agent cytotoxicity by the potent poly(ADP-ribose) polymerase inhibitors NU1025 and NU1064. Br J Cancer. 1998;78:1269–77.
228. Rouleau M, Patel A, Hendzel MJ, Kaufmann SH, Poirier GG. PARP inhibition: PARP1 and beyond. Nat Rev Cancer. 2010;10:293–301.
229. Ashworth A. A synthetic lethal therapeutic approach: poly (ADP) ribose polymerase inhibitors for the treatment of cancers deficient in DNA double-strand break repair. J Clin Oncol. 2008;26:3785–90.
230. Patel AG, Sarkaria JN, Kaufmann SH. Nonhomologous end joining drives poly(ADP-ribose) polymerase (PARP) inhibitor lethality in homologous recombination-deficient cells. Proc Natl Acad Sci U S A. 2011;108:3406–11.
231. Menear KA, Adcock C, Boulter R, et al. 4-[3-(4-cyclopropanecarbonylpiperazine-1-carbonyl)-4-fluorobenzyl]-2H-phth alazin-1-one: a novel bioavailable inhibitor of poly(ADP-ribose) polymerase-1. J Med Chem. 2008;51:6581–91.
232. Donawho CK, Luo Y, Penning TD, et al. ABT-888, an orally active poly(ADP-ribose) polymerase inhibitor that potentiates DNA-damaging agents in preclinical tumor models. Clin Cancer Res. 2007;13:2728–37.

233. O'Shaughnessy J, Osborne C, Pippen JE, et al. Iniparib plus chemotherapy in metastatic triple-negative breast cancer. N Engl J Med. 2011;364:205–14.
234. O'Shaughnessy J, Schwartzberg LS, Danso MA, et al. A randomized phase III study of iniparib (BSI-201) in combination with gemcitabine/carboplatin (G/C) in metastatic triple-negative breast cancer (TNBC). J Clin Oncol. 2011;29(suppl):1007. 2011 ASCO Annual Meeting.
235. Wooster R, Weber BL. Breast and ovarian cancer. N Engl J Med. 2003;348:2339–47.
236. Brose MS, Rebbeck TR, Calzone KA, Stopfer JE, Nathanson KL, Weber BL. Cancer risk estimates for BRCA1 mutation carriers identified in a risk evaluation program. J Natl Cancer Inst. 2002;94: 1365–72.
237. Ford D, Easton DF, Bishop DT, Narod SA, Goldgar DE. Risks of cancer in BRCA1-mutation carriers. Breast Cancer Linkage Consortium. Lancet. 1994;343:692–5.
238. Cancer risks in BRCA2 mutation carriers. The breast cancer linkage consortium. J Natl Cancer Inst. 1999; 91:1310–16.
239. Turner N, Tutt A, Ashworth A. Hallmarks of "BRCAness" in sporadic cancers. Nat Rev Cancer. 2004;4:814–9.
240. Venkitaraman AR. Cancer susceptibility and the functions of BRCA1 and BRCA2. Cell. 2002;108:171–82.
241. Lord CJ, Garrett MD, Ashworth A. Targeting the double-strand DNA break repair pathway as a therapeutic strategy. Clin Cancer Res. 2006;12: 4463–8.
242. Stark JM, Pierce AJ, Oh J, Pastink A, Jasin M. Genetic steps of mammalian homologous repair with distinct mutagenic consequences. Mol Cell Biol. 2004;24:9305–16.
243. Tutt A, Bertwistle D, Valentine J, et al. Mutation in Brca2 stimulates error-prone homology-directed repair of DNA double-strand breaks occurring between repeated sequences. EMBO J. 2001;20:4704–16.
244. Moynahan ME, Pierce AJ, Jasin M. BRCA2 is required for homology-directed repair of chromosomal breaks. Mol Cell. 2001;7:263–72.
245. Moynahan ME, Chiu JW, Koller BH, Jasin M. Brca1 controls homology-directed DNA repair. Mol Cell. 1999;4:511–8.
246. Zhuang J, Zhang J, Willers H, et al. Checkpoint kinase 2-mediated phosphorylation of BRCA1 regulates the fidelity of nonhomologous end-joining. Cancer Res. 2006;66:1401–8.
247. Rodon J, Iniesta MD, Papadopoulos K. Development of PARP inhibitors in oncology. Expert Opin Investig Drugs. 2009;18:31–43.
248. Haber JE. DNA recombination: the replication connection. Trends Biochem Sci. 1999;24:271–5.
249. Saleh-Gohari N, Bryant HE, Schultz N, Parker KM, Cassel TN, Helleday T. Spontaneous homologous recombination is induced by collapsed replication forks that are caused by endogenous DNA single-strand breaks. Mol Cell Biol. 2005;25:7158–69.
250. Gottipati P, Vischioni B, Schultz N, et al. Poly(ADP-ribose) polymerase is hyperactivated in homologous recombination-defective cells. Cancer Res. 2010;70:5389–98.

Psychological Aspects of Hereditary and Non-hereditary Ovarian Cancer

13

Kate Absolom, Elena Takeuchi, Geoff Hall, and Galina Velikova

Introduction

The psychological implications of cancer are an essential consideration for professionals as the importance of holistic care in oncology continues to be recognised. Throughout this chapter the phrase psychological distress will be used as an overarching term for the range of emotional problems patients may experience including anxiety, depression and post-traumatic stress. The term distress has been adopted by the National Cancer Comprehensive Network (NCCN) [1] and defined as:

> a multifactorial unpleasant emotional experience of a psychological (cognitive, behavioural, emotional), social, and/or spiritual nature that may interfere with the ability to cope effectively with cancer, its physical symptoms and its treatment. Distress extends along a continuum, ranging from common normal feelings of vulnerability, sadness, and fears to problems that can become disabling, such as depression, anxiety, panic, social isolation, and existential and spiritual crisis

Understandably a cancer diagnosis will routinely be coupled with the occurrence of psychological distress for patients and their families though feelings and reactions vary in their levels of intensity and impact on individual coping. In the general cancer population, reported levels of distress are wide ranging and can depend on the method and timing of measurement. Current estimates suggest that a third of patients may develop depressive or anxiety disorders [2], but levels of distress vary across the trajectory of the cancer experience from diagnosis through to long-term survivorship. Importantly distress has been shown to impact negatively on patient's adherence to treatment [3], survival [4] and health service utilisation [5, 6]. These findings underline the importance of a whole-person approach to cancer care for both the individual and healthcare organisations.

Patients affected by ovarian cancer are potentially a particularly vulnerable group given the nature of the disease. Sixty per cent of women diagnosed present with advanced disease (stages III or IV) for which current 5-year survival figures are less than 30 % [7]. Consequently these patients face difficult news about prognosis from the outset of their disease. Treatment typically aims to control the disease and its symptoms with the hope that prolonged periods of remission can be

K. Absolom, PhD, BSc (Hons) (✉)
Psychosocial Oncology and Clinical Practice Research Group, Leeds Institute of Molecular Medicine, Division of Cancer Studies and Pathology, University of Leeds, Leeds, UK
e-mail: k.l.absolom@leeds.ac.uk

E. Takeuchi, MB ChB, MRCP
Psychosocial Oncology and Clinical Practice Research Group, St. James's Institute of Oncology, Level 3, Bexley Wing, Beckett Street, Leeds LS9 7TF, UK
e-mail: e.takeuchi@leeds.ac.uk

G. Hall, MD ChB, MRCP, PhD, FRCP
G. Velikova, BMBS(MD), PhD, FRCP
Department of Oncology, University of Leeds/St. James' Institute of Oncology, Level 4, Bexley Wing, Beckett Street, Leeds LS9 7TF, UK
e-mail: g.hall@leeds.ac.uk; g.velikova@leeds.ac.uk

S.A. Farghaly (ed.), *Advances in Diagnosis and Management of Ovarian Cancer*,
DOI 10.1007/978-1-4614-8271-0_13, © Springer Science+Business Media New York 2014

achieved. Recurrence is however to be expected, and therefore, the cancer is characteristically regarded as incurable [8]. The majority of patients with ovarian cancer experience several relapses and are treated with repeated courses of chemotherapy (and increasingly biological therapy) over long periods of time, typically several years. The psychological impact surrounding diagnosis and managing the ongoing uncertainty about prognosis during periods of remission are challenges common to many ovarian cancer patients.

The intensive treatment regimens for ovarian malignancies include chemotherapy and radical cytoreductive surgery and may have consequences for psychological well-being. Common side effects of the cancer and treatment include pain, fatigue, nausea, vomiting and insomnia [8–13] which will impair physical functioning and patients' ability to continue with routine activities to varying degrees. As with other gynaecological cancers, ovarian malignancies also have the potential to cause negative feelings about body image, sexual functioning, reproduction, femininity and relationships. In addition, patients may need to make difficult treatment decisions about whether or not to continue with medical interventions which have the potential to prolong life but can significantly impair its quality. All these issues can be considered as possible risk factors for impaired psychological functioning.

For a subset of ovarian cancer patients and their family, additional concerns will occur surrounding the risk of hereditary disease. Around 5–10 % of ovarian cancers are believed to be the result of gene mutations in BRCA1 and BRCA2. Whereas the risk of the developing ovarian cancer in general population is around 1–2 %, women carrying a gene mutation are at a 14–40 % risk [14]. Additionally, hereditary non-polyposis colorectal cancer (HNPCC) is an autosomal dominant condition [15], associated with a 10–36 % lifetime risk of ovarian cancer risk [16]. Therefore, exploring and potentially discovering a hereditary risk to ovarian cancer creates another opportunity for stressful decision making for patients and the wider family in addition to the cancer diagnosis.

This chapter will explore findings from the research literature on the degree and nature of psychological distress reported by ovarian cancer patients. A number of studies have explored the psychological well-being of patients diagnosed with ovarian cancer, though in comparison with other more prevalent cancers (e.g. breast), ovarian malignancies are far less well represented in the literature. Evidence from recent research will be drawn on to describe the key variables found to be associated with distress in the ovarian patient population. Guidance for detecting and managing distress and interventions to support psychological well-being in ovarian cancer will also be discussed along with recommendations for improving the psychological care provided for this group.

Psychological Distress and Ovarian Cancer: The Extent of the Problem and Risk Factors

Overview of Research to Date

In 2008, a systematic review of 18 studies was published describing psychological distress in ovarian cancer and associated variables [17]. To be included in the review, studies were required to present data exclusively from ovarian patients or as a clearly separate component of a wider gynaecological sample and to have used standardised and validated tools for measuring psychological distress. From the 18 papers identified, overall levels of depression were found to be higher for ovarian populations than normative groups with those scoring above clinical cut-offs ranging from 21 to 33 %. Anxiety was more prevalent than depression with clinical levels reaching 47 % at 3 months after treatment in one study [18].

The review highlights some key variables associated with distress levels. One of the main findings was the substantial evidence linking physical functions and symptoms with psychological well-being. This link was described in one of the earliest studies by Kornblith and colleagues [19] who investigated 151 ovarian cancer patients on treatment every 3 months for a year using a battery of quality of life measures (including the Mental Health Inventory, MHI, and the

Memorial Symptom Assessment Scale, MSAS). At the first time point, a third or more of patients were reporting symptoms in the moderate to very severe range for anxiety and depression on the MSAS. Using the MHI scores, 33 % had high global distress with 22 % being highly anxious and 17 % highly depressed. Distress was associated with worse physical symptomatology, worse physical functioning and advanced disease. Demographic variables (age and marital status and disease stage) were not significant. Over the course of the study, around 23 % of patients appeared resilient to distress, and at 12 months a subset of the cohort had a relatively good quality of life despite advanced disease.

The results from subsequent studies add to these findings from Kornblith and colleagues [19]. In Bodurka-Bevers et al.'s [20] cross-sectional exploration of anxiety and depression in ovarian cancer, 246 patients completed measures of quality of life, anxiety and depression. The majority of the samples (74 %) were diagnosed with advanced disease, and approximately half were receiving treatment at the time of data collection. Worse emotional function was reported by the patients on active treatment compared to those receiving posttreatment surveillance. Twenty-one per cent of patients met the clinical cut-off for depression warranting a full clinical evaluation, and 29 % were in the 75th percentile for anxiety. Performance status was linked to both forms of distress, with worse scores on the Zubrod scale of symptoms (self-reported by patients) being associated with worse distress and overall quality of life. Younger women were more likely to be depressed than older patients. Compared to the general population, the participant group reported greater levels of depression and anxiety. However, when considered in the context of their performance status, those with worse symptoms reported levels of depression twice that of the general population and four times that of the women in the study with few or no symptoms. A similar pattern was observed for anxiety.

So two of the first studies to explore psychological distress in ovarian cancer both concluded that a considerable proportion of women report clinically significant levels of anxiety and depression. Poor physical function and symptoms are shown to play an integral role. There has been further convincing support demonstrating the importance of physical impairments as a predictor of distress in ovarian cancer [21–25]. However, the interaction between the range of stressors contributing to psychological well-being is complex and challenging to extricate. Norton et al. [24] investigated the relationship between physical impairment and psychological distress along with the role of patients' personal feelings of illness control. Drawing on findings from the chronic illness literature which suggests an apparent link between better physical functioning and greater perceived control, Norton and colleagues tested the hypothesis with patients undergoing chemotherapy or radiotherapy for ovarian cancer. Overall, the sample reported significantly higher distress levels compared to normative data, with older patients reporting less anxiety and depression. Worse physical impairment was significantly correlated with higher distress. As predicted, patients who believed they had less control over their treatment reported worse distress. This suggests the stress of impaired physical functioning which can result in individuals not being able to perform usual activities serves as a means to reduce feelings of personal control over their illness. This potential ongoing stressor can then lead to increased psychological distress as the patient is unable to continue their normal life. Interventions to promote personal feelings of control in the event of functional difficulty are recommended by the authors.

Researchers have also been interested in exploring the role social support plays in women's distress when faced with a diagnosis of ovarian cancer [18, 24, 26]. When the relationship between psychological function and social support was assessed in 63 ovarian cancer patients at the completion of chemotherapy (a time believed to be associated with fear and anxiety about the withdrawal of medical care) and 3 months later, poor perceived emotional support was associated with worse anxiety [18]. Clinical and physical variables, including performance status, stage of disease and time since diagnosis were not significant. In addition an interesting pattern of psychological distress was detected. At time 1, 33 % of the sample scored in the clinical range for anxiety and 38 % did so for depression (with 17 % of individuals being cases for both anxiety and depression). At time 2, 47 % scored in the clinical range for anxiety and 19 % for depression. So whereas cases of anxiety increased over time, depression decreased. These results are explained by the authors in relation to the vulnerability patients' feel at the cessation of treatment when the safety of regular medical attention stops or becomes less frequent and fears about detecting disease progression are commonplace.

Few studies with longitudinal assessments of psychological functioning during and beyond ovarian cancer treatment have been conducted. A study from the UK [21] followed patients (diagnosed at any stage of disease) from the beginning of chemotherapy until 3 months posttreatment. The role of social support on anxiety and depression was explored along with levels of neuroticism. Measures were completed by the sample at four time points. Throughout the period of assessment, the authors predicted identifying three morbidity profiles: (1) stable cases of distress, (2) occasional cases and (3) non-cases. Poor social support and high neuroticism were anticipated to be associated with distress. The results (from 85 women who complete the measures across all time points) showed that women were most commonly categorised into the occasional case profile for anxiety (52 %). For depression the majority were non-cases (55 %). Thus, depression was not prevalent in the group, and anxiety was intermittent. More detailed analysis revealed that stable cases of anxiety were associated with younger age, being married and higher neuroticism. Being a non-case for depression was associated with better health status and being further from diagnosis. Cases of depression were associated with a diagnosis of advanced disease. Perceived social support was not associated with psychological morbidity. Although the role of social support was not endorsed, younger women were again shown to fare worse psychologically in line with other studies [18, 23, 24, 27–30] and highlight the potential vulnerability of this group who appear to experience greater adjustment problems when faced with their diagnosis and coping with its impact on their life.

Post-traumatic stress disorder (PTSD) is classified as an anxiety disorder and can develop following a life-threatening experience [31]. Symptoms of PTSD may emerge months or years after the event and include re-experiencing the trauma and avoiding people and places which are reminiscent of the experience. PTSD has been investigated in the wider cancer population, and a few studies have specifically examined post-traumatic stress in ovarian cancer patients [22, 30, 32–35]. When a measure of PTSD was included as part of a longitudinal assessment of ovarian cancer [32], it appeared that patients experienced PTSD across the early phases of the cancer trajectory with cases rising from 36 % at the beginning of treatment to 45 % after the completion of chemotherapy at 3-month follow-up. Only 30 % of the sample was not found to have PTSD at some point during the study. Younger women emerge again as the most susceptible, but medical characteristics were not associated with cases of PTSD. Even years after treatment, 26 % of long-term survivors of early-stage ovarian cancer gave scores on the Post-Traumatic Stress Disorder Checklist which were indicative of PTSD [33]. PTSD may become more prevalent in women over time as the extent of the disease and its consequences become apparent; however, it is possible for the condition to occur at different points throughout the cancer experience.

Although many women with ovarian cancer will have later-stage malignancy at the time of diagnosis, around a third present with stage I or II disease and the possibility of positive long-term prognosis [7]. A recent study compared women who had been diagnosed (at least 3 years previously) with either early ($n=58$) or advanced ($n=42$) ovarian disease [34]. No difference between the two groups was found on the quality of life or mental health variables assessed. Other researches specifically focusing on the psychological well-being of early-stage ovarian cancer patients in the years after treatment suggests the majority of women cope well emotionally with their experience and enjoy good quality of life [25, 33, 36]. However, fear of recurrence is still reported by many women and is associated with distress [33]. Elevated levels of anxiety are also documented years after treatment [36] with fears surrounding follow-up and test results being common [25]. Menopausal status appears to be a significant variable associated with distress [25, 36]. As early-stage ovarian cancer patients are typically younger than their later-stage counterparts, these women may face different challenges as a consequence of their disease experience. For example, the impact of disease and treatment on ability to conceive and fears about long-term prognosis for those with a young family are more common problems for women in younger age categories. In addition, symptoms of the menopause may be particularly more challenging to deal with in women who are premenopausal at the time of diagnosis.

Regardless of disease stage issues surrounding the disclosure of medical information and the provision of clinical care can be a source of distress for patients. There are a number of uncertainties surrounding the best way to follow up patients after treatment for ovarian cancer [37]. In particular concern has been raised about the potential negative impact of routine surveillance of the cancer antigen 125 (CA-125) tumour marker on patients' distress levels [38, 39]. This marker is routinely used as an indicator of disease progression, but patient's preoccupation with the results has been associated with depression and anxiety [29, 38, 40]. Although the value of the marker has been questioned, patients are very keen to obtain the test results even when they are informed of its limitations [41]. The results of a recent systematic review of follow-up care for ovarian cancer patients highlight the paucity of data on the psychological implications of different follow-up strategies following primary treatment [42].

Powers et al. [43] conducted a qualitative study with women from different stages of the ovarian cancer trajectory to explore patient perspectives on disease-related distress and coping. Women reported experiencing distress associated to a number of different issues linked to their medical care such as the gap in support between cancer diagnosis and initial appointments with oncologists and poor communication at times with medical staff. Some also expressed a feeling that ovarian cancer is under researched and therefore a 'forgotten cancer' in comparison with other tumour groups. As a result they believed the signs and symptoms of their illness had not readily been detected by primary care physicians and led to a delay in their diagnosis.

Population-Based Studies

Data from population-based research are now becoming available and provide insight into the psychological functioning of large numbers of affected patients. Recent data from the quality of life component of the Australian Ovarian Cancer Study [44] explores distress in ovarian cancer patients (n=798) and caregivers (n=373, 72 % male spouses). Using mailed questionnaires, information on distress (Hospital Anxiety and Depression Scale, HADS), symptom burden, social support, optimism and use of mental treatment and supportive services was collected [45]. The patients compared favourably with normative HADS data for anxiety (15.0 % of patients reached reported clinical levels vs 16.0 % in the general population). Levels of depression were however double that of the normative population (5.9 % vs 3.0 %). These levels are still considerably lower than reports in the earlier studies mentioned above. Higher levels of distress were associated with worse perceived social support, lower optimism and worse symptom burden. Caregivers were found to have significantly more cases of clinical anxiety in comparison with norms (18.8 % vs 12.6 %). A similar pattern was reported for clinical levels of depression in this group (5.1 % vs 3.6 %). Comparisons between the patient and caregivers showed that distress was significantly lower for patients. The significant predictors of distress in caregivers were younger age, worse perceived social support and lower scores of optimism. Being the offspring of the patient was associated with worse distress in comparison to caregivers who were spouses. The authors speculate the lower levels of distress found in patients may be indicative of the larger and more representative sample size recruited and the possibility that mental health problems are now better recognised in the community. Indeed, many patients who acknowledged having mental health problems were receiving specialist treatment. Caregivers certainly appear to experience considerable burden and anxiety related to looking after a loved one with ovarian cancer. The extent of distress found in the carer group is concerning and demonstrates the need for wider support mechanisms that extend beyond the patient.

Although the findings from Australia depict a favourable picture of distress levels in ovarian cancer patients, sub-analysis of a large epidemiological study in the USA provides a stark warning message about the psychological vulnerability of some women [46]. Data from the US Surveillance, Epidemiology and End Results (SEER) Program of the National Cancer Institute for the period of 1988–2007 were analysed to investigate suicide rates and associated risk factors in patients diagnosed with gynaecologic cancers (ovarian, uterine, cervical, vulvar and vaginal). For the period, 252,235 patients with gynaecologic cancer were identified of whom 100 committed suicide. Overall the suicide rate was significantly higher than the general population, specifically in the ovarian group, principally during the first year after diagnosis (though relative suicide risks persisted over time). The need for implementing effective strategies to detect unrecognised distress and provide psychological support is again evident, particularly for women with ovarian malignancies.

Positive Psychological Consequences of Ovarian Cancer

It is understandable that researchers have principally focussed attention on the negative consequences of cancer given its potential to effect function and well-being. There is however an appreciation that the experience of a chronic or life-threatening condition can have a positive impact on patient's lives and emotional outlook [47, 48]. A number of different terms have been used to describe this phenomenon including benefit finding, post-traumatic growth, stress-related growth and found or discovered meaning. From the ovarian literature, Molassiotis et al. [28] found that of early-stage patients who completed a measure of post-traumatic growth, 66 % appreciated the value of life and 59 % recognised a change in life priorities as a result of their cancer. Ovarian patients have also reported positive reactions to their experience by acknowledging altered perspectives including their relationships and an ability to take greater pleasure in different aspect of their lives that they had not done previously [49]. In Hodgkinson et al.'s [22] assessment of long-term survivors of gynaecologic cancers (27.1 % ovarian), around half of the sample felt they had grown up as a person, valued life and appreciated relationships with others more. Husbands of ovarian cancer patients have also acknowledged the disease can result in positive changes in the relationship with their partner [50].

Lutgendorf et al. [51] assessed quality of life, mood and coping style in 98 gynaecological cancer patients (25 % of whom had ovarian malignancies) at initial clinic visits and a year later. They discovered that women who used active coping skills including positive reframing and acceptance of their illness reported better emotional, functional and physical well-being and higher quality of life overall. Being able to positively reframe their diagnosis and come to terms with the cancer may help individuals to feel an enhanced sense of control over the illness experience, a similar concept to that previously described above in Norton et al.'s [24] exploration of the role of perceived control on physical function and distress.

Ponto et al. [30] investigated predictors of adjustment and growth in 60 women with recurrent ovarian cancer. Although the variables with most significance to better adjustment appeared to be older age, better performance status and less symptom distress, finding positive meaning in the illness experience also had a significant, if weak, association. Overall, the women reported having grown from their illness experience. Data of this kind lends support to the idea of developing psychological interventions which assist women in positively reframing their illness experience.

Summary of the Research and Study Limitations

The research described above demonstrates that a range of psychological assessments in the ovarian cancer population have been conducted, and although most women cope well with their disease, a subset will experience significant distress that may warrant intervention. Psychological distress is common around diagnosis, but anxiety, depression and PTSD can occur at later points when the full impact of the disease and treatment are realised. Anxieties about follow-up and the threat of recurrence make the ovarian cancer group vulnerable even when long-term survivorship status is achieved. Arden-Close et al. [17] concluded from their systematic view that anxiety was more prevalent than depression in the ovarian cancer, and although depression decreases with time since diagnosis, it remains a problem for a subset of patients even years after treatment.

In Arden-Close et al.'s [17] review, the 18 studies were rated for methodological quality in terms of rationale, disease variables reported, study design, statistical analysis, quality of measures and conclusions drawn. Based on these criteria, studies were rated as either methodologically good ($n = 12$), average ($n = 5$) or poor ($n = 1$). This allowed an assessment to be made of the level of evidence for each variable associated with distress based on the standard of the studies from which findings originated. The significant variables associated with distress and the degree of evidence for each are summarised in Table 13.1. As mentioned throughout this chapter, younger age has been consistently associated with higher levels of distress in a range of good quality studies. A strong verification for the link between distress and advanced disease, worse performance status and physical impairments are also well established in the literature. Of the other clinical variables, only time since diagnosis had strong evidence to support a link with distress, with three good quality studies indicating distress is worse around the time of diagnosis. The extent to which being on active treatment and experiencing a cancer recurrence are risk factors for distress remains unclear. Though both have the potential to have psychological repercussions, some women will find the follow-up phases of medical care anxiety provoking as they wait for signs of disease progression. Although recurrence has negative connotations for prognosis, women do not necessarily experience heightened distress. This may be because they have previous experience of the disease and have had time to adapt to their circumstances and recurrence risk.

The studies reviewed here provide insight into the distress associated with ovarian malignancies,

Table 13.1 Factors correlated with distress in ovarian cancer

Level of evidence	Factor	Most frequently observed observation
Strong	Age	Younger age—more distress
	Disease stage	More advanced disease—more distress
	Time since diagnosis	Shorter—more distress
	Disability status	Worse—more distress
	Physical symptoms	More symptoms—more distress
	Quality of life	Poorer quality of life—more distress
Some	Perceived social support	More social support—less distress
Inconclusive	Active chemotherapy/follow-up	Chemotherapy—more distress
	Phase of treatment: initial/recurrence	Recurrence—more distress
	Site of cancer	Ovarian more distress
	Previous level of depression	More—more distress
	Previous level of anxiety	More—more distress
	Previous level of intrusive thoughts	More—more distress

Adapted from Arden-Close et al. [17]

but it is important to acknowledge limitations in the research. These include medical information not being systematically reported in psychological studies (e.g. type of treatment). Where it is reported, patients have often been asked to provide this information which may result in the collection of erroneous data. Vice versa, in medical studies with a psychological component, sociodemographic information about the sample is often excluded [17]. In addition there is considerable variation in measures of distress used with some emotional subscales of general quality of life assessment being used as reports of psychological well-being. Debate surrounds the value of popular assessment tools including what the clinical cut-offs should be and which measures are most appropriate for which stage of the cancer trajectory [52, 53]. Also no studies used formal psychiatric interviews to determine distress in patients though this is regarded as the gold standard for diagnosing depression.

Although larger-scale ovarian population data is becoming available from some countries [45, 46], many of the studies of ovarian cancer have involved small sample sizes without control groups; instead, data has mostly been compared to general population data available for the specific measures of distress used [17].

Further research is needed to explore the variables associated with distress related to ovarian cancer which rectify the issues outlined above. In particular more longitudinal studies would be a valuable addition. In addition, a systematic review [42] of follow-up care strategies following primary treatment for ovarian cancer points to the need for randomised trials with an emphasis on quality of life and psychological well-being in addition to survival outcomes and cost-effectiveness.

Detecting and Managing Psychological Distress Related to Ovarian Cancer

Although the emotional challenges associated with cancer have been well documented, many patients continue to express a need for psychological support [54–57]. In the UK, USA and Australia, international guidelines have been developed to provide recommendations and evidence-based advice on supporting cancer patients and their families throughout the disease trajectory [1, 58, 59]. These all outline the need for cancer services to regularly assess patients' distress levels and for any detected problems to be addressed by staff with the appropriate degree of training skills and knowledge.

The guidance documents also recommend stepped care or triaged systems where patients are referred when appropriate to the most suitable specialist support (e.g. psychologist, counsellor, social worker). This approach highlights the role that all health-care professionals caring for cancer patients can have in the detection and management of cancer patients' distress. Although more specialist psychological care should be provided by trained individuals, members of nursing staff, health-care workers and doctors can all assist with low- or mid-level distress by communicating effectively and compassionately with patients, being vigilant to any signs that warrant exploration and referring to other professionals where necessary. In England, advanced communication skills training is mandatory for all staff involved with cancer and palliative care [60]. In concordance with the general supportive guidance for all cancer populations, specific recommendations for gynaecological cancers call for oncology teams to practise a high standard of communication and information provision to minimise patient anxiety. Along with patients being given the name of a nurse trained in counselling, the maintenance of close links with psychology and psychiatry is advised to ensure psychological support is available at every stage of care.

Determining which patients require support for psychological distress can be challenging for a number of reasons. Patients can be unwilling to disclose problems, and professionals may focus on the medical management of cancer [61]. The guidance documents described above recommend the routine use of screening for psychological distress, and a number of studies show that standardised self-reported tools correctly identify a larger proportion of distressed patients than health professionals [61–63]. There is also evidence from randomised trials indicating that the provision of screening tool information to oncologists leads to improvements in patient's emotional well-being [64–67]. However, translating the value of systematic screening for distress into routine cancer practice is not simple. Stumbling blocks to routine implementation include practical considerations related to resource and financial limitations and the ability to utilise new technologies of data collection (such as using touch screen computers to collect information from patients). Surveys from the USA and UK show that many cancer centres and professionals are not using screening tools to detect distress [68, 69]. A recent qualitative study of cancer professionals found that feelings of reticence to use screening tools centred on the perceived costs to services and the ability to successfully cope with identified distress [70]. There is also continued debate about the most appropriate screening measure for cancer distress across the disease trajectory [53]. The NCCN endorse the use of the distress thermometer (DT) as a practical and simple approach to routine screening [1]. The DT assesses distress on a 0–10 scale with a problem list to indicate reasons contributing to distress levels. It has been widely validated and used in a variety of cancer populations including gynaecological patients [71–73].

In terms of managing distress, there is a question as to the degree to which limited psychological resources should focus on those exhibiting persistent distress or if interventions should more generally target patients early in stages of treatment to prevent psychological morbidity developing in at-risk groups. The results from studies demonstrating the positive impact of ovarian cancer have led to the idea of interventions to promote well-being via supporting the mechanisms for development of positive meaning from a diagnosis of ovarian cancer. Recently the Meaning-Making intervention (MMi) has been pilot tested in a small number of newly diagnosed advanced-stage ovarian cancer patients [74]. In this randomised controlled trial (RCT), 12 patients received an intervention consisting of three to four sessions with a therapist which focussed on (1) reviewing the impact and meaning of the cancer diagnosis, (2) exploring past significant life events and successful ways of coping and (3) discussing life priority and goal changes that give meaning to one's life. At the end of the trial, compared to controls the intervention group reported a better sense of meaning in life. There was some evidence that fewer women in intervention group met the clinical cut-off for anxiety and depression on the HADS, but further large-scale assessment of the clinical impact of the MMi is required. Consideration into how resource intensive interventions of this kind might be modified for use with large numbers of patients in routine practice would also be necessary.

A recent review of psychosocial interventions for gynaecological cancer patients assessed findings from 22 controlled trials [75]. Emotional adjustment was assessed in all the studies, and interventions included psychotherapy, counselling, relaxation/complementary therapies and provision of education and support. The results were inconclusive due to limitations in research design; however, there was some evidence that counselling and psychoeducation were beneficial for mood and distress. As with Arden-Close et al.'s [17] systematic review, Hersch and colleagues found that many studies were weakened by small sample sizes and a lack of longitudinal research, meaning the longer-term impact of interventions, remains unknown. Kew et al.'s [42] review of follow-up care strategies in ovarian cancer services concludes there is a need for prospective trials to evaluate interventions during follow-up that may help reduce anxiety and promote return to normal functioning.

Psychological Distress and Hereditary Ovarian Cancer

The Impact of Genetic Counselling and Screening

Alongside the distress associated with a diagnosis of ovarian cancer and coping with the disease and treatment, women with a family history of the disease and an increased hereditary risk are confronted with challenging decisions about managing the threat. Initially focus can centre on whether or not to receive genetic counselling and screening. Choices also need to be made about whether or not to disclose information to or involve other family members who may also be at risk. These issues can place increased burden on the patients and family members, and if a genetic predisposition is found to be present, additional potentially stressful medical care decisions are required. A range of unique emotional consequences for people at hereditary cancer risk are possible with feelings of uncertainty sadness, worry, anxiety, anger and guilt being commonplace [76].

There has been substantial research conducted in the area of the psychological impact of screening for hereditary cancer perhaps because the *BRCA1/2* genes are linked to the development of both breast and ovarian cancers. Although the positive implications of screening include being able to encourage informed health choices for managing cancer risk, researchers have been conscious that being faced with this threatening information may have adverse consequences on psychological functioning [77]. Although not all individuals tested for genetic mutations will be identified as carriers, the process of testing in itself can still be emotionally demanding. In addition a subset of people will receive inconclusive results where neither *BRCA* gene is identified, but there may still be a hereditary cancer risk, the genetic cause of which being unknown. How these people process and understand their test results and how this affects them emotionally is not well understood as the population has been identified as being particularly under researched [78].

Women with a family history of ovarian cancer who seek advice and genetic screening have been found to have higher levels of anxiety and depression compared to the general population [79–81]. The levels of distress observed in these groups highlight the importance of providing emotional and psychological support integrated as standard in screening programmes. A variety of studies have used measures specifically designed to assess distress related to cancer risk or genetic testing, and perhaps unsurprisingly many have shown that women found to test positive for genetic mutations report greater distress than those with negative results [82–84].

Other studies have however not routinely produced comparable findings regarding the impact of testing on distress levels. Inconsistencies in research results led to a meta-analysis of data to ascertain the extent of general anxiety and cancer-related distress in people undergoing *BRCA1/2* mutation screening and to explore differences between carriers, non-carrier groups and those with inconclusive results [85]. Hamilton and colleagues synthesised the data from 20 studies that had all prospectively assessed distress before genetic testing and up to 1 year after. Collectively the studies included data from 2,171 participants, the majority were female (95.2 %), 664 were gene mutation carriers, 794 non-carriers and 713 were given inconclusive test results. In line with past findings and Baum et al.'s [86] framework for interpreting responses to genetic testing from a stress and coping perspective, the authors predicted that non-carriers would experience a decrease in distress after receiving results and that carriers and those with inconclusive results would experience stable or increased distress with levels lessening with time as individuals adapted. The findings showed the importance of time for all groups. As predicted, distress levels of carriers increased slightly after receipt of test results but returned to pretest levels over time. Carriers with a personal history of cancer experienced less distress than carriers who had not. Non-carriers reported decreases in general and cancer-specific distress soon after testing, only the latter persisted over time. Most surprisingly, the group with inconclusive results showed decreases in cancer-related distress similar in magnitude to that reported by non-carriers. This led Hamilton et al. to question if this group is misinterpreting their results and considering themselves to be at a reduced cancer risk. Indeed, qualitative interviews with women with a previous diagnosis of breast or ovarian cancer who had undergone *BRCA1/2* screening found that those with inconclusive results did not correctly comprehend its meaning and thought the hereditary risk was not present in their family [87]. Further research is required in this area to clarify the emotional impact of inconclusive genetic testing and how this is associated with individual perceptions of cancer risk.

Hamilton et al.'s [85] meta-analysis also provides evidence of some national variation in carrier distress levels. Specifically, carriers in the USA reported greater decreases in distress compared to those in Europe or Australia. This may be an indication of the impact of the varying health services available in different countries. In the USA, issues surrounding health insurance and the costs associated with any ongoing follow-up care by those found to be at risk of a hereditary cancer may add to concerns and anxieties about personal health. Thus, the non-carrier group may experience an enhanced sense of relief on receiving test results. Overall the results show that genetic testing for *BRCA1/2* mutations does have emotional consequences, but these appear to be minimised with time. It is important to note that the authors highlight that the participants in the samples analysed had typically received extensive genetic counselling which will have played a role in supporting the challenges and consequences of the testing process.

How families as a whole communicate and manage issues surrounding genetic risk is an important consideration with considerable implications for how personal risk is understood and for the psychological health of individual members. Within the cancer population generally more open communication has been linked with less distress in patient and family members [88, 89]. Less openness to discuss genetic test results with family members has been associated with more cancer worry and distress in female *BRCA1/2* carriers 5 years after tests were conducted [90]. Mellon and colleagues [91] explored communication and decision making about inherited cancer risk in a series of focus groups involving family pairs consisting of breast or ovarian cancer patients with increased hereditary risk and a close female relative. The women reported using different communication strategies to cope with the cancer experience; some openly discussed it, whereas others avoided conversations due to fear of making the risk too real. Many women were misinformed or unknowledgeable about the role genetics and heredity play in cancer risk and their understanding centred on their own personal experiences of cancer in the family. Concerns centred on the health of other family members, increased vigilance for detecting any signs of cancer, and in some cases the fear of finding out their cancer risk prevented them pursuing testing. Similar responses from families uncertain about testing were also detected in a qualitative study conducted by Dancyger et al. [92]. The challenge for clinicians caring for at-risk patients is in understanding the psychological variables and family context in which individuals are making personal decisions about testing.

Psychological Implications of the Medical Management of Hereditary Risk

For women found to carry the genetic mutations putting them at risk of ovarian cancer, the two major medical strategies available are increased surveillance to improve the chances of early cancer detection (routine assessment of CA-125 levels and transvaginal ultrasound) or risk-reducing salpingo-oophorectomy (RRSO, surgical removal of the healthy ovaries and fallopian tubes) [93]. Surveillance has not to date proven to be a highly successful option, as it has led to an increased number of false-positive test results or the detection of ovarian cancer at later stages [94–96].

Many women are reluctant to take the RRSO option and in the UK Familial Ovarian Cancer Screening Study (UK FOCSS) [97] is an ongoing trial due to close in 2013 assessing the clinical effectiveness of familial ovarian cancer screening using CA-125 markers (measured every 4 months) and annual ultrasound scans. The trial also includes a psychosocial component to explore the psychological impact of screening (PsyFOCS). A recently published study from this psychosocial arm explored the factors associated with women dropping out of the screening programme in order to have RRSO [98]. Lifford and colleagues found that both clinical and psychological variables were associated with women opting for surgery; specifically women who had in the past been recalled for further tests (as a result of participating in the screening programme) and greater cancer-specific distress were both significant variables in the uptake of surgery. In a recent review of factors associated with women opting for RRSO [99], a range of significant demographic and psychological variables were identified. Women who were older, had children, had a family history of ovarian cancer or a personal history of breast cancer, had prophylactic mastectomy and were *BRCA1/2* mutation carriers were all more likely to undergo RRSO. Greater perceived risk of ovarian cancer and cancer-related anxiety were also predictive. The authors conclude the design of decisions aids for women considering prophylactic surgery should cover a range of issues to ensure that demographic and medical background of women are addressed along with psychosocial variables surrounding views of cancer risk.

The guidelines for RRSO promote the use of surgery in at-risk women who have completed child bearing [100]. The negative consequences of surgery include the general risks associated with the procedure, the impact of hormone deprivation, leading to immediate menopause, as well as the continued risk of breast and peritoneal cancer which RRSO cannot completely eliminate. These reasons are likely to lead to a high percentage of women who choose not to undergo the procedure [99]. The impact of RRSO on psychological well-being is uncertain. Researchers in the UK found that women who have surgery reported worse emotional and physical symptoms than those remaining on screening programmes, whereas the levels of cancer worry were comparable between the two groups [101]. This small study (which retrospectively investigated 29 women who had received RRSO and compared them to 28 on screening) also reported that problems were worse in women who were premenopausal at the time of RRSO which may be a reflection of the impact of coping with unfamiliar and debilitating menopausal symptoms. Younger age at the time of RRSO has also been associated with greater anxiety. There is however also evidence of psychological benefit of RRSO despite the physical side effects and potential risk of impairments to quality of life and body image [90, 99]. Michelsen et al.'s [102] observational questionnaire study of 361 Norwegian women who had undergone RRSO found that that women reported more somatic morbidity (including osteoporosis, palpitations, constipation and pain) but comparable anxiety and lower depression (measured using the HADS) compared to age-matched population data. Although many women report a high degree of satisfaction with their decision to go ahead with RRSO [99, 103], the need for ongoing counselling, support and information for women who choose to either undergo RRSO or screening is essential [104].

Conclusions

Many women diagnosed with ovarian cancer cope well with the experience of their disease and treatment, even finding some positive benefit to their outlook on life and relationships in response to the disease. A subset of approximately a third of women, however, are at risk of significant distress, and this appears to be particularly related to worse physical function, younger age, proximity to diagnosis and advanced disease. Although the recent large and representative population study from Australia suggests ovarian cancer patients may experience less distress than previously documented [45], it is of concern that levels of suicide appear to be particularly high in this group in comparison with other gynaecological cancers [46]. Over time women's distress levels may improve as they adapt to the shock of their diagnosis, but as many will experience disease progression and worsening physical symptoms, professionals should remain vigilant to distress at all stages of the disease. The conclusions of much of the literature covered in this chapter call for strategic and routine screening for distress in ovarian cancer, but despite the cancer guidelines also recommending such strategies, the actual implementation into services is not well established, and many barriers exist. The future challenge for researchers is to promote the value of routine screening and help support their systematic use into cancer services.

Limitations in the studies exploring psychological distress in ovarian cancer and those assessing interventions to improve psychosocial well-being include the lack of longitudinal studies, mixed methods in assessing distress and small sample sizes. Ovarian cancer is less well investigated in the literature compared to more prevalent cancer groups, and researchers should work towards conducting well-designed studies which add greater clarity on how distress changes over time for patients and how and when supportive interventions might be best used to limit the levels of distress in at-risk groups (such as those with worse physical symptoms and women in younger age categories).

Continued treatment developments for ovarian malignancies means that women are living for longer periods following diagnosis. Decisions about long-term follow-up and medical surveillance for disease progression continue to be an important issue for patients given the anxieties and fears about disease recurrence reported by many. As pointed out in a recent review [42], more randomised trials of follow-up care strategies are required that incorporate assessments of psychological and quality of life outcomes.

Patients and families affected by hereditary ovarian cancer are susceptible to additional distress. The need for supportive genetic counselling and the monitoring of psychological well-being in this patient group is also essential. Interestingly the findings from Hamilton's systematic review showed that people receiving inconclusive tests results reported the same levels of distress than those found not to be carriers of the *BRCA1/2* genes. This is an example of how measuring distress can be useful in determining how cancer risk is being comprehended or misinterpreted by different groups. Individuals at risk of hereditary disease face many complex decisions in relation to deciding whether or not to receive genetic testing and choosing medical surveillance options when a genetic predisposition is discovered. The provision of well-designed information and excellent communication skills among the professionals involved in the care of these patients is vital to limit distress as far as possible.

Many challenges remain in our understanding of the psychological implications of ovarian cancer. Future changes to the care and treatment patients receive will continue to influence how patients cope with the disease. For example, results from studies evaluating the value of ovarian cancer screening in the general population are expected in coming years [105]. If shown to be successful, screening may result in ovarian cancer routinely being diagnosed at less advanced stages which will undoubtedly be of benefit for the life expectancy and the psychological well-being of patients. In the meantime the focus should be on developing strategies to successfully detect distress and support affected patients throughout all the stages of their treatment and follow-up.

References

1. National Comprehensive Cancer Network Clinical Practice Guidelines in Oncology: Distress Management Version 2.2013. http://www.nccn.org/professionals/physician_gls/f_guidelines.asp. Accessed 9 Aug 2013
2. Zabora J, BrintzenhofeSzoc K, Curbow B, Hooker C, Piantadosi S. The prevalence of psychological distress by cancer site. Psychooncology. 2001;10(1):19–28.
3. Fann JR, Thomas-Rich AM, Katon WJ, et al. Major depression after breast cancer: a review of epidemiology and treatment. Gen Hosp Psychiatry. 2008;30(2):112–26.
4. Watson M, Haviland JS, Greer S, Davidson J, Bliss JM. Influence of psychological response on survival in breast cancer: a population-based cohort study. Lancet. 1999;354(9187):1331–6.
5. Carlson LE, Bultz BD. Benefits of psychosocial oncology care: improved quality of life and medical cost offset. Health Qual Life Outcomes. 2003;1:8.
6. Simpson JS, Carlson LE, Trew ME. Effect of group therapy for breast cancer on healthcare utilization. Cancer Pract. 2001;9(1):19–26.
7. Cancer Research UK. Ovarian cancer survival statistics. http://info.cancerresearchuk.org/cancerstats/types/ovary/survival/#stage. Accessed 01 Dec 2011.

8. Hennessy BT, Coleman RL, Markman M. Ovarian cancer. Lancet. 2009;374(9698):1371–82.
9. Casey C, Chen LM, Rabow M. Symptom management in gynecologic malignancies. Expert Rev Anticancer Ther. 2011;11(7):1077–89.
10. Kayl AE, Meyers CA. Side-effects of chemotherapy and quality of life in ovarian and breast cancer patients. Curr Opin Obstet Gynecol. 2006;18(1):24–8.
11. Portenoy RK, Kornblith AB, Wong G, et al. Pain in ovarian-cancer patients - prevalence, characteristics, and associated symptoms. Cancer. 1994;74(3):907–15.
12. Price MA, Zachariae R, Butow PN, et al. Prevalence and predictors of insomnia in women with invasive ovarian cancer: anxiety a major factor. Eur J Cancer. 2009;45(18):3262–70.
13. Sun CC, Bodurka DC, Donato ML, et al. Patient preferences regarding side effects of chemotherapy for ovarian cancer: do they change over time? Gynecol Oncol. 2002;87(1):118–28.
14. National Cancer Institute. PDQ® Cancer Information Summary Genetics of Breast and Ovarian Cancer (PDQ®) - Health Professional. http://www.cancer.gov/cancertopics/pdq/genetics/breast-and-ovarian/healthprofessional. Accessed 01 Dec 2011.
15. Vasen HFA, Stormorken A, Menko FH, et al. MSH2 mutation carriers are at higher risk of cancer than MLH1 mutation carriers: a study of hereditary nonpolyposis colorectal cancer families. J Clin Oncol. 2001;19(20):4074–80.
16. Manchanda R, Menon U, Michaelson-Cohen R, Beller U, Jacobs I. Hereditary non-polyposis colorectal cancer or Lynch syndrome: the gynaecological perspective. Curr Opin Obstet Gynecol. 2009;21(1):31–8.
17. Arden-Close E, Gidron Y, Moss-Morris R. Psychological distress and its correlates in ovarian cancer: a systematic review. Psychooncology. 2008;17(11):1061–72.
18. Hipkins J, Whitworth M, Tarrier N, Jayson G. Social support, anxiety and depression after chemotherapy for ovarian cancer: a prospective study. Br J Health Psychol. 2004;9(Pt 4):569–81.
19. Kornblith AB, Thaler HT, Wong G, et al. Quality of life of women with ovarian cancer. Gynecol Oncol. 1995;59(2):231–42.
20. Bodurka-Bevers D, Basen-Engquist K, Carmack CL, et al. Depression, anxiety, and quality of life in patients with epithelial ovarian cancer. Gynecol Oncol. 2000;78(3 Pt 1):302–8.
21. Goncalves V, Jayson G, Tarrier N. A longitudinal investigation of psychological morbidity in patients with ovarian cancer. Br J Cancer. 2008;99(11):1794–801.
22. Hodgkinson K, Butow P, Fuchs A, et al. Long-term survival from gynecologic cancer: psychosocial outcomes, supportive care needs and positive outcomes. Gynecol Oncol. 2007;104(2):381–9.
23. Norton TR, Manne SL, Rubin S, et al. Prevalence and predictors of psychological distress among women with ovarian cancer. J Clin Oncol. 2004;22(5):919–26.
24. Norton TR, Manne SL, Rubin S, et al. Ovarian cancer patients' psychological distress: the role of physical impairment, perceived unsupportive family and friend behaviors, perceived control, and self-esteem. Health Psychol. 2005;24(2):143–52.
25. Wenzel LB, Donnelly JP, Fowler JM, et al. Resilience, reflection, and residual stress in ovarian cancer survivorship: a gynecologic oncology group study. Psychooncology. 2002;11(2):142–53.
26. Petersen RW, Graham G, Quinlivan JA. Psychologic changes after a gynecologic cancer. J Obstet Gynaecol Res. 2005;31(2):152–7.
27. Boscaglia N, Clarke DM, Jobling TW, Quinn MA. The contribution of spirituality and spiritual coping to anxiety and depression in women with a recent diagnosis of gynecological cancer. Int J Gynecol Cancer. 2005;15(5):755–61.
28. Molassiotis A, Chan CW, Yam BM, Chan SJ. Quality of life in Chinese women with gynaecological cancers. Support Care Cancer. 2000;8(5):414–22.
29. Parker PA, Kudelka A, Basen-Engquist K, Kavanagh J, de Moor J, Cohen L. The associations between knowledge, CA125 preoccupation, and distress in women with epithelial ovarian cancer. Gynecol Oncol. 2006;100(3):495–500.
30. Ponto JA, Ellington L, Mellon S, Beck SL. Predictors of adjustment and growth in women with recurrent ovarian cancer. Oncol Nurs Forum. 2010;37(3):357–64.
31. American Psychiatric Association. Diagnostic and statistical manual of mental disorders. 4th ed. Washington, DC: APA; 1994. DSM–IV.
32. Goncalves V, Jayson G, Tarrier N. A longitudinal investigation of posttraumatic stress disorder in patients with ovarian cancer. J Psychosom Res. 2011;70(5):422–31.
33. Matulonis UA, Kornblith A, Lee H, et al. Long-term adjustment of early-stage ovarian cancer survivors. Int J Gynecol Cancer. 2008;18(6):1183–93.
34. Mirabeau-Beale KL, Kornblith AB, Penson RT, et al. Comparison of the quality of life of early and advanced stage ovarian cancer survivors. Gynecol Oncol. 2009;114(2):353–9.
35. Posluszny DM, Edwards RP, Dew MA, Baum A. Perceived threat and PTSD symptoms in women undergoing surgery for gynecologic cancer or benign conditions. Psychooncology. 2011;20(7):783–7.
36. Bisseling KCHM, Kondalsamy-Chennakesavan S, Bekkers RLM, Janda M, Obermair A. Depression, anxiety and body image after treatment for invasive stage one epithelial ovarian cancer. Aust N Z J Obstet Gynaecol. 2009;49(6):660–6.
37. Miller RE, Rustin GJ. How to follow-up patients with epithelial ovarian cancer. Curr Opin Oncol. 2010;22(5):498–502.

38. Jordens CF, Morrell B, Harnett P, Hobbs K, Mason C, Kerridge IH. Cancergazing? CA125 and post-treatment surveillance in advanced ovarian cancer. Soc Sci Med. 2010;71(9):1548–56.
39. Karam AK, Karlan BY. Ovarian cancer: the duplicity of CA125 measurement. Nat Rev Clin Oncol. 2010;7(6):335–9.
40. Oskay-Oezcelik G, du Bois A, Fasching PA, et al. What do patients think about CA-125 monitoring in the follow-up? Results from a multicenter trial in 1,060 patients with ovarian cancer. J Clin Oncol. 2009;27(15s):5522.
41. Markman M, Peterson J, Belland A, Burg K. CA-125 monitoring in ovarian cancer: patient survey responses to the results of the MRC/EORTC CA-125 surveillance trial. Oncology. 2010;78:1–2.
42. Kew F, Galaal K, Bryant A, Naik R. Evaluation of follow-up strategies for patients with epithelial ovarian cancer following completion of primary treatment. Cochrane Database Syst Rev. 2011;(6):CD006119.
43. Power J, Brown L, Ritvo P. A qualitative study examining psychosocial distress, coping, and social support across the stages and phases of epithelial ovarian cancer. Health Care Women Int. 2008;29(4):366–83.
44. Australian Ovarian Cancer Study. http://www.aoc-study.org/hp_programme.aspl. Accessed 01 Dec 2011.
45. Price MA, Butow PN, Costa DSJ, et al. Prevalence and predictors of anxiety and depression in women with invasive ovarian cancer and their caregivers. Med J Aust. 2010;193(5):S52–7.
46. Mahdi H, Swensen RE, Munkarah AR, et al. Suicide in women with gynecologic cancer. Gynecol Oncol. 2011;122(2):344–9.
47. Jansen L, Hoffmeister M, Chang-Claude J, Brenner H, Arndt V. Benefit finding and post-traumatic growth in long-term colorectal cancer survivors: prevalence, determinants, and associations with quality of life. Br J Cancer. 2011;105(8):1158–65.
48. Mols F, Vingerhoets AJJM, Coebergh JWW, van de Poll-Franse LV. Well-being, posttraumatic growth and benefit finding in long-term breast cancer survivors. Psychol Health. 2009;24(5):583–95.
49. Stewart DE, Wong F, Duff S, Melancon CH, Cheung AM. "What doesn't kill you makes you stronger": an ovarian cancer survivor survey. Gynecol Oncol. 2001;83(3):537–42.
50. Ponto JA, Barton D. Husbands 'perspective of living with wives' ovarian cancer. Psychooncology. 2008;17(12):1225–31.
51. Lutgendorf SK, Anderson B, Ullrich P, et al. Quality of life and mood in women with gynecologic cancer: a one year prospective study. Cancer. 2002;94(1):131–40.
52. Carey M, Noble N, Sanson-Fisher R, Mackenzie L. Identifying psychological morbidity among people with cancer using the Hospital Anxiety and Depression Scale: time to revisit first principles? Psychooncology. 2011;21(3):229–38. doi:10.1002/pon.2057. Early view (online version).
53. Ziegler L, Hill K, Neilly L, et al. A systematic review of self-report measure performance at key stages of the cancer illness trajectory. J Pain Symptom Manage. 2011;41(3):619–36.
54. Armes J, Crowe M, Colbourne L, et al. Patients' supportive care needs beyond the end of cancer treatment: a prospective, longitudinal survey. J Clin Oncol. 2009;27(36):6172–9.
55. Beesley V, Eakin E, Steginga S, Aitken J, Dunn J, Battistutta D. Unmet needs of gynaecological cancer survivors: implications for developing community support services. Psychooncology. 2008;17(4):392–400.
56. Harrison JD, Young JM, Price MA, Butow PN, Solomon MJ. What are the unmet supportive care needs of people with cancer? A systematic review. Support Care Cancer. 2009;17(8):1117–28.
57. Merckaert I, Libert Y, Messin S, Milani M, Slachmuylder JL, Razavi D. Cancer patients' desire for psychological support: prevalence and implications for screening patients' psychological needs. Psychooncology. 2010;19(2):141–9.
58. National Institute of Health & Clinical Excellence. Improving supportive and palliative care for adults with cancer: the manual. London: National Institute for Clinical Excellence; 2004.
59. National Breast Cancer Centre and the National Cancer Control Initiative. Clinical practice guidelines for the psychosocial care of adults with cancer. Camperdown: National Breast Cancer Centre; 2003.
60. National Cancer Action Team. Connected: National communication skills training. 2011; http://www.connected.nhs.uk/.
61. Sharpe M, Strong V, Allen K, et al. Major depression in outpatients attending a regional cancer centre: screening and unmet treatment needs. Br J Cancer. 2004;90(2):314–20.
62. Passik SD, Dugan W, McDonald MV, Rosenfeld B, Theobald DE, Edgerton S. Oncologists' recognition of depression in their patients with cancer. J Clin Oncol. 1998;16(4):1594–600.
63. Fallowfield L, Ratcliffe D, Jenkins V, Saul J. Psychiatric morbidity and its recognition by doctors in patients with cancer. Br J Cancer. 2001;84(8):1011–5.
64. McLachlan SA, Allenby A, Matthews J, et al. Randomized trial of coordinated psychosocial interventions based on patient self-assessments versus standard care to improve the psychosocial functioning of patients with cancer. J Clin Oncol. 2001;19(21):4117–25.
65. Velikova G, Booth L, Smith AB, et al. Measuring quality of life in routine oncology practice improves communication and patient well-being: a randomized controlled trial. J Clin Oncol. 2004;22(4):714–24.
66. Strong V, Waters R, Hibberd C, et al. Management of depression for people with cancer (SMaRT oncology 1): a randomised trial. Lancet. 2008;372(9632):40–8.

67. Detmar SB, Muller MJ, Schornagel JH, Wever LDV, Aaronson NK. Health-related quality-of-life assessments and patient-physician communication - a randomized controlled trial. JAMA. 2002;288(23): 3027–34.
68. Jacobsen PB, Ransom S. Implementation of NCCN distress management guidelines by member institutions. J Natl Compr Canc Netw. 2007;5(1):99–103.
69. Mitchell AJ, Kaar S, Coggan C, Herdman J. Acceptability of common screening methods used to detect distress and related mood disorders-preferences of cancer specialists and non-specialists. Psychooncology. 2008;17(3): 226–36.
70. Absolom K, Holch P, Pini S, et al. The detection and management of emotional distress in cancer patients: the views of health care professionals. Psychooncology. 2011;20(6):601–8.
71. Gessler S, Low J, Daniells E, et al. Screening for distress in cancer patients: is the distress thermometer a valid measure in the UK and does it measure change over time? A prospective validation study. Psychooncology. 2008;17(6):538–47.
72. Johnson RL, Gold MA, Wyche KF. Distress in women with gynecologic cancer. Psychooncology. 2010; 19(6):665–8.
73. McCorkle R, Dowd M, Ercolano E, et al. Effects of a nursing intervention on quality of life outcomes in post-surgical women with gynecological cancers. Psychooncology. 2009;18(1):62–70.
74. Henry M, Cohen SR, Lee V, et al. The Meaning-Making intervention (MMi) appears to increase meaning in life in advanced ovarian cancer: a randomized controlled pilot study. Psychooncology. 2010; 19(12):1340–7.
75. Hersch J, Juraskova I, Price M, Mullan B. Psychosocial interventions and quality of life in gynaecological cancer patients: a systematic review. Psychooncology. 2009;18(8):795–810.
76. McAllister M, Davies L, Payne K, Nicholls S, Donnai D, MacLeod R. The emotional effects of genetic diseases: implications for clinical genetics. Am J Med Genet A. 2007;143A(22):2651–61.
77. Hopwood P. Psychosocial aspects of risk communication and mutation testing in familial breast-ovarian cancer. Curr Opin Oncol. 2005;17(4):340–4.
78. Vadaparampil ST, Wey JP, Kinney AY. Psychosocial aspects of genetic counseling and testing. Semin Oncol Nurs. 2004;20(3):186–95.
79. Cull A, Fry A, Rush R, Steel CM. Cancer risk perceptions and distress among women attending a familial ovarian cancer clinic. Br J Cancer. 2001;84(5): 594–9.
80. Erlick Robinson G, Rosen BP, Bradley LN, et al. Psychological impact of screening for familial ovarian cancer: reactions to initial assessment. Gynecol Oncol. 1997;65(2):197–205.
81. Wardle FJ, Collins W, Pernet AL, Whitehead MI, Bourne TH, Campbell S. Psychological impact of screening for familial ovarian cancer. J Natl Cancer Inst. 1993;85(8):653–7.
82. Schwartz MD, Peshkin BN, Hughes C, Main D, Isaacs C, Lerman C. Impact of BRCA1/BRCA2 mutation testing on psychologic distress in a clinic-based sample. J Clin Oncol. 2002;20(2):514–20.
83. Watson M, Foster C, Eeles R, et al. Psychosocial impact of breast/ovarian (BRCA1/2) cancer-predictive genetic testing in a UK multi-centre clinical cohort. Br J Cancer. 2004;91(10):1787–94.
84. Wood ME, Mullineaux L, Rahm AK, Fairclough D, Wenzel L. Impact of BRCA1 testing on women with cancer: a pilot study. Genet Test. 2000;4(3):265–72.
85. Hamilton JG, Lobel M, Moyer A. Emotional distress following genetic testing for hereditary breast and ovarian cancer: a meta-analytic review. Health Psychol. 2009;28(4):510–8.
86. Baum A, Friedman AL, Zakowski SG. Stress and genetic testing for disease risk. Health Psychol. 1997;16(1):8–19.
87. Hallowell N, Foster C, Eeles R, Ardern-Jones A, Watson M. Accommodating risk: responses to BRCA1/2 genetic testing of women who have had cancer. Soc Sci Med. 2004;59(3):553–65.
88. Germino BB, Fife BL, Funk SG. Cancer and the partner relationship: what is its meaning? Semin Oncol Nurs. 1995;11(1):43–50.
89. Pistrang N, Barker C. The partner relationship in psychological response to breast-cancer. Soc Sci Med. 1995;40(6):789–97.
90. van Oostrom I, Meijers-Heijboer H, Lodder LN, et al. Long-term psychological impact of carrying a BRCA1/2 mutation and prophylactic surgery: a 5-year follow-up study. J Clin Oncol. 2003;21(20):3867–74.
91. Mellon S, Berry-Bobovski L, Gold R, Levin N, Tainsky MA. Communication and decision-making about seeking inherited cancer risk information: findings from female survivor-relative focus groups. Psychooncology. 2006;15(3):193–208.
92. Dancyger C, Smith JA, Jacobs C, Wallace M, Michie S. Comparing family members' motivations and attitudes towards genetic testing for hereditary breast and ovarian cancer: a qualitative analysis. Eur J Hum Genet. 2010;18(12):1289–95.
93. Griffiths SE, Lopes T, Edmondson RJ. The role of prophylactic salpingo-oophorectomy in women who carry mutations of the BRCA genes. Obstet Gynecol. 2005;7:23–7.
94. Oei AL, Massuger LF, Bulten J, Ligtenberg MJ, Hoogerbrugge N, de Hullu JA. Surveillance of women at high risk for hereditary ovarian cancer is inefficient. Br J Cancer. 2006;94(6):814–9.
95. Van Nagell Jr JR, DePriest PD, Reedy MB, et al. The efficacy of transvaginal sonographic screening in asymptomatic women at risk for ovarian cancer. Gynecol Oncol. 2000;77(3):350–6.
96. Woodward ER, Sleightholme HV, Considine AM, Williamson S, McHugo JM, Cruger DG. Annual surveillance by CA125 and transvaginal ultrasound for ovarian cancer in both high-risk and population risk women is ineffective. BJOG. 2007;114(12):1500–9.

97. UK Familial Ovarian Cancer Screening Study (UK FOCSS). 2011; http://www.instituteforwomenshealth.ucl.ac.uk/academic_research/gynaecologicalcancer/gcrc/ukfocss. Accessed 25 Nov 2011.
98. Lifford KJ, Fraser L, Rosenthal AN, et al. Withdrawal from familial ovarian cancer screening for surgery: findings from a psychological evaluation study (PsyFOCS). Gynecol Oncol. 2011; 124(1):158–63.
99. Miller SM, Roussi P, Daly MB, Scarpato J. New strategies in ovarian cancer: uptake and experience of women at high risk of ovarian cancer who are considering risk-reducing salpingo-oophorectomy. Clin Cancer Res. 2010;16(21):5094–106.
100. NIH consensus conference. Ovarian cancer. Screening, treatment, and follow-up. JAMA. 1995; 273:491–7.
101. Fry A, Busby-Earle C, Rush R, Cull A. Prophylactic oophorectomy versus screening: psychosocial outcomes in women at increased risk of ovarian cancer. Psychooncology. 2001;10(3):231–41.
102. Michelsen TM, Dorum A, Dahl AA. A controlled study of mental distress and somatic complaints after risk-reducing salpingo-oophorectomy in women at risk for hereditary breast ovarian cancer. Gynecol Oncol. 2009;113(1):128–33.
103. Touboul C, Uzan C, Ichante JL, et al. Factors associated with altered long-term well-being after prophylactic salpingo-oophorectomy among women at increased hereditary risk for breast and ovarian cancer. Oncologist. 2011;16(9):1250–7.
104. Scottish Intercollegiate Guidelines Network. Epithelial ovarian cancer: a national clinical guideline. Edinburgh: Royal College of Physicians; 2003.
105. UK Collaborative Trial of Ovarian Cancer Screening (UKCTOCS). 2011; http://www.instituteforwomenshealth.ucl.ac.uk/academic_research/gynaecologicalcancer/gcrc/ukctocs. Accessed 25 Nov 2011.

Quality of Life in Patients with Ovarian Cancer

14

Sally E. Jensen and David Cella

Introduction

Traditionally, the goals of treatment for ovarian cancer[1] have included increasing progression-free and overall survival and minimizing symptom burden due to disease and treatment. However, in recent years, research examining clinically meaningful patient-centered outcomes has increasingly focused on maximizing quality of life (QOL)[2] as an important end point. With a greater emphasis on QOL as a clinically meaningful patient-centered outcome, a growing body of research has detailed the impact of disease and treatment on QOL. Given the realization that certain clinical benefits of treatment for ovarian cancer may compromise QOL, decision-making regarding anti-neoplastic treatment often involves a consideration of the balance between efficacy and safety or benefit and harm. On the other hand, a clinical benefit from therapy may also provide a parallel QOL benefit, essentially increasing the value of that therapy beyond the clinical measures of response, disease-free survival, progression-free survival, and overall survival. This chapter provides an overview of the QOL issues faced by women with ovarian cancer, advances in the measurement of patient-reported QOL in ovarian cancer, state-of-the-art medical intervention trials and their QOL outcomes, and future directions in interventions to optimize QOL in women with ovarian cancer.

Quality of Life

QOL is a subjective, multidimensional concept that has been defined as an individual's typical physical, functional, emotional, and social well-being and how it is influenced by medical conditions and treatments [1]. QOL encompasses a number of domains, including physical, functional, demographics, spiritual, social, psychological, and cognitive [2, 3]. The World Health Organization (WHO) also broadly defines QOL as inclusive of culture, personal value systems, goals, standards, and concerns [4]. Figure 14.1 depicts the domains of QOL. Unlike most clinical treatment outcomes, QOL is a patient-reported outcome and thus reflects the patient's perception of the impact of disease

[1]Unless otherwise specified, the term "ovarian cancer" is used to refer to epithelial ovarian cancer throughout this chapter.

[2]We use this term to refer to quality of life in the context of ovarian cancer and its treatment, what many have termed "health-related quality of life."

S.E. Jensen, PhD (✉)
Department of Medical Social Sciences and Department of Surgery, Division of Organ Transplantation, Northwestern University Feinberg School of Medicine, Chicago, IL, USA
e-mail: sally-jensen@northwestern.edu

D. Cella, PhD
Department of Medical Social Sciences, Northwestern University Feinberg School of Medicine, Chicago, IL 60611, USA
e-mail: d-cella@northwestern.edu

S.A. Farghaly (ed.), *Advances in Diagnosis and Management of Ovarian Cancer*,
DOI 10.1007/978-1-4614-8271-0_14, © Springer Science+Business Media New York 2014

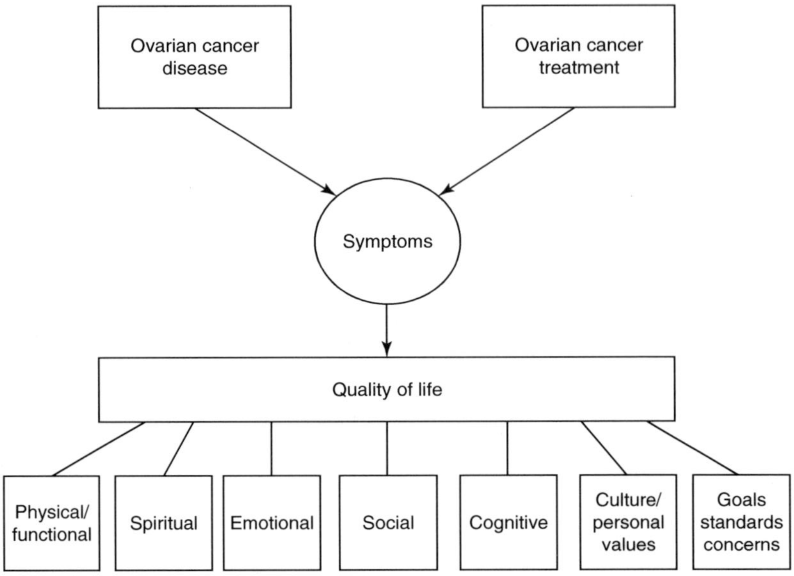

Fig. 14.1 Conceptual model of QOL in ovarian cancer (Adapted from Kornblith et al. [2] and [3])

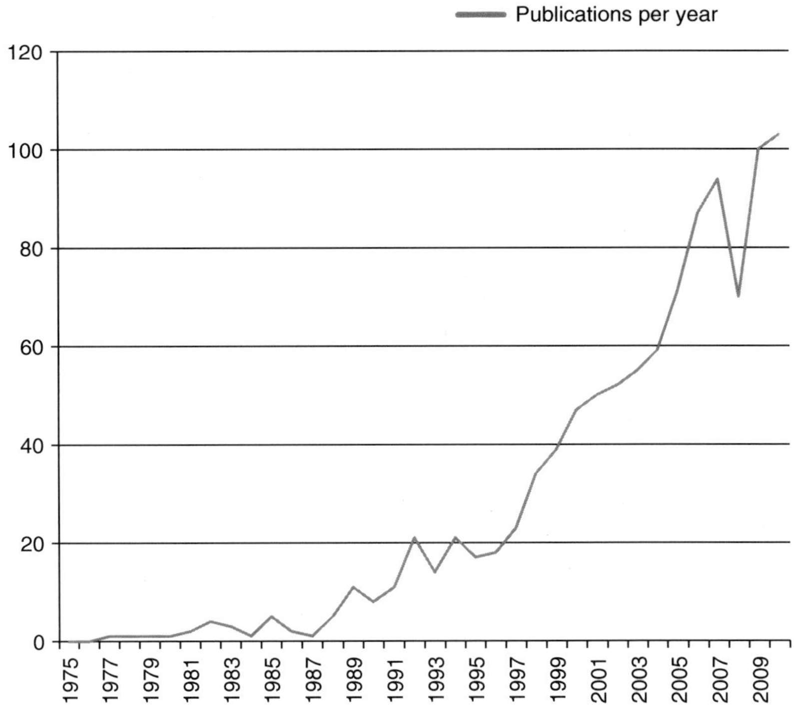

Fig. 14.2 Number of references with "quality of life" and "ovarian cancer" in Pubmed search from 1975–2010

and treatment. The assessment of QOL can help to inform treatment decision-making and symptom management. Furthermore, QOL measurement has been incorporated into most Gynecologic Oncology Group (GOG) trials and is increasingly considered an emerging standard of care [5].

As recognition of the importance of QOL as a patient-centered outcome has increased over time (see Fig. 14.2), the measurement of QOL as a patient-reported outcome has evolved. Numerous measures that ask patients to rate their response to questions about specific domains of QOL currently

Fig. 14.3 QOL measurement tools (Adapted from Arriba et al. [86])

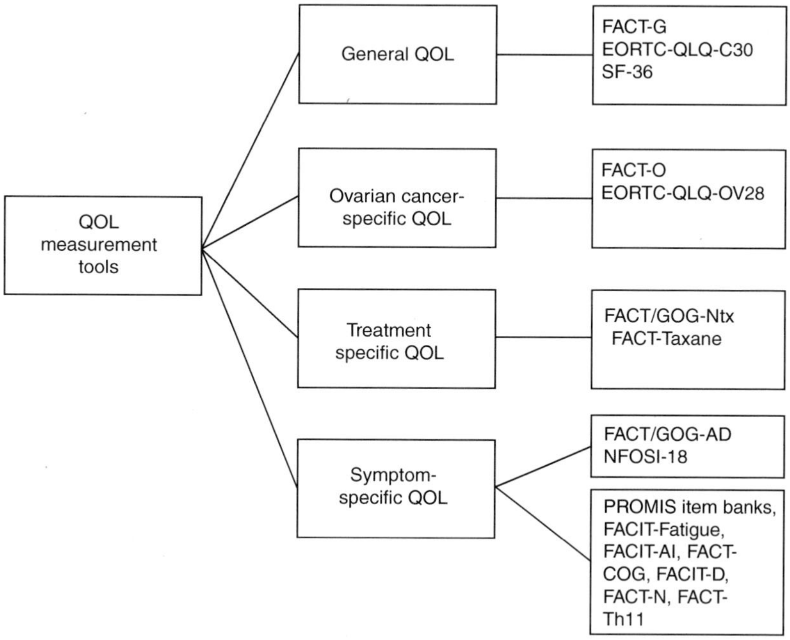

exist. However, the value of the information provided by measures of QOL is contingent upon the quality of the measure. Good measures of QOL should be validated, have good reliability, be sensitive to change, and be accepted by clinicians and patients. In an effort to regulate claims of drug effectiveness in improving QOL, the Food and Drug Administration (FDA) has further addressed concerns about QOL measurement [6]. According to the FDA Oncologic Drug Advisory Committee Quality of Life Subcommittee, pharmaceutical company claims of improved QOL must be specific to the QOL domain that was measured, with the recommendation that assessment of specific symptoms is an appropriate way to improve measurement of QOL domains [7].

The validated instruments most commonly used to assess QOL in ovarian cancer include both general measures of QOL as well as ovarian cancer-specific measures of QOL. Additionally, a number of symptom-specific measures of QOL have recently been developed for use in women with ovarian cancer and provide a focused assessment of disease- and treatment-related symptoms. Figure 14.3 displays the categories of QOL measures and measures most commonly used in ovarian cancer.

General QOL Measures

Several psychometrically sound general measures of QOL have been used to assess QOL in ovarian cancer. The Functional Assessment of Cancer Therapy-General (FACT-G [1]) is a 27-item general measure of QOL in cancer that assesses four domains of well-being: physical well-being, functional well-being, emotional well-being, and social well-being. The FACT-G can be used alone or in combination with disease and/or treatment-specific subscales. The European Organization for the Research and Treatment of Cancer QLQ-C30 (EORTC QLQ-C30 [8]) is a 30-item general measure of QOL in cancer that is comprised of five functional subscales, three symptom subscales and a global health and QOL scale. Like the FACT-G, it can be used alone or combined with cancer-specific modules. Finally, the Short-Form 36 health survey (SF-36 [9]) is a generic measure of QOL that has been widely used in numerous disease and treatment conditions. It consists of 36 items comprising eight subscales which form two higher-order scales: the Physical Component Summary (PCS) and the Mental Component Summary (MCS).

Ovarian Cancer-Specific QOL Measures

Several instruments have been developed to measure aspects of QOL specific to women with ovarian cancer. The Functional Assessment of Cancer Therapy-Ovarian (FACT-O [10]) consists of the FACT-G plus an ovarian cancer-specific subscale. The 11-item ovarian subscale was developed with input from ovarian cancer patients and gynecologic oncology clinical experts. The FACT-O provides a reliable and valid assessment of QOL in ovarian cancer that is sensitive to change. The Physical Well-Being scale, Functional Well-Being scale, and the Ovarian Cancer Subscale can be combined to create the Trial Outcome Index (TOI), which is frequently used in clinical trials to assess change in physical/functional outcomes. In addition to the FACT-O, the European Organization for the Research and Treatment of Cancer Quality of Life Ovarian Cancer (QLQ-OV28 [11]) is a 28-item ovarian cancer symptom-specific questionnaire module developed to supplement the EORTC QLQ-C30. The EORTC QLQ-OV28 measures abdominal/gastrointestinal symptoms, neurotoxicity, chemotherapy side effects, hormonal symptoms, body image, perception of disease/treatment, and sexual functioning and demonstrates good reliability and validity [11].

Treatment-Specific QOL Measures

A number of valid and reliable instruments have been developed to assess the QOL issues associated with specific types of treatment. The 11-item Functional Assessment of Cancer Therapy/Gynecologic Oncology Group-Neurotoxicity (FACT/GOG-Ntx [12, 13]) questionnaire measures peripheral neuropathy secondary to platinum/paclitaxel chemotherapy. Similarly, the Functional Assessment of Cancer Therapy-Taxane (FACT-Taxane [14]) is a 16-item questionnaire that measures the symptoms and QOL effects associated with the taxane class of chemotherapeutic agents. Although these measures were not developed for specific use among women with ovarian cancer, given that platinum/paclitaxel is a common chemotherapy regimen for ovarian cancer, they provide an opportunity to assess treatment impact on QOL in ovarian cancer.

Ovarian Cancer Symptom-Specific QOL Measures

In response to the FDA's statement that pharmaceutical company claims of improved QOL must be specific to the QOL domain measured, several valid and reliable instruments have recently been developed to measure ovarian cancer-specific symptoms and their impact on QOL. The Functional Assessment of Cancer Therapy/Gynecologic Oncology Group-Abdominal Discomfort (FACT/GOG-AD [15]) is a four-item measure of abdominal discomfort that was created in an effort to more accurately measure patients' perceptions of abdominal discomfort and its impact on QOL. The FACT/GOG-AD was created in response to evidence suggesting greater pain among intraperitoneal chemotherapy recipients [16]. It can be used to measure differences in treatment response as well as symptoms and complications resulting from both disease and treatment in ovarian cancer.

A recent addition to the measures of ovarian cancer-specific symptoms and QOL is the National Comprehensive Cancer Network-Functional Assessment of Cancer Therapy Ovarian Symptom Index-18 (NFOSI-18 [17]). The NFOSI-18 is an 18-item symptom index that reflects the symptoms rated as highest priority by both oncology clinical experts and women with advanced ovarian cancer (see Table 14.1). It was developed to address the potential discrepancy between symptoms reported as high priority by oncologists and patients in an effort to provide a more comprehensive perspective on symptoms and QOL in advanced ovarian cancer. It is comprised of three subscales: disease-related symptoms, treatment-related symptoms, and general function/well-being. Preliminary evidence suggests good reliability and validity [17].

In addition to these ovarian cancer-specific symptom indices, several non-disease-specific

Table 14.1 Rankings of top five symptoms/concerns[a] by advanced ovarian cancer patients with comparison to oncology clinician symptom ratings

Symptom/concern	Patient overall rank	% Patients endorsed top 5	Oncology clinician overall rank
Lack of energy (fatigue)	1	61	1
Able to sleep well	2	37	–
Able to enjoy life	3	25	–
Content with current QOL	4	24	7
Able to get around by myself	5	22	–
Constipation	5	22	–
Nausea	5	22	4
Pain	8	20	3
Worry that condition will get worse	8	20	5
Feeling ill	10	18	–

Data from Jensen et al. [17]
[a]Includes only those items endorsed at a probability greater than chance

Table 14.2 Non-disease-specific symptom measures from the Functional Assessment of Chronic Illness Therapy (FACIT) Measurement System

Symptom domain	Measure	Number of items
Fatigue	Functional Assessment of Chronic Illness Therapy-Fatigue Scale (FACIT-Fatigue [87])	13
Ascites	Functional Assessment of Chronic Illness Therapy-Ascites Scale (FACIT-AI [88])	13
Diarrhea	Functional Assessment of Chronic Illness Therapy-Diarrhea Scale (FACIT-D [88])	11
Cognitive function	Functional Assessment of Cancer Therapy-Cognitive Function Issues Scale (FACT-Cog [88])	13
Neutropenia	Functional Assessment of Cancer Therapy-Neutropenia Scale (FACT-N [89])	19
Thrombocytopenia	Functional Assessment of Cancer Therapy-Thrombocytopenia (FACT-Th11 [36])	11
Anemia	Functional Assessment of Cancer Therapy-Anemia/Fatigue (FACT-An [90])	20

instruments measure symptoms of relevance among women with ovarian cancer. Table 14.2 lists instruments from the Functional Assessment of Chronic Illness Therapy-Fatigue Scale (FACIT) Measurement System which can be administered individually or in combination with the FACT-O. Additionally, the National Institutes of Health (NIH) Patient-Reported Outcomes Measurement Information System (PROMIS) initiative has resulted in the development of a host of item banks measuring QOL-related domains in chronic illness, such as physical function [18], pain [19, 20], sleep [21], emotional distress [22], and social health [23]. The availability of psychometrically sound measures, such as those described, enables a better understanding of the impact of symptoms on QOL in ovarian cancer.

Symptoms and QOL in Ovarian Cancer

Women with ovarian cancer are at risk for diminished QOL due to the disease itself, as well as aggressive treatments such as abdominal surgeries and chemotherapy [2, 24]. While these therapies may have antineoplastic benefits, they can also result in a host of toxicities, which, along with disease-related symptoms, have the potential to adversely affect a variety of QOL domains. Table 14.3 lists common symptoms affecting QOL in ovarian cancer.

Physical Symptoms

QOL is adversely affected by ovarian cancer symptoms; in fact they are a part of the QOL concept itself in the context of ovarian cancer.

Table 14.3 Ovarian cancer symptoms affecting quality of life

Symptom category	Symptoms
Physical	Fatigue
	Neurotoxicity
	Neutropenia
	Abdominal pain/discomfort
	Alopecia
	Nausea/vomiting
	Thrombocytopenia
	Anemia
	Cognitive changes
Sexual and reproductive	Decreased interest in sexual activity
	Decreased sexual pleasure
	Increased sexual discomfort
	Increased fertility concerns
Psychological	Depression
	Anxiety
	Anger
	Changes in social functioning
	Impaired sleep quality

Disease, treatment, and psychological factors can result in elevated rates of fatigue among women with ovarian cancer [25], which is the most consistently endorsed high-priority symptom by women with advanced disease [17]. Fatigue has been defined as a persistent, distressing, subjective sense of tiredness related to cancer treatment that is not in proportion to recent activity and which interferes with typical functioning [26]. Fatigue may continue to present difficulties even well after the completion of treatment, as indicated by the finding that 32.7 % of ovarian cancer survivors at least 6 months posttreatment continued to report difficulty due to fatigue [27]. This finding highlights the importance of ongoing monitoring of fatigue even among women no longer actively receiving treatment for ovarian cancer.

Neurotoxicity represents another common physical symptom that negatively impacts QOL in women with ovarian cancer. Neurotoxicity is a symptom often associated with cisplatin or taxane chemotherapy regimens. Neurotoxicity symptoms associated with these chemotherapy regimens include burning, numbness, tingling, and shooting sensations in the extremities [28] and may interfere with functional abilities and activities of daily living. Neurotoxicity may also persist beyond the completion of chemotherapy. A recent randomized controlled trial revealed that one-third of women receiving cisplatin and paclitaxel had persistent neuropathy 12 months after starting treatment [29], and neurotoxicity was significantly greater at 12 months among women who received intraperitoneal chemotherapy compared to those who only received intravenous chemotherapy. At the present time, there is a paucity of therapies that have been effective in preventing or treating neurotoxicity [30, 31], although novel taxanes may offer promise of reduced neurotoxicity, compared to paclitaxel [32].

Abdominal discomfort and pain may also adversely impact QOL in women with ovarian cancer. Abdominal symptoms are common in ovarian cancer and may be related to disease-related factors, such as bloating and ascites [5], or treatments such as surgery or intraperitoneal chemotherapy [33]. A recent randomized controlled trial found that patients receiving only intravenous chemotherapy had significantly more improvement in abdominal discomfort from baseline to cycle four when compared to patients receiving chemotherapy via both intravenous and intraperitoneal administration [15]. However, it should also be noted that no differences in abdominal discomfort existed between intravenous-only and intravenous/intraperitoneal patients by 1 year follow-up [34].

Myelosuppression, including anemia, neutropenia, and thrombocytopenia, represents another physical symptom that may negatively affect QOL in ovarian cancer. Myelosuppression is a common toxicity associated with the platinum-based chemotherapies, as well as paclitaxel. Anemia may also be related to disease-related factors and is associated with numerous symptoms impacting QOL, including fatigue, dizziness, dyspnea, activity intolerance, headaches, concentration difficulties, and sleep disturbance [35]. Severe anemia may require treatment with erythropoietin or red blood cell transfusion, which may delay treatment and confer additional threat to QOL. Neutropenia related to cancer enhances susceptibility to infection and may result in fever and hospitalization. Neutropenia is a common

Table 14.4 Studies that have assessed cognitive functioning in women with ovarian cancer

Author	Design	*N*	Participants	Cognitive domains assessed	Findings
Correa et al. [44]	Cross-sectional	48	Long-term ovarian cancer survivors who were either in remission or with recurrent disease	Attention Executive function Learning Memory	There were no significant differences between the two groups in any cognitive domain. Although group mean cognitive scores were in the average range, 28 % of participants met criteria for cognitive impairment
Hess et al. [41]	Prospective	27	Women with ovarian cancer receiving platinum-based chemotherapy	Attention Processing speed Reaction time	92 % of participants demonstrated cognitive impairment from baseline to cycle 3. 86 % demonstrated cognitive impairments from baseline to cycle 6
Hensley et al. [43]	Prospective	27	Women with ovarian cancer receiving combination therapy with paclitaxel, carboplatin, and gemcitabine	Attention Concentration Cognitive flexibility Psychomotor speed	Scores on cognitive function tests ranged from average to high average on all tests across time, with no decline in cognitive function
Mayerhofer et al. [42]	Prospective	28	Women with ovarian cancer receiving combination paclitaxel/carboplatin	Motor skills Short-term attention Numerical memory	Scores on a test assessing short-term attention significantly improved from pre- to post-chemotherapy. There were no other significant changes over time in scores from the other cognitive tests administered

dose-limiting toxicity of taxane [5], and may also result in delay of chemotherapy administration. Thrombocytopenia is associated with concerns such as bruising, bleeding, fatigue, and worry, which may, in turn, affect activity level [36]. Thrombocytopenia is standardly treated with platelet transfusions and may be associated with delays in treatment and dose reductions.

Impaired cognitive functioning can also have an adverse effect upon QOL. Although research has begun to explore changes in cognitive functioning in ovarian cancer, it is not well understood and is likely due to multiple etiologies. Proposed mechanisms of cognitive impairment in individuals receiving chemotherapy include chemotherapy-induced neurotoxicity associated with demyelination, secondary inflammatory response, and microvascular injury [37]; chemotherapy-induced disruption of hippocampal neurogenesis [38] is associated with decreased cerebral gray and white matter volume; [39] anemia, fatigue, and neuroimmunologic changes [40]; and comorbid psychiatric or neurologic conditions [41]. Recent research has begun to explore cognitive functioning in women undergoing treatment for ovarian cancer using objective, cognitive, and neuropsychological assessments (See Table 14.4). Several of these studies found no evidence of a decline in cognitive functioning [42, 43]; one noted a significant improvement in short-term attention from baseline to posttreatment [42], and several found that scores on cognitive tests ranged from average to high average when compared with published normative values [43, 44]. This is in contrast to the findings of Hess and colleagues, who reported a decline in cognitive functioning over time in the majority of participants [41]. The reason for the variability in these findings remains unclear; however, it is possible that the use of different measures or domains of cognitive functioning may account for these contrasting findings. Questions remain about the discrepancy between patient-reported cognitive

Table 14.5 Comparison of reproductive and sexual functioning in survivors of ovarian germ cell tumors and matched controls

	Ovarian germ cell tumor survivors ($N = 132$)		Matched controls ($N = 137$)		
Reproductive/sexual domain	Mean	SD	Mean	SD	p
Menstrual/gynecological symptoms	18.2	6.8	17.0	4.6	.123
Reproductive concerns[a]	15.7	12.1	8.5	7.1	<.0001
Sexual pleasure[b]	9.9	5.5	11.8	4.3	.017
Sexual discomfort[b]	1.3	1.7	1.0	1.3	.154
Sexual self schema[c]	55.8	13.4	55.8	11.8	.983

Data from Gershenson et al. [48]
Note. Analyses after controlling for income, partnership, and perception of fertility
[a]Measured by the Reproductive Concerns scale
[b]Measured by the Sexual Activity questionnaire
[c]Measured by the Sexual Self Schema scale

impairment and results from neuropsychological assessments suggesting little impairment.

Sexual and Reproductive Symptoms

Disease- and treatment-related factors are commonly associated with sexual and reproductive symptoms that impair QOL in women with ovarian cancer. Specifically, nerve damage from surgery, removal of tissues important for sexual activity, surgical menopause, and estrogen deficiency may negatively impact sexual activity and functioning in women with ovarian cancer [5]. Findings suggest that approximately half of ovarian cancer survivors are sexually active [45, 46]. Among ovarian cancer survivors who were not sexually active, a lack of interest/desire in sex and physical problems were cited significantly more frequently as reasons for sexual inactivity, when compared to a normative sample [45, 46]. Moreover, sexually active ovarian cancer survivors reported significantly greater levels of sexual discomfort and significantly lower levels of sexual pleasure compared to a normative sample [45]. These findings are noteworthy, given recent evidence from Von Gruenigen and colleagues that the majority of participants with ovarian cancer indicated significantly impaired interest and satisfaction with sexual activity [47].

Survivors of ovarian germ cell tumors may experience a slightly different profile of sexual symptoms than survivors of epithelial ovarian cancer. Ovarian germ cell tumors are typically diagnosed in younger women of childbearing age and are associated with more favorable treatment outcomes and cure rates [48]. Table 14.5 displays the results from a recent comparison of sexual and reproductive functioning among survivors of ovarian germ cell tumors and matched controls. Although survivors of ovarian germ cell tumors did not differ from matched controls in menstrual/gynecologic difficulties or sexual discomfort, they reported significantly less sexual pleasure [48]. In addition, the fertility impact of cancer may be especially salient in survivors of ovarian germ cell tumors. Gershenson and colleagues found that the majority of survivors of ovarian germ cell tumors who received fertility-sparing surgery followed by combination chemotherapy reported experiencing regular menstrual cycles [48]. However, compared to age-, race-, and education-matched controls, survivors of ovarian germ cell tumors had significantly more reproductive concerns, and, as expected, infertile survivors of germ cell tumors had significantly greater reproductive concerns than fertile survivors [48].

Psychological Symptoms

The psychological sequelae of ovarian cancer, which is described in greater detail in a separate chapter of this book, may also pose a threat to QOL. For example, in one study, 21 % of a sample of women with ovarian cancer met clinical cutoff for depression, and 29 % scored above the 75th percentile for anxiety [49]. Indeed, there is some evidence to suggest that anxiety poses a greater problem than depression among women with ovarian cancer [47, 50]. For example, women with advanced ovarian cancer rated "worry that condition would worsen" among their highest-priority symptoms [17], and in one sample of women with ovarian cancer, 55 % reported a fear of dying [51]. It is possible that treatment-related factors may impact anxiety symptoms in ovarian cancer. For example, a greater proportion of women who underwent suboptimal debulking reported more severe anxious symptoms compared to women who underwent optimal debulking [47].

Implications of QOL Assessment

Given the impact of symptoms on QOL, QOL is an important end point when assessing the effects of cancer treatment. Measuring QOL provides the ability to examine how well treatment ameliorates disease-related symptoms, as well as whether treatment-related toxicities outweigh the potential clinical benefits. The assessment of QOL may also serve as a prognostic factor across the disease trajectory. For example, two independent randomized controlled trials have found QOL to be predictive of survival outcomes in ovarian cancer. In a randomized controlled trial of interval secondary cytoreduction, Wenzel and colleagues found that QOL at the third chemotherapy cycle predicted overall survival in women with advanced ovarian cancer [29]. In a randomized trial comparing cisplatin/cyclophosphamide and cisplatin/paclitaxel chemotherapy, Carey and colleagues found that better baseline global QOL predicted longer progression-free survival and overall survival, independent of performance status [52]. These findings suggest that perhaps QOL may also serve as an indicator of which patients may not respond well to treatment. Another clinical implication of assessing QOL is the opportunity for enhanced patient-provider communication surrounding treatment decision-making and symptom management. As previously noted, patients and oncology clinicians may differ in terms of the symptoms and aspects of QOL they perceive as most important [17]. Thus, assessing and discussing QOL enables oncology providers to develop a better understanding of the patients' perception of QOL as it pertains to their treatment. Incorporating QOL into discussions regarding treatment decision-making is especially important in situations where different treatments demonstrate similar survival benefits but different toxicity profiles.

In addition to the benefits of QOL assessment in the clinical setting, there are also benefits of incorporating QOL measurement into ovarian cancer research. This is reinforced by the National Cancer Institute (NCI) and the FDA, both of which have recently asserted that the improvement of survival and QOL should be the aims of cancer research [53]. Given that approximately three-fourths of women with ovarian cancer are diagnosed with advanced disease [54], as well as the limited curative treatment options for advanced disease, the improvement and maintenance of QOL is an important outcome in clinical trials. Clinical trials that include QOL as an outcome can measure treatment success by the extent to which the treatment manages or improves ovarian cancer-specific symptoms affecting QOL.

QOL and Recent Advances in the Treatment of Ovarian Cancer

The preservation and improvement of QOL represents an important aim of clinical trials investigating advances in treatment modalities for ovarian cancer. The development of validated QOL measurement tools has enabled clinical trials to collect and report on QOL data in the context of newly emerging treatment modalities. In recent years, a number of treatment advances have emerged, including new chemotherapeutic agents, innovations in the timing and mode of chemotherapy administration, and new surgical

Table 14.6 Measures of QOL used in recent clinical trials of treatment for ovarian cancer

Study	QOL measure	QOL outcomes
Greimel et al. [58]	EORTC QLQ-C30	Paclitaxel/carboplatin arm experienced better QOL than paclitaxel/cisplatin arm
Pokrzywinski et al. [55]	FACT-O	Sequential treatment arm experienced better QOL than combination treatment arm
Wenzel et al. [34]	FACT-O FACT/GOG-Ntx FACT/GOG-AD	Intraperitoneal arm experienced worse QOL during and shortly after treatment, compared to the intravenous-only arm. No significant differences in QOL between groups at 1 year
Vergote et al. [64]	EORTC QLQ-C30 EORTC QLQ-Ov28	No significant difference in QOL between primary debulking and neoadjuvant chemotherapy arms
Wenzel et al. [29]	FACT-O	No significant difference in QOL between participants who underwent interval secondary cytoreduction and those that did not

Note. *EORTC QLQ-C30* European Organization for the Research and Treatment of Cancer Quality of Life Questionnaire, Core Module, *FACT-O* Functional Assessment of Cancer Therapy-Ovarian, *FACT/GOG-Ntx* Functional Assessment of Cancer Therapy/Gynecologic Oncology Group-Neurotoxicity, *FACT/GOG-AD* Functional Assessment of Cancer Therapy/Gynecologic Oncology Group-Abdominal Discomfort, *EORTC QLQ-Ov28* European Organization for the Research and Treatment of Cancer Quality of Life Questionnaire, Ovarian Cancer Module

procedures. Research has increasingly sought to identify how these new treatment strategies affect QOL in women with ovarian cancer, and efforts are necessary to continue to more comprehensively incorporate measures of QOL in trials assessing novel therapies. Table 14.6 summarizes recent research evaluating new treatment modalities that has included QOL as an end point.

Maintenance Chemotherapy

Despite improvements in treatment, the majority of women with ovarian cancer will recur within 5 years of treatment [55], and there is evidence to suggest that most women will relapse within 18 months of completion of first-line treatment [32]. Despite the availability of chemotherapeutic agents for relapsed disease, response rates diminish with each relapse due to drug resistance over time [32]. Maintenance chemotherapy has been proposed as a potential solution; however, the potential for improved survival with maintenance chemotherapy must be considered in light of additional toxicity from prolonged treatment and its potential impact on QOL. It has been proposed that symptoms associated with maintenance therapy such as fatigue, myalgias, myelosuppression, alopecia, and neuropathy may impact QOL [32]. Although maintenance therapy using novel taxanes may confer benefit with less impact on QOL, no studies to date have reported on QOL in maintenance therapy in ovarian cancer, and though toxicity data has been used as a proxy measure of QOL, it does not fully capture patients' perceptions of QOL [32]. An ongoing phase 3 trial examining monthly taxane maintenance therapy includes QOL as a secondary end point [56], and future research on the QOL outcomes in maintenance chemotherapy trials is needed.

Combination Chemotherapy

The combination of paclitaxel and cisplatin as a first-line therapy for ovarian cancer historically demonstrated better survival outcomes than regimens that did not contain taxanes [57]. However, given that carboplatin was associated with fewer toxicities than cisplatin, a prospective randomized controlled trial examined QOL as a secondary end point in women with ovarian cancer randomized to receive either paclitaxel/cisplatin or paclitaxel/carboplatin first-line chemotherapy [58]. There were no differences in progression-free or overall survival outcomes between the paclitaxel/cisplatin and paclitaxel/carboplatin groups; however, women randomized to the paclitaxel/carboplatin arm experienced better overall posttreatment QOL, physical functioning, role functioning, and cognitive functioning when compared to the paclitaxel/cisplatin arm [58]. The findings of this trial had important implications in terms of treatment decision-making, as carboplatin demonstrated a clear QOL advantage over cisplatin in combination therapy with paclitaxel, despite equivalent survival outcomes.

A recent prospective phase two randomized clinical trial examined QOL as a secondary outcome in women with recurrent platinum-sensitive ovarian cancer randomized to either docetaxel in combination with carboplatin or single-agent docetaxel followed sequentially by carboplatin [55]. Although there was no difference in overall survival, there was significantly longer progression-free survival, more neurotoxicity, and more neutropenia in the combination arm [59]. However, the sequential treatment had significantly less impact on QOL outcomes. Specifically, the sequential arm had less impact on the FACT-O treatment outcome index over the course of the trial, compared to the combination arm [55]. Moreover, physical well-being was preserved in the sequential arm, whereas it decreased in the combination arm [55]. There was, however, no difference between groups in median time to QOL deterioration [55]. These findings highlight a trade-off between better progression-free survival and greater toxicity and poorer QOL in the combination chemotherapy arm. Given that there was no significant difference in overall survival between the combination and sequential chemotherapy strategies, discussion of toxicity and QOL issues will likely be an important focus in treatment decision-making.

Intraperitoneal Chemotherapy

There is ongoing controversy [60, 61] surrounding findings suggesting that intraperitoneal (IP) chemotherapy confers a survival advantage to women with advanced ovarian cancer [16, 62, 63]. Although a phase three randomized trial found that intravenous paclitaxel plus IP cisplatin and paclitaxel significantly increased progression-free and overall survival when compared to intravenous-only (IV) paclitaxel and cisplatin [16], QOL was significantly worse in the IP group before cycle 4 and 3–6 weeks after treatment [34]. Patients receiving IP therapy reported significantly and clinically meaningfully more physical, functional, and ovarian cancer-specific problems during treatment and shortly after, compared to IV-treated patients [34]. Moreover, although patient-reported neurotoxicity worsened for both groups after baseline, IP-treated patients had significantly greater worsening even 12 months after cycle six [34]. Both groups reported improved QOL over time, and there were no QOL differences between the IP arm and the IV arm at 1 year [34]. Additionally, QOL and abdominal discomfort improved in both groups by 6 weeks after treatment [34]. These findings highlight the fact that the peritoneal catheter and greater dose intensity of IP chemotherapy are associated with toxicities that adversely impact QOL. Discussions about treatment decision-making must balance the potential survival advantages of IP chemotherapy with the (mostly) short-term QOL decrements associated with it.

Neoadjuvant Chemotherapy

In advanced ovarian cancer, primary debulking surgery before beginning chemotherapy has been the standard of care. However, a recent prospective randomized controlled trial in women with advanced ovarian cancer explored whether there may be an advantage to neoadjuvant chemotherapy. Specifically, women were randomized to either primary debulking surgery followed by at least six courses of platinum-based chemotherapy or three courses of neoadjuvant platinum-based chemotherapy followed by interval debulking surgery followed by at least three courses of platinum-based chemotherapy [64]. The trial found similar progression-free and overall survival between the primary debulking and neoadjuvant chemotherapy arms. Moreover, there was no difference in QOL [64].

Interval Secondary Cytoreduction

Although the standard treatment for advanced ovarian cancer is radical cytoreduction surgery followed by chemotherapy [65], research has begun to examine whether interval debulking, a second surgery that is preceded and followed by chemotherapy, might improve outcomes. Although a previous study reported that interval cytoreduction improved survival by one-third in advanced ovarian patients [66], a more recent randomized trial found no survival benefit associated with interval secondary cytoreduction [67]. In this trial that compared patients who did and did not undergo interval secondary cytoreduction, QOL was examined as a secondary end point, with no group differences at any time point [29]. While scores across both groups reflected impaired QOL at the first two time points, with the greatest impact on the functional and physical well-being, there was a clinically significant improvement after completing treatment [29]. However, because pretreatment QOL was not assessed, it is not possible to determine whether the improvement reflects the results of acute toxicity during treatment or improvement from treatment benefits. Interestingly, the same trial reported that patients who underwent interval secondary cytoreduction had significantly less neurotoxicity 6 months after the start of treatment, which may reflect a benefit resulting from the time off chemotherapy following surgery [29].

Novel Biologic Therapies

Despite improvements in surgical and chemotherapeutic treatment strategies for women with ovarian cancer, curative options remain limited, thus prompting a search for alternative therapeutic agents, such as novel biologic therapies. Among the novel biologic therapies under development and investigation, bevacizumab has been the most studied. Bevacizumab is an antiangiogenic monoclonal antibody that targets VEGF and shows preliminary promise for use in recurrent ovarian cancer [30, 68]. The preliminary results of several ongoing phase three clinical trials suggest that bevacizumab, as an adjunct to standard chemotherapy, may be associated with more favorable outcomes [68]. However, no studies to date have reported on QOL outcomes associated with bevacizumab in ovarian cancer. Prospective QOL assessment in patients receiving bevacizumab is needed to enhance understanding of its effect on QOL, particularly given findings from one phase two trial in which a higher than expected incidence of gastrointestinal perforation was observed in ovarian cancer patients receiving bevacizumab [69].

Palliative Chemotherapy

Outcomes in women with refractory and recurrent ovarian cancer receiving palliative chemotherapy have not been widely examined. Difficulty arises in assessing whether palliative chemotherapy actually palliates disease-related symptoms affecting QOL given that symptoms could also be attributed to prior surgical and chemotherapy treatments. In a small pilot study, Doyle and colleagues assessed QOL and patient expectations among women with refractory and recurrent ovarian cancer undergoing palliative chemotherapy [70]. Although only one-fourth of the women experienced objective clinical response to palliative chemotherapy, after two cycles of palliative chemotherapy, global function and emotional function improved and were sustained for a median of 2 and 3 months, respectively [70]. However, 65 % of the women expressed their belief that the palliative chemotherapy would extend their life, and 42 % believed that it would cure them [70]. These findings highlight the importance of delineating QOL and survival benefits in discussions of treatment decision-making pertaining to palliative chemotherapy.

Future Directions: Improving QOL in Ovarian Cancer

Although our understanding of how emerging treatments affect QOL in women with ovarian cancer is far from complete, efforts have also begun to explore the specific symptoms and QOL domains that account for overall diminished QOL during treatment, as well as associations among clusters of QOL domains that may serve as targets for future intervention. For example, Von Gruenigen and colleagues sought to identify which specific QOL symptoms and concerns were associated with lower overall QOL, as measured by the FACT-O, during chemotherapy [47]. Domain item responses from women in the lowest quartile of overall QOL were compared with those from women in the upper three quartiles of overall QOL to determine which individual items were associated with lower total FACT-O scores. Table 14.7 summarizes the symptoms/concerns associated with lower QOL in this sample. The identification of the symptoms that are most disruptive to overall QOL has important implications, as many of these symptoms may be amenable to intervention via supportive therapies. The implementation of supportive interventions to target these symptoms may serve to improve overall QOL, although randomized controlled trials are needed to assess the impact of supportive interventions on QOL in ovarian cancer.

Table 14.7 QOL symptoms and concerns associated with lower QOL as measured by the FACT-O

QOL Domain	QOL symptom/concern
Physical well-being	I have a lack of energy
	I have nausea
	I have trouble meeting the needs of my family
	I have pain
	I am bothered by the side effects of treatment
	I feel ill
	I am forced to spend time in bed
Social well-being	I am satisfied with my sex life
Emotional well-being	I feel sad
	I feel nervous
	I worry about dying
Functional well-being	I am able to work
	My work is fulfilling
	I am able to enjoy life
	I am sleeping well
	I am enjoying the things I usually do for fun
	I am content with the quality of my life right now
Ovarian cancer-specific	I have a good appetite
	I like the appearance of my body
	I am able to feel like a woman

Data from von Gruenigen et al. [47]

Recent research has also begun to explore associations among clusters of QOL domains that may serve as targets for future intervention. Findings suggest that women undergoing chemotherapy for ovarian cancer have lower functional well-being and physical well-being scores, but higher social well-being scores when compared to the US female adult normative scores on the FACT-G [71]. Von Gruenigen and colleagues combined the physical and functional well-being domains and the social and emotional well-being domains in order to create clusters of conceptually similar QOL domains [71]. Preliminary findings revealed that the functional/physical well-being cluster was significantly positively associated with the social/emotional well-being cluster [71]. This may reflect the possibility that women with lower functional/physical well-being may experience lower social/emotional well-being, as well as the possibility that women with lower social/emotional well-being are more vulnerable to the effects of treatment on their functional/physical well-being [71]. The relationship between these two QOL domain clusters suggests the possibility that supportive interventions targeting the functional/physical well-being domain may also improve the social/emotional well-being domain and overall QOL.

Supportive interventions to enhance specific domains of QOL affected during ovarian cancer treatment could have the potential to lessen the QOL impact associated with treatments that improve survival but confer numerous toxicities. To date, no multisite randomized controlled trial of a multidisciplinary QOL intervention has been conducted. Such a trial would be necessary in order to determine whether intervention effects on specific QOL concerns and symptoms would also improve overall QOL or survival outcomes. However, several evidence-based treatments currently exist to address many of the specific concerns that have been identified as contributing to diminished overall QOL, such as pain, nausea, and sleep. In addition, psychotherapeutic interventions may be implemented to target symptoms of anxiety and concerns about body image.

A growing number of single-site studies have begun to explore the feasibility of employing interventions to improve QOL in women with ovarian cancer. Although the studies differ in their approach to intervention and their findings are still in need of replication in larger, multisite randomized controlled trials, they provide preliminary evidence suggesting that targeted QOL interventions are feasible and may yield QOL benefits (See Table 14.8 for a summary).

Several intervention feasibility studies have focused on enhancing health-promoting behaviors as a means to improve QOL in ovarian cancer. Von Gruenigen and colleagues recently reported on the findings from a single-group, prospective study to assess the feasibility of a lifestyle intervention to enhance health-promoting behaviors during chemotherapy for women with ovarian cancer [72]. Specifically, participants were seen individually for 30 minutes at each chemotherapy session by a registered dietitian, as well as given pedometers which they were encouraged to use [72]. They found that emotional well-being, functional well-being, and overall QOL improved significantly from baseline to cycle six of chemotherapy. Moreover, an increase in moderate to strenuous physical activity was significantly associated with better physical well-being during chemotherapy [72]. Donnelly and colleagues also investigated whether physical activity may positively impact QOL in ovarian cancer [73]. They carried out a single-site, randomized controlled trial to determine the feasibility and efficacy of a home-based moderate intensity physical activity intervention in the management of fatigue of a sample of ovarian and endometrial cancer patients [73]. Women assigned to the physical activity group had a significant decrease in fatigue post-intervention and at 6 months, compared to the contact control group [73]. Additionally, qualitative findings revealed that psychological benefits was identified as the most commonly perceived benefit of the physical activity intervention, suggesting that improvements in physical activity may act as a potential mediator of the link between fatigue and psychological well-being [73]. Although the physical activity intervention and contact control groups did not differ significantly in QOL over time, the study was likely insufficiently powered to detect significant differences in secondary outcomes [73]. Newton and colleagues also recently reported on the findings from their non-randomized phase two study that assessed the safety and feasibility of an individualized walking intervention for women with ovarian cancer during chemotherapy [74]. In this study, the walking intervention was individualized by an exercise physiologist who met with participants (face to face or via phone)weekly for 20–60 min for the duration of their chemotherapy treatments [74]. The findings revealed statistically significant improvements in functional well-being and ovarian-specific concerns, and clinically meaningful improvements in physical well-being and ovarian-specific concerns [74]. There was no change over time in social or emotional well-being [74]. Collectively, the findings from these three feasibility studies suggest that physical activity interventions may have the potential to improve certain domains of QOL, although these findings are in need of replication in adequately powered, randomized controlled trials.

In addition to physical activity intervention feasibility studies, several single-site studies have investigated the feasibility of integrative medicine (also known as complementary and alternative medicine) interventions to improve QOL in women with ovarian cancer. A recent prospective, single-site randomized controlled pilot trial examined the effects of an integrative medicine intervention on QOL, toxicity, and immune profiles in ovarian cancer [75]. Women who were randomized to receive the integrative medicine intervention received clinical hypnosis, therapeutic massage, and healing touch with each

Table 14.8 Studies investigating interventions to enhance QOL in women with ovarian cancer

Intervention	Design	*N*	QOL measure	QOL outcome
Lifestyle intervention (physical activity and diet) [72]	Single group	27	FACT-G	QOL, emotional and functional well-being significantly increased at follow-up
Physical activity intervention [73]	Randomized controlled trial	33	Multidimensional Fatigue Symptom Inventory-Short Form, FACIT-Fatigue	Significantly less post-intervention fatigue in the intervention group. No significant group differences over time
Individualized walking intervention [74]	Single group	17	FACT-O	Significant improvements in functional well-being and ovarian-specific concerns from baseline to follow-up
Combined modality integrative medicine intervention [75]	Randomized trial	43	FACT-O	No group differences in QOL over time
Traditional Chinese medicine intervention [76]	Double-blind, placebo-controlled randomized trial	81	EORTC-QLQ C30	No group differences in QOL over time
Psychoeducational intervention [77]	Randomized trial	33	QOL-Ovarian Cancer Tool	No group differences in QOL over time
Meaning-making intervention [78]	Randomized controlled trial	24	McGill Quality of Life Questionnaire, FACIT-Sp-12 [79]	There was a non-statistically significant trend toward greater QOL in the intervention group at 3 months
Nursing intervention [80]	Single-blind, randomized clinical trial	123	SF-12	Intervention group experienced significantly better physical and mental QOL over time, compared to control group

Note. *FACT-G* Functional Assessment of Cancer Therapy-General, *FACIT-Fatigue* Functional Assessment of Chronic Illness Therapy-Fatigue Scale, *FACT-O* Functional Assessment of Cancer Therapy-Ovarian, *EORTC QLQ-C30* European Organization for the Research and Treatment of Cancer Quality of Life Questionnaire, Core Module, *FACIT-Sp-12* Functional Assessment of Chronic Illness Therapy-Spiritual Well-being, *SF-12* Short-Form 12 health survey

chemotherapy cycle. The findings revealed no significant differences between groups in QOL at any time point, which may reflect true lack of intervention effects or that the study design was underpowered to detect QOL effects [75]. Another recent study utilized a randomized placebo-controlled trial to examine traditional Chinese medicine's effects on QOL, side effects, and immune functioning in women undergoing treatment for ovarian cancer [76]. This study also found no differences in QOL between groups over time and no improvement in symptoms in the Chinese medicine intervention group [76]. Moreover, emotional function, cognitive function, and nausea/vomiting were found to be worse or less improved among women assigned to the Chinese medicine group [76]. Although the findings from these studies suggest that integrative medicine interventions are feasible in women with ovarian cancer, they do not provide evidence of QOL benefit.

Several recent QOL intervention feasibility studies in ovarian cancer have employed a psychosocial/psychoeducational approach to QOL intervention. In a randomized study to assess the QOL effect of an ovarian cancer psychoeducational intervention, both the intervention and control group received written psychoeducational materials, and the intervention group also received four one-hour teaching visits from a licensed registered nurse or social worker, which covered physical well-being, psychological well-being, social concerns, and spiritual well-being

[77]. The authors report that there were no significant QOL differences between groups and attribute the lack of significant intervention effects to methodological concerns given the wide variability in the length with which participants had been coping with ovarian cancer and participants' previous familiarity with material covered in the psychoeducational intervention [77]. Recently, Henry and colleagues described the results of their randomized controlled trial to examine the acceptability and usefulness of a meaning-making intervention to improve QOL in ovarian cancer [78]. The meaning-making intervention, which was compared with a with usual care waitlist control group, consisted of an individual brief existential intervention delivered by a psychologist ranging from one to four sessions that systematically addressed situational, global, and existential meaning [78]. Specifically, the meaning-making intervention reviewed the impact and meaning of diagnosis, reviewed past life events and strategies for coping related to the cancer experience, and discussed priority and goal changes that enhance meaning, in balance with limitations secondary to cancer [78]. The findings demonstrated a non-statistically significant trend toward greater QOL at 3 months for the intervention group; however, the authors state that the feasibility trial was not powered to detect significant differences between groups in QOL. Adequately powered randomized trials are needed to elucidate whether psychosocial/psychoeducational interventions may positively impact QOL in women with ovarian cancer.

One recent randomized clinical trial examined the QOL effects of a nursing intervention among women with ovarian cancer during the postsurgical transition period [80]. The nursing intervention consisted of 6 months of individually tailored care by an advanced practice nurse to assist patients with self-management skills after surgery and to foster active participation in medical decision-making [80]. The advanced practice nurse assisted with referrals, coordination of care, and symptom management. In addition, participants who met the threshold for distress at baseline received an assessment from the psychiatric consult-liaison nurse [80]. Participants assigned to the nursing intervention received a total of 18 contacts divided among home visit, phone calls, and clinic visits, and those seen by the psychiatric consult-liaison nurse received an additional one to two visits. Participants assigned to the attention control group received eight contacts divided amongst home visit and telephone in which a trained research assistant assessed and addressed symptom management [80]. Women who received the combined intervention had significantly better mental and physical QOL over time compared to the attention control [80]. The results of this intervention provide preliminary evidence that nursing interventions targeting symptom management may be associated with improvement in multiple QOL domains.

The majority of recent QOL intervention feasibility studies in ovarian cancer have employed interventions targeting individual women with ovarian cancer, as opposed to group-based interventions. Group-based interventions are more common in breast cancer research. Further study is needed to establish whether group-based QOL interventions would be an acceptable format for women with ovarian cancer, particularly given the prevalence of advanced disease. Results from a recent qualitative study exploring perceptions of supportive expressive group therapy among women with advanced ovarian cancer described challenges perceived by participants related to the discussion of distressing emotions and the observation of other group members' physical decline and death [81]. However, qualitative themes also suggested that coping with these difficult emotions was part of the adjustment to the disease, and in that sense, the opportunity to participate in supportive expressive group therapy was described as helpful by participants [81].

Few of the QOL intervention feasibility studies in ovarian cancer have directly focused on the social and emotional aspects of QOL. QOL intervention studies in other female cancer populations suggest potential promise in this area. For example, a randomized trial comparing a 10-session group-based Cognitive Behavioral Stress Management (CBSM) intervention with a 1-day CBSM seminar resulted in improvements in social and emotional aspects of QOL for up to

1 year among women with nonmetastatic breast cancer who were randomized to the CBSM group [82]. Additionally, in a randomized controlled trial of an 18-session group-based multicomponent biobehavioral intervention (targeting stress management, adaptive coping, and health-promoting behaviors related to diet and exercise) among stage II or III breast cancer awaiting adjuvant therapy, women randomized to the intervention experienced more improvement in social and emotional aspects of QOL post-intervention than women randomized to an assessment-only control condition [83]. Moreover, several recent randomized controlled trials have reported QOL benefits following group-based Mindfulness-Based Stress Reduction interventions in women with newly diagnosed early-stage breast cancer [84] and survivors of breast cancer [85]. Taken together, these findings support the feasibility of group-based interventions targeting the social and emotional aspects of QOL in women with ovarian cancer. Furthermore, given the relationships between the physical/functional well-being and social/emotional well-being, QOL domains in ovarian cancer [71], a multimodal approach to intervention which directly targets both the physical/functional, as well as the social/emotional aspects of QOL, may be merited. As the feasibility and acceptability of QOL interventions in ovarian cancer are established, multisite randomized controlled trials will be needed to examine the efficacy of interventions to improve QOL in ovarian cancer, particularly given evidence for the association between QOL and outcomes such as survival [29, 52].

Conclusion

A growing body of research reflects the fact that QOL is an important outcome in its own right, as well as in relation to other outcomes, such as survival, in ovarian cancer. Given that QOL is affected by both disease- and treatment-related factors, improved measurement of the aspects of QOL relevant to ovarian cancer and more frequent inclusion of QOL as an outcome in clinical trials examining novel therapeutic modalities have resulted in an enhanced understanding of the QOL issues faced by women with ovarian cancer. As antineoplastic and supportive treatments evolve, QOL considerations will continue to play an important role in treatment decision-making. Furthermore, ongoing research to develop and assess the efficacy of QOL interventions may provide additional opportunity to ameliorate symptoms and concerns that confer a threat to QOL in women with ovarian cancer. Ongoing multidisciplinary collaboration will remain vital to optimizing QOL among women with ovarian cancer in both the research and clinical settings.

References

1. Cella DF, Tulsky DS, Gray G, et al. The Functional Assessment of Cancer Therapy scale: development and validation of the general measure. J Clin Oncol. 1993;11(3):570–9.
2. Kornblith AB, Thaler HT, Wong G, et al. Quality of life of women with ovarian cancer. Gynecol Oncol. 1995;59(2):231–42.
3. Ferrell B, Smith SL, Cullinane CA, Melancon C. Psychological well being and quality of life in ovarian cancer survivors. Cancer. 2003;98(5):1061–71.
4. Study protocol for the World Health Organization project to develop a Quality of Life assessment instrument (WHOQOL). Qual Life Res. 1993;2(2):153–9.
5. Grzankowski KS, Carney M. Quality of life in ovarian cancer. Cancer Control. 2011;18(1):52–8.
6. Rothermich EA, Pathak DS. References for health-related quality-of-life claims in prescription drug advertisements. Am J Health Syst Pharm. 1997; 54(22):2596–9.
7. Food and Drug Administration Oncologic Drugs Advisory Committee (ODAC) Quality of Life Subcommittee Meeting Transcript, February 10, 2000.
8. Aaronson NK, Ahmedzai S, Bergman B, et al. The European Organization for Research and Treatment of Cancer QLQ-C30: a quality-of-life instrument for use in international clinical trials in oncology. J Natl Cancer Inst. 1993;85(5):365–76.
9. Ware Jr JE, Sherbourne CD. The MOS 36-item short-form health survey (SF-36). I. Conceptual framework and item selection. Med Care. 1992;30(6):473–83.
10. Basen-Engquist K, Bodurka-Bevers D, Fitzgerald MA, et al. Reliability and validity of the functional assessment of cancer therapy-ovarian. J Clin Oncol. 2001;19(6):1809–17.
11. Greimel E, Bottomley A, Cull A, et al. An international field study of the reliability and validity of a disease-specific questionnaire module (the QLQ-OV28) in assessing the quality of life of patients with ovarian cancer. Eur J Cancer. 2003;39(10):1402–8.

12. Calhoun EA, Welshman EE, Chang CH, et al. Psychometric evaluation of the Functional Assessment of Cancer Therapy/Gynecologic Oncology Group-Neurotoxicity (Fact/GOG-Ntx) questionnaire for patients receiving systemic chemotherapy. Int J Gynecol Cancer. 2003;13(6):741–8.
13. Huang HQ, Brady MF, Cella D, Fleming G. Validation and reduction of FACT/GOG-Ntx subscale for platinum/paclitaxel-induced neurologic symptoms: a gynecologic oncology group study. Int J Gynecol Cancer. 2007;17(2):387–93.
14. Cella D, Peterman A, Hudgens S, Webster K, Socinski MA. Measuring the side effects of taxane therapy in oncology: the functional assessment of cancer therapy-taxane (FACT-taxane). Cancer. 2003;98(4): 822–31.
15. Wenzel L, Huang HQ, Cella D, Walker JL, Armstrong DK. Validation of FACT/GOG-AD subscale for ovarian cancer-related abdominal discomfort: A Gynecologic Oncology Group study. Gynecol Oncol. 2008;110(1):60–4.
16. Armstrong DK, Bundy B, Wenzel L, et al. Intraperitoneal cisplatin and paclitaxel in ovarian cancer. N Engl J Med. 2006;354(1):34–43.
17. Jensen SE, Rosenbloom SK, Beaumont JL, et al. A new index of priority symptoms in advanced ovarian cancer. Gynecol Oncol. 2011;120(2):214–9.
18. Rose M, Bjorner JB, Becker J, Fries JF, Ware JE. Evaluation of a preliminary physical function item bank supported the expected advantages of the patient-reported outcomes measurement information system (PROMIS). J Clin Epidemiol. 2008;61(1): 17–33.
19. Amtmann D, Cook KF, Jensen MP, et al. Development of a PROMIS item bank to measure pain interference. Pain. 2010;150(1):173–82.
20. Revicki DA, Chen WH, Harnam N, et al. Development and psychometric analysis of the PROMIS pain behavior item bank. Pain. 2009;146(1–2):158–69.
21. Buysse DJ, Yu L, Moul DE, et al. Development and validation of patient-reported outcome measures for sleep disturbance and sleep-related impairments. Sleep. 2010;33(6):781–92.
22. Pilkonis PA, Choi SW, Reise SP, Stover AM, Riley WT, Cella D. Item banks for measuring emotional distress from the patient-reported outcomes measurement information system (PROMIS(R)): depression, anxiety, and anger. Assessment. 2011;18(3):263–83.
23. Hahn EA, Devellis RF, Bode RK, et al. Measuring social health in the patient-reported outcomes measurement information system (PROMIS): item bank development and testing. Qual Life Res. 2010;19(7):1035–44.
24. Wenzel L, Vergote I, Cella D. Quality of life in patients receiving treatment for gynecologic malignancies: special considerations for patient care. Int J Gynaecol Obstet. 2003;83 Suppl 1:211–29.
25. Houck K, Avis NE, Gallant JM, Fuller Jr AF, Goodman A. Quality of life in advanced ovarian cancer: identifying specific concerns. J Palliat Med. 1999;2(4):397–402.
26. National Comprehensive Cancer Network (NCCN). NCCN clinical practice guidelines in oncology (TM): cancer-related fatigue. http://www.nccn.org/professionals/physician_gls/pdf/fatigue.pdf. Accessed 10 Nov 2011.
27. Holzner B, Kemmler G, Meraner V, et al. Fatigue in ovarian carcinoma patients: a neglected issue? Cancer. 2003;97(6):1564–72.
28. Cavaletti G, Bogliun G, Marzorati L, et al. Early predictors of peripheral neurotoxicity in cisplatin and paclitaxel combination chemotherapy. Ann Oncol. 2004;15(9):1439–42.
29. Wenzel L, Huang HQ, Monk BJ, Rose PG, Cella D. Quality-of-life comparisons in a randomized trial of interval secondary cytoreduction in advanced ovarian carcinoma: a Gynecologic Oncology Group study. J Clin Oncol. 2005;23(24):5605–12.
30. Penson RT, Wenzel LB, Vergote I, Cella D. Quality of life considerations in gynecologic cancer. FIGO 26th Annual Report on the Results of Treatment in Gynecological Cancer. Int J Gynaecol Obstet. 2006;95 Suppl 1:S247–57.
31. Chase DM, Wenzel L. Health-related quality of life in ovarian cancer patients and its impact on clinical management. Expert Rev Pharmacoecon Outcomes Res. 2011;11(4):421–31.
32. Herzog TJ, Coleman RL, Markman M, Cella D, Thigpen JT. The role of maintenance therapy and novel taxanes in ovarian cancer. Gynecol Oncol. 2006;102(2):218–25.
33. Goff BA, Mandel LS, Melancon CH, Muntz HG. Frequency of symptoms of ovarian cancer in women presenting to primary care clinics. JAMA. 2004;291(22):2705–12.
34. Wenzel LB, Huang HQ, Armstrong DK, Walker JL, Cella D. Health-related quality of life during and after intraperitoneal versus intravenous chemotherapy for optimally debulked ovarian cancer: a Gynecologic Oncology Group Study. J Clin Oncol. 2007;25(4): 437–43.
35. Holzner B, Kemmler G, Greil R, et al. The impact of hemoglobin levels on fatigue and quality of life in cancer patients. Ann Oncol. 2002;13(6):965–73.
36. Cella D, Beaumont JL, Webster KA, Lai JS, Elting L. Measuring the concerns of cancer patients with low platelet counts: the Functional Assessment of Cancer Therapy–thrombocytopenia (FACT-Th) questionnaire. Support Care Cancer. 2006;14(12):1220–31.
37. Tuxen MK, Hansen SW. Neurotoxicity secondary to antineoplastic drugs. Cancer Treat Rev. 1994;20(2): 191–214.
38. Dietrich J, Han R, Yang Y, Mayer-Proschel M, Noble M. CNS progenitor cells and oligodendrocytes are targets of chemotherapeutic agents in vitro and in vivo. J Biol. 2006;5(7):22.
39. Inagaki M, Yoshikawa E, Matsuoka Y, et al. Smaller regional volumes of brain gray and white matter demonstrated in breast cancer survivors exposed to adjuvant chemotherapy. Cancer. 2007;109(1): 146–56.

40. Kayl AE, Meyers CA. Side-effects of chemotherapy and quality of life in ovarian and breast cancer patients. Curr Opin Obstet Gynecol. 2006;18(1): 24–8.
41. Hess LM, Chambers SK, Hatch K, et al. Pilot study of the prospective identification of changes in cognitive function during chemotherapy treatment for advanced ovarian cancer. J Support Oncol. 2010;8(6):252–8.
42. Mayerhofer K, Bodner-Adler B, Bodner K, et al. A paclitaxel-containing chemotherapy does not cause central nervous adverse effects: a prospective study in patients with ovarian cancer. Anticancer Res. 2000;20(5C):4051–5.
43. Hensley ML, Correa DD, Thaler H, et al. Phase I/II study of weekly paclitaxel plus carboplatin and gemcitabine as first-line treatment of advanced-stage ovarian cancer: pathologic complete response and longitudinal assessment of impact on cognitive functioning. Gynecol Oncol. 2006;102(2):270–7.
44. Correa DD, Zhou Q, Thaler HT, Maziarz M, Hurley K, Hensley ML. Cognitive functions in long-term survivors of ovarian cancer. Gynecol Oncol. 2010;119(2):366–9.
45. Liavaag AH, Dorum A, Bjoro T, et al. A controlled study of sexual activity and functioning in epithelial ovarian cancer survivors. A therapeutic approach. Gynecol Oncol. 2008;108(2):348–54.
46. Carmack Taylor CL, Basen-Engquist K, Shinn EH, Bodurka DC. Predictors of sexual functioning in ovarian cancer patients. J Clin Oncol. 2004;22(5):881–9.
47. von Gruenigen VE, Huang HQ, Gil KM, et al. Assessment of factors that contribute to decreased quality of life in Gynecologic Oncology Group ovarian cancer trials. Cancer. 2009;115(20):4857–64.
48. Gershenson DM, Miller AM, Champion VL, et al. Reproductive and sexual function after platinum-based chemotherapy in long-term ovarian germ cell tumor survivors: a Gynecologic Oncology Group Study. J Clin Oncol. 2007;25(19):2792–7.
49. Bodurka-Bevers D, Basen-Engquist K, Carmack CL, et al. Depression, anxiety, and quality of life in patients with epithelial ovarian cancer. Gynecol Oncol. 2000;78(3 Pt 1):302–8.
50. Liavaag AH, Dorum A, Fossa SD, Trope C, Dahl AA. Controlled study of fatigue, quality of life, and somatic and mental morbidity in epithelial ovarian cancer survivors: how lucky are the lucky ones? J Clin Oncol. 2007;25(15):2049–56.
51. Shinn EH, Taylor CL, Kilgore K, et al. Associations with worry about dying and hopelessness in ambulatory ovarian cancer patients. Palliat Support Care. 2009;7(3):299–306.
52. Carey MS, Bacon M, Tu D, Butler L, Bezjak A, Stuart GC. The prognostic effects of performance status and quality of life scores on progression-free survival and overall survival in advanced ovarian cancer. Gynecol Oncol. 2008;108(1):100–5.
53. National Cancer Institute. Ovarian cancer: National Cancer Institute. http://www.cancer.gov/cancertopics/types/ovarian/. Accessed 15 Oct 2009
54. Benedet JL, Bender H, Jones 3rd H, Ngan HY, Pecorelli S. FIGO staging classifications and clinical practice guidelines in the management of gynecologic cancers. FIGO Committee on Gynecologic Oncology. Int J Gynaecol Obstet. 2000;70(2):209–62.
55. Pokrzywinski R, Secord AA, Havrilesky LJ, et al. Health-related quality of life outcomes of docetaxel/carboplatin combination therapy vs. sequential therapy with docetaxel then carboplatin in patients with relapsed, platinum-sensitive ovarian cancer: results from a randomized clinical trial. Gynecol Oncol. 2011;123(3):505–10.
56. Paclitaxel or polyglutamate paclitaxel or observation in treating patients with stage III or stage IV ovarian epithelial or peritoneal cancer or fallopian tube cancer. http://clinicaltrials.gov/ct2/show/NCT00108745?term=Paclitaxel+or+polyglutamate+paclitaxel&rank=1. Accessed 2 Nov 2011.
57. McGuire WP, Hoskins WJ, Brady MF, et al. Cyclophosphamide and cisplatin compared with paclitaxel and cisplatin in patients with stage III and stage IV ovarian cancer. N Engl J Med. 1996;334(1):1–6.
58. Greimel ER, Bjelic-Radisic V, Pfisterer J, Hilpert F, Daghofer F, du Bois A. Randomized study of the Arbeitsgemeinschaft Gynaekologische Onkologie Ovarian Cancer Study Group comparing quality of life in patients with ovarian cancer treated with cisplatin/paclitaxel versus carboplatin/paclitaxel. J Clin Oncol. 2006;24(4):579–86.
59. Alvarez Secord A, Berchuck A, Higgins R, Nycum L, Kohler M, Puls L, Holloway R, Lewandowski G, Valea F, Havrilesky L. A multicenter, randomized, phase II study evaluating the efficacy and safety of combination docetaxel and carboplatin and sequential therapy with docetaxel then carboplatin in patients with recurrent platinum-sensitive ovarian cancer. Gynecol Oncol. 2010;166(3, Supplement):1.
60. Gore M, du Bois A, Vergote I. Intraperitoneal chemotherapy in ovarian cancer remains experimental. J Clin Oncol. 2006;24(28):4528–30.
61. Armstrong DK, Brady MF. Intraperitoneal therapy for ovarian cancer: a treatment ready for prime time. J Clin Oncol. 2006;24(28):4531–3.
62. Alberts DS, Liu PY, Hannigan EV, et al. Intraperitoneal cisplatin plus intravenous cyclophosphamide versus intravenous cisplatin plus intravenous cyclophosphamide for stage III ovarian cancer. N Engl J Med. 1996;335(26):1950–5.
63. Markman M, Bundy BN, Alberts DS, et al. Phase III trial of standard-dose intravenous cisplatin plus paclitaxel versus moderately high-dose carboplatin followed by intravenous paclitaxel and intraperitoneal cisplatin in small-volume stage III ovarian carcinoma: an intergroup study of the Gynecologic Oncology Group, Southwestern Oncology Group, and Eastern Cooperative Oncology Group. J Clin Oncol. 2001;19(4):1001–7.
64. Vergote I, Trope CG, Amant F, et al. Neoadjuvant chemotherapy or primary surgery in stage IIIC or IV ovarian cancer. N Engl J Med. 2010;363(10):943–53.

65. Pecorelli S, Odicino F, Favalli G. Interval debulking surgery in advanced epithelial ovarian cancer. Best Pract Res Clin Obstet Gynaecol. 2002;16(4):573–83.
66. van der Burg ME, van Lent M, Buyse M, et al. The effect of debulking surgery after induction chemotherapy on the prognosis in advanced epithelial ovarian cancer. Gynecological Cancer Cooperative Group of the European Organization for Research and Treatment of Cancer. N Engl J Med. 1995;332(10): 629–34.
67. Rose PG, Nerenstone S, Brady MF, et al. Secondary surgical cytoreduction for advanced ovarian carcinoma. N Engl J Med. 2004;351(24):2489–97.
68. Eskander RN, Randall LM. Bevacizumab in the treatment of ovarian cancer. Biologics. 2011;5:1–5.
69. Cannistra SA, Matulonis UA, Penson RT, et al. Phase II study of bevacizumab in patients with platinum-resistant ovarian cancer or peritoneal serous cancer. J Clin Oncol. 2007;25(33):5180–6.
70. Doyle C, Crump M, Pintilie M, Oza AM. Does palliative chemotherapy palliate? Evaluation of expectations, outcomes, and costs in women receiving chemotherapy for advanced ovarian cancer. J Clin Oncol. 2001;19(5):1266–74.
71. von Gruenigen VE, Huang HQ, Gil KM, et al. A comparison of quality-of-life domains and clinical factors in ovarian cancer patients: a Gynecologic Oncology Group study. J Pain Symptom Manage. 2010;39(5):839–46.
72. von Gruenigen VE, Frasure HE, Kavanagh MB, Lerner E, Waggoner SE, Courneya KS. Feasibility of a lifestyle intervention for ovarian cancer patients receiving adjuvant chemotherapy. Gynecol Oncol. 2011;122(2):328–33.
73. Donnelly CM, Blaney JM, Lowe-Strong A, et al. A randomised controlled trial testing the feasibility and efficacy of a physical activity behavioural change intervention in managing fatigue with gynaecological cancer survivors. Gynecol Oncol. 2011;122(3): 618–24.
74. Newton MJ, Hayes SC, Janda M, et al. Safety, feasibility and effects of an individualised walking intervention for women undergoing chemotherapy for ovarian cancer: a pilot study. BMC Cancer. 2011;11: 389.
75. Judson PL, Dickson EL, Argenta PA, et al. A prospective, randomized trial of integrative medicine for women with ovarian cancer. Gynecol Oncol. 2011;123(2):346–50.
76. Chan KK, Yao TJ, Jones B, et al. The use of Chinese herbal medicine to improve quality of life in women undergoing chemotherapy for ovarian cancer: a double-blind placebo-controlled randomized trial with immunological monitoring. Ann Oncol. 2011;22(10):2241–9.
77. Otis-Green S, Ferrell B, Sun V, Spolum M, Morgan R, Macdonald D. Feasibility of an ovarian cancer quality-of-life psychoeducational intervention. J Cancer Educ. 2008;23(4):214–21.
78. Henry M, Cohen SR, Lee V, et al. The Meaning-Making intervention (MMi) appears to increase meaning in life in advanced ovarian cancer: a randomized controlled pilot study. Psychooncology. 2010; 19(12):1340–7.
79. Cohen SR, Mount BM, Bruera E, Provost M, Rowe J, Tong K. Validity of the McGill Quality of Life Questionnaire in the palliative care setting: a multicentre Canadian study demonstrating the importance of the existential domain. Palliat Med. 1997;11(1): 3–20.
80. McCorkle R, Dowd M, Ercolano E, et al. Effects of a nursing intervention on quality of life outcomes in post-surgical women with gynecological cancers. Psychooncology. 2009;18(1):62–70.
81. Walker LM, Bischoff TF, Robinson JW. Supportive expressive group therapy for women with advanced ovarian cancer. Int J Group Psychother. 2010;60(3): 407–27.
82. Antoni MH, Lechner SC, Kazi A, et al. How stress management improves quality of life after treatment for breast cancer. J Consult Clin Psychol. 2006; 74(6):1143–52.
83. Andersen BL, Farrar WB, Golden-Kreutz DM, et al. Psychological, behavioral, and immune changes after a psychological intervention: a clinical trial. J Clin Oncol. 2004;22(17):3570–80.
84. Henderson VP, Clemow L, Massion AO, Hurley TG, Druker S, Hebert JR. The effects of mindfulness-based stress reduction on psychosocial outcomes and quality of life in early-stage breast cancer patients: a randomized trial. Breast Cancer Res Treat. 2011;131(1):99–109.
85. Lengacher CA, Johnson-Mallard V, Post-White J, et al. Randomized controlled trial of mindfulness-based stress reduction (MBSR) for survivors of breast cancer. Psychooncology. 2009;18(12):1261–72.
86. Arriba LN, Fader AN, Frasure HE, von Gruenigen VE. A review of issues surrounding quality of life among women with ovarian cancer. Gynecol Oncol. 2010;119(2):390–6.
87. Yellen SB, Cella DF, Webster K, Blendowski C, Kaplan E. Measuring fatigue and other anemia-related symptoms with the Functional Assessment of Cancer Therapy (FACT) measurement system. J Pain Symptom Manage. 1997;13(2):63–74.
88. Functional Assessment of Chronic Illness Therapy (FACIT). FACIT Questionnaires. http://www.facit.org/FACITOrg/Questionnaires. Accessed 2 Nov 2011.
89. Wagner LI, Beaumont JL, Ding B, et al. Measuring health-related quality of life and neutropenia-specific concerns among older adults undergoing chemotherapy: validation of the Functional Assessment of Cancer Therapy-Neutropenia (FACT-N). Support Care Cancer. 2008;16(1):47–56.
90. Cella D. The Functional Assessment of Cancer Therapy-Anemia (FACT-An) Scale: a new tool for the assessment of outcomes in cancer anemia and fatigue. Semin Hematol. 1997;34(3 Suppl 2):13–9.

Index

DOI 10.1007/978-1-4614-8271-0,

E

F

Printed by Printforce, the Netherlands